Veterinary
Guide
Animal
Owners,

2nd Edition

Completely New and Revised!

Veterinary *Guide* for Animal *Owners,*

2nd Edition

Caring for Cats, Dogs, Chickens, Sheep, Cattle, Rabbits, and More

C.E. Spaulding, D.V.M.
and Jackie Clay

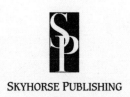

SKYHORSE PUBLISHING

Skyhorse Publishing books may be purchased in bulk at special discounts for sales promotion, corporate gifts, fund-raising, or educational purposes. Special editions can also be created to specifications. For details, contact the Special Sales Department, Skyhorse Publishing, 555 Eighth Avenue, Suite 903, New York, NY 10018 or info@skyhorsepublishing.com.

www.skyhorsepublishing.com

10 9 8 7 6 5 4 3 2 1

Library of Congress Cataloging-in-Publication Data is available on file.
ISBN: 978-1-61608-139-3

Printed in Canada

*F*or all the animals and for the veterinarians, animal health professionals, and owners who love and care for them.

Contents

POULTRY—*Continued*

RABBITS

DOGS

CATS

INTRODUCTION

*A*ccording to statistics, nearly every family today owns at least one animal, whether it is a cat or small dog in an apartment in New York City or a hundred milk cows on a farm in Nebraska. Couple that with a tremendous movement toward rural, or at least semi-rural living and we see even more animals enter the picture. People are stressed by too-hurried lives, worried about just where their family's food is coming from and the care it received along the way and seeking a more self-reliant lifestyle. Suddenly, living a more simple life, like Grandma's and Grandpa's in a quiet rural area, having a large garden, raising a few goats, a milk cow, a flock of chickens and perhaps a horse looks very attractive.

However, many of these people (and maybe you're one of them) have had little or no experience raising animals at all. Unlike Grandma and Grandpa, who were raised up from children, taking care of farmstead animals. They were taught what to look for, guarding against sickness and what to do, should it happen. But, along the way, even Grandma and Grandpa picked up a few old wives' tales and what I call "helpful untruths," which, unfortunately, still prevail today in some areas. How does a person, even an experienced farmer, sort out the solid veterinary information from the sometimes ineffective untruths and downright harmful old wives' tales? The new rural dweller often asks, "How do I know how to keep my animals well?" and

"How do I know when I can take care of animals myself and when I should call my vet?"

A *Veterinary Guide for Animal Owners* attempts to answer these questions by providing an easy-to-understand book, giving animal owners a quick, illustrated reference to help prevent many pet and livestock health problems, to quickly spot and treat developing conditions before they get serious and to correctly handle a crisis situation. This book covers most common pet and farmstead animals, from dogs and cats through goats, sheep, chickens, and cattle. As veterinary care can be costly, the book also teaches you to perform routine animal care procedures, such as dehorning, castrations, and giving medication. In addition, it aids your decision of when to call your veterinarian.

CHOOSING THE RIGHT VETERINARIAN

If you live in an area where there are several veterinarians, it is usually relatively easy to find one that you believe in. Veterinarians, after all, are people, and like people in any profession, some are better at it than others. When trying to pick a veterinarian for your animals, ask around. If several neighbors recommend one veterinarian over others, you might consider this choice first. Try not to let personality or bedside manner (stallside manner?) affect your choice. A good veterinarian doesn't necessarily have to cuddle your cat or hug your goat to do an excellent job doctoring it. On the other hand, you wouldn't trust someone who kicks your dog or swats your steer with a 2 × 4, vet or not.

It's a good idea to pick a veterinarian just as you do a family doctor: by results and attitude rather than by superfluous details. A million-dollar clinic can house a poor veterinarian. Those impressive banks of stainless-steel operating lights, X-ray units, and counters full of scary-looking instruments and testing devices are no good if they are used more to impress clients than to help sick or injured animals. But you can't have much luck with a veterinarian who uses only a stethoscope and a bottle of penicillin, either.

Look for a veterinarian who seems interested in your problems and who will, when you ask, explain the trouble and tell you what he's doing. Keep in mind that many veterinarians will not explain things without being asked, for the simple reason that a lot of people won't bother to listen.

Watch out for a veterinarian who tries too hard to be superprofessional. His every word sounds like a tape-recorded medical dictionary; his clinic and office help are an exact copy of an M.D.'s office; he wants to run tests for everything, on every visit; everything is perfect. Fine—he may well be a supervet, but usually his fees are super, too.

Better this type, though, than a veterinarian who is a slob. Very, very few modern veterinarians use dirty needles, obviously reused syringes, or unwashed surgical instruments, but occasionally you may be unfortunate enough to run into one. Don't make the mistake of judging a veterinarian by the inside of his car or truck, however. Eighty percent of the busy large animal practitioners' rigs look pretty cruddy at times, mine included. Rough, dusty roads, rutted fields, and bumpy driveways can quickly shake loose those neatly packed bags and boxes, dump drawers upside down, and spill used throwaway syringes, empty vials, bags, and boxes all over the place. An hour's ride can dust-cover the outside of bags and boxes that were previously clean and shining.

Throughout this book you'll notice that I refer to veterinarians as "he" (rather than the awkward "he/she") to make the text easier to read. However, this is in no way meant to imply that all veterinarians are men. In today's veterinary fields, there are nearly as many women veterinarians as men. And these dedicated women make just as good veterinarians as their male counterparts—not just in small animal clinics but in large animal practices, as well. I personally know of several women who specialize in treating large animals, and they excel in their field. So, do not let the sex of a veterinarian influence your choice!

In brief, you should look for an interested, honest, up-to-date veterinarian who works on your animal as if it were his own. By honest, I mean a person who, if he doesn't know the answer, will say so and try to find out—not snow you with medical jargon and bypass the question. Veterinarians are called to treat such a wide variety of animals that it is impossible to be totally informed on all species. One day it may be cattle and sheep; another day, a canary, deer, and llama; and still another day, a goat, monkey, and turtle. No veterinarian knows all animals equally well. He may be an authority on sheep and cattle yet be in the dark on llamas. But he can brush up if he knows he's going to have a client with llamas. Remember: interested, honest, and up-to-date.

Okay, let's say you've found "your" veterinarian. Now, when you have a problem with one of your large animals and make arrangements for the vet to come out, have the animal in the barn or tied up, and be there yourself. It is frustrating for a veterinarian, late on rounds, to have to wait while a cow is herded in from a hundred-acre pasture by a neighbor who doesn't know anything about the animal or the signs of illness that it has shown.

Next, let your veterinarian diagnose the problem, choose the method of restraint, and treat the animal. This is why you called him. Offer help, such as describing symptoms and temperature or assisting in restraint. Ask any questions you have, and listen to the answers. Most veterinarians are overjoyed to go to a place where the owners are truly interested in learning and in following care instructions closely. After all, good nursing can be as important as drugs or surgery. It's truly a pleasure for a vet to go through a rough operation or serious illness with an animal and then return the next day to see everything just the way he had told the owner to have it, with the animal munching its feed and on its way to a good recovery.

It's always a good idea to have your veterinarian refer you to another veterinarian you can call in case yours is out of town or ill. This eases the panic you feel when your pet goat is down with milk fever and you find out Dr. Smith won't be back until next Tuesday. With a prior referral, you can simply dial Dr. Jones and know you're in good hands.

Okay, you say, fine, but I live in the "boonies," and the nearest veterinarian is 60 miles away. What do I do for veterinary care? In this case make an appointment, and then take a drive, in advance of any animal problems, to visit that veterinarian. Explain your distance problem, and ask if you may call for over-the-phone advice. It is not as good as having a veterinarian out, but it might save the animal you could lose without help. Many veterinarians are very good at talking an owner through an injury or illness via phone conversations. (A hint: When calling long-distance, call person-to-person; since most large animal practitioners are in and out all day, you could save several dollars by doing this.) In cases where surgery is needed, most animals can be hauled to the veterinarian, if necessary.

THE IMPORTANCE OF PREVENTIVE MEDICINE

I can't stress the importance of preventive medicine and care enough. If more people practiced preventive medicine, there would be a lot less work for veterinarians and a lot more healthy animals and happy owners.

The most important "drug" you can give your animals is good husbandry. This means having a warm, dry, well-ventilated, draft-free shelter in the winter, a cool, shady, rainproof shelter in the summer, and room to exercise in the sunshine and fresh air. It also means having different-sized animals separated to prevent injuries and giving them all the correct amount of the right food.

A daily check of every animal is a key part of good care. If you notice any problems, such as lack of appetite, listlessness, weight loss, diarrhea, constipation, noises of pain (grunting, whining, etc.), swellings, or other unusual symptoms, give the animal a thorough examination at once. Tomorrow may be too late.

Remember to check things like teeth, ears, eyes, and feet. Cleaning or floating (filing) teeth will prevent a lot of dental problems that can waste feed, cause infection, and even eventually kill the animal. Cleaning dirt and wax from the ear canals can prevent ear mites and discourage bacterial or fungal infections. While checking the ears, you may also discover, and thus be able to remove, ticks in the ear canal. The eyes are important, too. Noticing and treating eye problems right away, such as foreign bodies, white spots, redness, or discharge, may save the sight in that eye. And it is a lot easier to trim a toenail or hoof regularly than to teach an animal to walk again after it has been crippled by one that grew too long, forcing the beast to walk abnormally. Likewise, it's easy to remove a stone from a horse's hoof or a thorn from a dog's pad in the early stages. But after it has caused severe pain, bruising, or infection, treatment can get expensive, lengthy, and frustrating.

To keep your animals in tip-top shape, a good general program of routine veterinary care is essential, too. Routine fecal examinations by your veterinarian and worming, if necessary, will increase your profits as well as the health of your animals. Even with a house dog, you will save money if your dollar buys food for your dog, not your dog's worms.

Talk to your veterinarian to find out what routine vaccinations are a good idea in your area. Don't be afraid that he will try to sell you a bunch of expensive, unnecessary vaccinations. But a small investment in the needed vaccinations can save your animal's life as well as prevent more extensive veterinary bills later on.

Also, have your animals tested for any diseases prevalent in your area. Cattle and goats, for instance, should receive yearly tuberculosis and brucellosis tests, while dogs should have a yearly heartworm test wherever this parasite is a very real danger. Horses that are moved about (for racing, showing, or breeding) benefit from a yearly test for equine infectious anemia. And always test new animals before adding them to your herd, flock, or homestead. Knowing that you have a healthy animal not only gives you peace of mind but protects your other animals (and your neighbors'), too.

It is also smart to isolate any sick or new animals—even your own animals that have been to shows. This simple precaution will prevent the spread of a disease like shipping fever.

If you're new to caring for animals, all this may sound like a lot of work. But once you get the hang of it, you'll see it's mainly just common sense. Regular attention, good general care, and routine checkups are the keys to healthy, rewarding animals and happy animal owners.

CATTLE

GENERAL CARE AND MANAGEMENT

*G*ood general care will go a long way to keeping your cattle healthy and productive. Providing proper housing and feed are simple but effective steps in good cattle husbandry. You'll also need to know how to restrain your animals so you can treat them yourself or assist your veterinarian. Other management considerations include breeding, delivering calves, castration, dehorning, and foot trimming.

Housing

Proper housing is one of the most important aspects of cattle care. Fortunately, good housing doesn't need to be elaborate or expensive.

Open, or Loose, Housing

Cattle are more likely to become sick due to too much shelter rather than too little. Therefore, I recommend open housing where it is possible. This consists of a barn or loafing shed, with an opening to the south (unless the prevailing winds come from this direction) where the cows can wander in and out at will. Even in the northern United States and Canada, the south side of the barn stays warm in the sunlight, and the cows love to lie out in the sun and chew their cud.

If you have dairy cows, you should have individual bedded stalls inside the barn. (Beef cattle do not need stalls since they don't have to be kept quite as clean as dairy animals do.) This system really saves labor and bedding because you have to clean manure only from the aisles, and it also helps keep the cows clean. These stalls should be raised 6 inches from the aisle by placing a 2 × 6 across the back of the stalls and filling them with sawdust and/or sand. This will also help to save cleanup time.

Stall sizes differ greatly, depending on the breed of cattle you are housing. For instance, a 600-pound Jersey needs a much shorter stall than a 1,400-pound Holstein. The stalls should be just long enough for your cattle to lie in comfortably, with the platform dropping off right behind the tail.

Remember, the cows should be free to come and go as they need. A hay rack outside encourages them to walk out for exercise, as does a salt-and-mineral lick. After all, exercise is one of the most important reasons for having loose housing. I have seen fairly young cows ruined after being confined to a cement stall with their

PARTS OF A COW

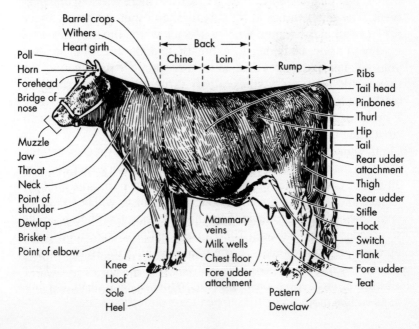

heads in a stanchion all winter. A combination of lack of exercise and lack of bedding, as well as having to lie and stand on an ungiving surface, has shortened many a cow's life by five or more years. These factors can also decrease a cow's milk production, owing to the pain of arthritis.

In the cold northern climates, there are a couple of things you have to watch with open housing in the winter months. First, make sure each cow's teats and bag are dry after milking before you turn her back outside. This will help prevent cracked and chapped teats. Also, try not to have your cows freshen (give birth and come into milk) during the coldest part of the winter: The full, tight bag, along with the cold, can cause frozen teats. If your loose housing shed gets too cold, you can partially close off the open south side. Sliding doors, nearly closed at night or during storms, and an overhang that is either solid or sided with clear fiberglass panels help to cut severe cold.

Confined Housing

If you have to confine your cattle, the animals are better off in comfort stalls. With comfort stalls the cows are kept on chains rather than in stanchions, thus giving them more freedom of movement. The temperature in your barn should not get much above 50°F (10°C) in the winter. When it gets too warm, the humidity goes up due to urine, body moisture, breath, and manure. This stresses your animals and makes them much more prone to pneumonia than they would be in a dry subzero barn. True, it's nice and comfy to work in a toasty barn, but I'm trying to limit your veterinarian bills. If necessary, invest in one or more ventilating fans to keep fresh air circulating through the barn.

If your cattle are on cement platforms with gutters behind, check to make sure that the manure is going in the gutter and that all of the cow is lying on the platform. If your barn was built for Jerseys and you have Holsteins now, the platforms will be too short; your cows will have to lie in the gutter, pressing their hocks on the sharp edge of the platform. This causes joint problems and will end up crippling your animals. If the barn was built for Holsteins and you have Jerseys, the platforms will be too long, and you will have a bunch of dirty cows. Besides being harder to keep clean, the animals will be more prone to chapped teats and urine scald.

Be sure to place plenty of bedding under cows when they have to be confined in stalls. If you can feel the hard cement under your feet, there isn't enough bedding. Shavings, sawdust, and straw all work fine. Bedding cows well is not wasteful: If your platforms are the right length, very little will be soiled or wet, and you can reuse all the clean, dry bedding. There is no use in trying to save money by skimping on bedding; you will just be shortening the useful, productive life of your cows.

Calf Housing

It's important to keep your calves separate from each other until they are past weaning age. This prevents them from sucking on each other's ears and udders. If they are kept separate, they will not be so apt to pass bacteria back and forth, lessening the chance of an outbreak of calf scours or pneumonia.

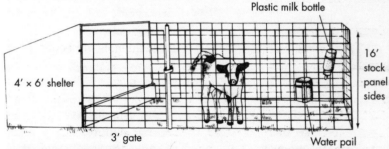

Calf hutch. Keep calves separated until they are past weaning age to help prevent the spread of diseases. Give each its own shelter and pen so it can see the other calves but not touch them.

Like adult cows, calves benefit from fresh air and sunshine as found in open housing. Calf hutches make a great place to raise several calves. Each calf can see the others but has its own little yard, with its own well-bedded, comfy house and its own water and food. With a little extra shelter from cold winds, calf hutches raise healthy calves even in the cold North.

General Housing Considerations

Whether you choose loose housing or comfort stalls, you should also have at least one sturdy stanchion or chute where you can restrain cattle for treatment. Trying to give a cow an injection is

First Aid Kit for Cattle

Here are some basic ingredients that belong in a bovine first aid kit. All of the items below are necessary if you keep a herd of cattle. If you have only one or two cows, you should at least keep those items that are marked with an asterisk. Of course, there is much more you can keep in your kit, but this is a good start. Ask your veterinarian for his advice for your situation. He might also be able to supply items that you can't find at your local farm supply store or in a farm veterinary supply catalog.

Balling gun*
Betadine*
Bloat medicine
Blood stopper
Calf bottle
Calf electrolytes*
Calf puller
California Mastitis Test
Clippers
Electric dehorner
Emasculatome
Forceps/needle holder
Hoof trimmers
Intravenous outfit
Mouth speculum
Nose lead
Obstetrical chains
Rectal veterinary thermometer*
Repeater syringe for vaccinating
Roll of cotton
Scarlet oil*
Stomach tube
Teat dip*
Three rolls of 4-inch gauze*
Three or four 18-gauge, 1½-inch needles*
Trochar and cannula
12-cc syringe*
Veterinarian's phone number*

quite challenging when she has free movement! A chute should not be over 28 inches wide, and some stockkeepers prefer 26 inches. This measurement holds true for all breeds of cattle, even large beef cattle. If the chute is built any wider, the animal can turn around, exploding chute planks in all directions. (For more information on building and using chutes, see "Restraint" on page 22.)

As much as you can, keep chickens and wild birds away from your cattle. Birds can carry avian tuberculosis (TB). This type of TB isn't transmissible to humans, but it can be picked up by cattle. When the cattle are tested for TB, they may react positively. I once tested a herd of cattle in Michigan and found several reactors to the TB test. Unfortunately, there is no way to differentiate avian TB from bovine TB in live animals. The cattle were shipped for slaughter, at some monetary loss and worry to the owner, and found to have "no visible lesions." I learned later that the farmer who owned this herd had a habit of throwing his dead chickens out on the manure pile, where the cattle had access, and evidently, the cows picked up avian TB. This is one of those lessons that are better to learn from someone else's mistake.

Feeding

During the summer cattle should have access to all the lush pasture grass they can consume. A word of caution here, though: Don't just turn cattle that have wintered on dry feeds and hay onto lush green pastures (especially legumes, such as alfalfa and clover) in spring, or you may have a bunch of very bloated cattle. It's important to provide a little extra attention at this time to help your animals make the adjustment. The first day, feed hay as usual in the morning, provide water, and then turn them out. Let the cattle graze for an hour or so; then drive them back to the barn. This is usually easier said than done as cattle don't like to leave the tasty green grass to go back to the barnyard. (Having a small fenced-off area and several assistants helps, but it's seldom easy.) Each day, extend their stay in the pasture by an hour. After a week it is usually safe to let them out full time. All this may sound like a lot of bother, but, believe me, it's worth it. I've seen several herds bloated by too much spring grass, and it's a big job for one veterinarian to treat dozens of affected cows at once!

In the winter a good, clean legume hay is best for cattle. By clean, I mean hay that is free of dust, mold, and weeds. This can be fed free-choice, giving them access to as much hay as they care to eat. As for recommending grains and grain rations for cattle, I'm going to pass the buck to your county Cooperative Extension Agent (usually located in your county seat). There's a wide geographic variation in grains available, costs of transportation involved, protein supplements, and other factors. Call your county agent for an appointment. He or she can give you several pamphlets describing the feeds available in your area and help you decide which will be best and most economical for you to use. The agent will also have numerous other free fliers and booklets on many aspects of animal care.

When you are formulating a ration, be extremely wary of using urea as a protein supplement. Personally, I would not use it at all. It's just too easy to make a mistake. Sometimes an elevator worker gets careless and dumps too much urea in a mix: The result is dead cows. Or you might use urea in your silage and then unknowingly buy dairy mix with urea in it, also. Uremic poisoning is tough to treat successfully. When fed at just a slightly toxic level, urea can cause a variety of problems, including sterility, lack of muscle coordination, and diarrhea.

To keep your cattle healthy, be sure to have fresh water available at all times, summer and winter. Snow is not good enough to supply water for cattle. Also, keep trace minerals and iodized salt accessible at all times. Your veterinarian will know what other supplements your animals might need and which you should avoid. There are areas throughout North America that are deficient in or have an overabundance of certain minerals, and it's a lot easier to prevent a deficiency or an overload than to treat it. A vitamin A and D supplement in the winter is a good idea because winter hay's vitamin A content is undependable and your animals won't be getting as much vitamin D during the less sunny winter months.

Feeds and Feeding by Frank B. Morrison is a must to read: It is the stock owner's bible of feeding. This book covers practically every feed available in the world and lets you know just what you are feeding, nutrition-wise. It discusses feeds for all livestock and poultry, and it is obtainable through most libraries.

Restraint

Here we get into perhaps the most important part of cattle raising; for without knowing and understanding the effective methods of restraining a bovine, you can become a bruised and bloody pulp trying to do some simple thing like pulling a splinter out of Bessie's hide. There are two ends to every cow: the butting, trample-you-into-the-manure end and the kicking, smash-you-into-the-wall and swat-your-face-with-the-tail end. First we'll restrain the front part, then the back.

Restraining Beef Cattle

The easiest way to restrain a beef animal, which is generally wilder and less often handled than a dairy cow, is to drive it into a funnel-shaped corral that leads to a 26- to 28-inch-wide chute. The sides of the chute should be either hardwood or pipe. If you choose a wooden chute, set the posts (railroad ties are best) 3 feet into the ground, and fasten the hardwood planks to the inside of the posts, ideally with bolts. When I say hardwood, I mean it: Cattle can smash pine 2 × 4s like matches if they get riled enough. If you prefer a pipe chute, set the posts in cement.

A few poles slid in close behind the cow, and a sturdy stanchion or squeeze chute with a head gate to hold the head in, wrap it up nicely. In a well-constructed chute, you can dehorn, deliver a calf, vaccinate, brand, sew up wounds, and perform other tasks in relative safety.

Restraining Dairy Cows

To restrain a dairy cow, drive her into a stanchion. If you have one, use a nose lead (also called a bull lead or nose clamp). This is a handy, inexpensive tool that is worth investing in, whether you have 1 cow or 50. Clamp the blunt, rounded ends in the cow's nostrils; then pull her head as far through the stanchion as possible and to one side, and tie it there. Make sure her shoulders are tight against the stanchion, or she can still jump around a lot and even get enough slack to shake the nose lead out of her nostrils. Someone is apt to be injured. If you don't have a nose lead, make a halter from a piece of rope, and pull the head around as with the nose lead. Either way, tie the rope with a knot

Restraint with a nose lead. Also known as a bull lead or nose clamp, this inexpensive tool is handy for restraint. Simply clamp the blunt, rounded ends into the nostrils, bring the handles together, and hold them shut with a rope.

that you can jerk loose in an emergency. This goes when tying any animal, anywhere!

A few more safety points: Don't wear gloves when working with ropes and live-stock—especially thick, fuzzy gloves, which can get tangled in ropes. Many fingers have been lost that way. Also, don't get between the rope and the post when tying an animal. It's a good way to get killed.

To restrain a cow's hind-quarters, the most readily available method is to grab her tail close to the base (yes, I know it's usually slimy with green stuff) and raise it straight up above her back. Really push, don't just hold it up, as that won't accomplish a thing. (Remember, the front end must be restrained first!) This nearly eliminates the chance of your getting kicked, because it puts pressure on the nerves and makes it hard for her to quickly raise her feet.

When working with a sore teat or an udder injury, you may need to place a figure eight around the hocks with a light but strong rope. Don't tie this rope, but have an assistant keep tension on it to prevent the cow from stepping around or kicking.

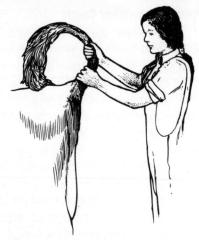

Restraint by holding the tail. *To prevent a cow from kicking during examination, medication, or treatment, grasp the base of the tail, and raise it firmly over the back of the cow.*

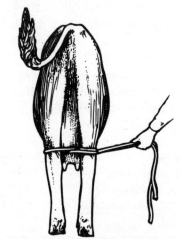

Restraint with a figure eight. *When working on the udder, you may need to have an assistant hold a figure eight of rope around the hocks. Keep the rope just tight enough to prevent kicking or stepping around. Do not tie the rope, or the cow may fall on you.*

Restraining Calves

To restrain a calf, the easiest one-person method is to straddle the calf's neck, facing the same way as the calf, grasp the chin, and raise the head for the bolus (pill) or drench. To give a bolus (pronounced bowl-us), coat it lightly with shortening. This makes it slide down easier. It's also smart to use a balling gun. This simple tool costs only a few dollars and makes dosing much easier, while also saving your hands from getting all skinned up on the calf's teeth. Shove the balling gun way in, past the hump in the tongue, and then pop the pill down. The same goes when drenching the calf with a dose syringe, only inject the liquid into the

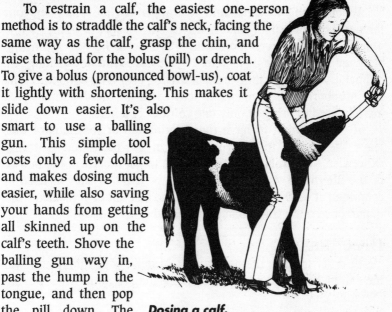

Dosing a calf.
The easiest way to restrain a calf for dosing or drenching is to straddle the calf's neck, facing the same way as the calf. Grasp the mouth, raise it slightly, and give the medication.

throat with more gentleness. You don't want the calf to choke and inhale the medication.

If you don't have a dose syringe to give liquid medication to a calf, use one of those plastic, squeeze-type bottles that shampoo or dishwashing liquid comes in. There is no danger of broken glass, and you can better gauge the size of the stream you are putting into the calf. Again, don't give it so fast that you choke the animal.

When you have to restrain a calf that's too big to straddle, tie the head, and push a knee firmly under the flank to force the animal against a wall or solid fence. With a large, active calf, it is best to have two people work with it: one to restrain and one to dose. If you don't have a helper, use either the chute method described in "Restraining Beef Cattle" or the stanchion method described in "Restraining Dairy Cows," both on page 23.

General Restraint Pointers

When trying to catch and restrain a bovine, don't let your temper show. Screaming and hollering don't help. They only rile the animal, making it even more wild or stubborn. Take your time; go slow, and do a little at a time. If you have trouble catching the animal, try offering a little grain or driving in several cows to get the one stubborn one. Remember that cows are herd animals: It's awfully hard to bring in only one cow out of a herd.

If you're going to have the veterinarian or inseminator out, leave the animal to be worked on in the barn that morning. Otherwise, you probably won't be able to get it back in the middle of the afternoon. Cattle are creatures of habit. If they're used to coming in at 6:00 to be fed or milked, no amount of persuasion will make those cattle think that they should go in at 2:30!

Breeding

In order to have the best supply of milk, your family cow will have to be bred each year. So keep breeding in mind when buying that milk cow.

When to Breed

Do not breed a heifer before she reaches 18 months of age or nearly all of her mature size. If you breed her earlier than this, she may have trouble calving or may never reach the potential she would have if not bred too early. For her first calf, it is wise to breed her to either a bull of her own breed known for small birth-weight calves or a breed known for small calves. These breeds are Jersey, Angus, Shorthorn, and Longhorn. Jersey and Angus calves are the smallest; but if you are after a calf to sell, choose Angus as they bring higher prices both as calves and as adults. Don't breed a small cow or first-calf heifer to a Charolais or Holstein unless that's what breed the heifer is; even then, choose a bull known for smaller birth-size calves. To disregard this advice is asking for trouble. Most of the really hard deliveries that veterinarians have to assist with are such cases. This is not to say that a Jersey heifer cannot have a Charolais calf, but the chances for trouble are greatly increased.

A heifer can begin coming into heat while she is still sucking on her mother or as young as 5 months. Therefore, it is best to keep bulls away from young heifers, even if they seem too young to breed. I have delivered calves from 15-month-old heifers, and it is usually a very rough job for all concerned.

Handling Bulls

When a heifer is old enough and large enough to breed, you have two alternatives: using a bull or using artificial insemination (AI). Turning the heifer in with a bull is the general practice with beef animals. However, if you have only one or two heifers to breed, keeping your own bull is not practical. He costs too much to buy and feed for the use you will get out of him. There is also quite a bit of risk involved with having a bull, especially if you have a dairy bull. No matter how tame a bull seems, you always have to remember that he is a bull. Most people are not hurt by a mean bull, because these bulls are watched constantly. It is the tame, friendly bull that is most dangerous. He may not mean to hurt you, but a 1,000-pound-plus playmate can get unintentionally rough in his play and smash you through the barn wall.

Never rub a bull's head or wrestle with his horns, even when he is a calf. This teaches him to use his head, and when he finds his strength, he will be very dangerous. I've seen a bull lift the front end of a tractor like a toy, and another push out the whole end of a barn, beams and all. I've seen one that walked through a five-strand barbed wire fence as if it were string, and another get a man down, kneel on him, and ignore pitchforks stuck into him in an effort to get him away from his victim. These are not scare stories but facts to consider before bringing a bull home.

If you do choose to have a bull, be sure you are prepared to handle him properly. Many handlers rely on a nose ring to control a bull. But a ring in his nose is no good unless you have a bull staff and use it. A bull staff is a pole with a snap in the end that clips to the bull ring. Leading a bull with a staff gives you a lot more handling power as the bull can't get any closer to you than the length of the staff allows. Leading him only by a chain in the ring lets him run over you at will. Even with a staff, it's smart to never completely trust the ring; I have seen bulls rip rings out of their noses when they got angry enough.

In most areas there are two alternatives to owning a bull. One is to use a nearby neighbor's bull, taking the cow to him and letting the neighbor deal with management responsibilities. The other is to use artificial breeding, or artificial insemination. The best ways to find out about a nearby good bull are to inquire of your neighbors with cattle, check with your county agent, and ask your veterinarian for recommendations.

Artificial Insemination

In most cases AI is the best choice, especially if you have only a few cows to breed. AI gives you several breeds to choose from and many choices for the bull, with complete information on the growth rate, production record, weight gain, and other traits of each bull. You can see what he looks like, what he's produced, and what his ancestry is. If you plan to keep the calves, this gives you a great chance to upgrade your herd at a really economical price. If you're determined to sell your calves, it gives you a chance to make a few dollars more by having the most salable calves possible.

The Heat Cycle

Most cows come into heat every 21 to 27 days, all year-round. If you have only one cow, you can tell she's in heat by several signs. She may bawl much more than usual—really roar. She may suddenly decide to wander off, looking for a bull. She will usually show strings of clear mucus on her tail or hindquarters. She may try to ride other cows, or even you. If your cow shows any of these signs but you are not sure she's in heat, jot down the date on your calendar, wait 21 to 27 days, and see if she repeats the same behavior. If so, chances are you were right. Most cows are in heat for 1 full day, some longer. The best time to breed is near the end of the heat cycle or, with some cows, just after they quit showing signs of heat, since some cows ovulate later than others.

Make arrangements with bull owners or inseminators before your cow actually comes into heat; then call them as soon as you can to tell them when you need your cow bred. Many bull owners like to have the cow at their place a few days before she is due in heat so she will be over her stress from hauling and more apt to settle (become pregnant).

After the cow is bred, just let her return to normal, and keep track of the date she would be due to come into heat in case she didn't conceive. Usually, the average cow settles with one or two services.

Pregnancy Exams

If you're not sure whether a cow is really bred, you can ask your veterinarian to do a pregnancy exam. He can examine her uterus rectally and give you a good guess as to whether or not she is pregnant. I say a good guess because at an early date, it often is only that: an educated guess. The fetus gains in size only during the last four months of pregnancy. (The gestation period for a cow is nine months.) The fetus at two months is about the size of a walnut. The veterinarian will, however, be able to tell whether the cow has any uterine problems or if she definitely is not bred.

When there is no veterinarian around, you just have to be patient and watch your cow carefully for signs of heat. At five or six months along in her pregnancy, you will, with some practice, be able to "bump" the calf. That is to say, make a fist and gently but firmly bump into the cow's right side in the flank region. If successful, you will feel a hard lump bump you back. This is your new calf.

Drying Up Cows

If you are milking the cow, it is best to dry her up six to eight weeks before she is due to calve. This gives her body a rest and gives her time to build a good, strong calf. There are many arguments over the best way to dry up a cow. These range from just stopping milking to milking only once daily or milking only when she looks uncomfortable. I firmly believe in just stopping milking and not touching her bag. She will look miserable for a couple of days but will then quickly dry up, usually uneventfully. Any milking just stimulates her to produce more milk, and this increases the time it takes her to dry up. If her bag gets too hard, a brief rub with warm bag balm will help; but if you spend too much time rubbing, this will also stimulate her milk production.

Several days after you stop milking her, you will notice quite a change in her udder. Where before you saw a nice round, full udder, there will now be only flabby skin. It's sort of like letting most of the air out of a balloon. Don't worry—that nice udder will return in a few weeks. Most cows start to spring bag (round out that udder) about a month before calving. It slowly fills out and soon starts to look beautiful again. Some cows don't bag up until they calve, so don't panic if Daisy looks as if she's going to give very little milk.

Wait until after she calves to start worrying. Even then, a veterinarian can give her a shot of oxytocin (a hormone) that will help force her to let the milk down—unless, of course, there is no milk to let down. Fortunately, this is rare.

Getting Ready for Calving

When a cow is heavy with calf, it is normal for her to throw off long strings of clear mucus, usually after she stands up. Many times people have thought this was the beginning of calving. It is not. I think it's a false alarm she gives just to see if you are watching her! When she's through fooling around and ready to give birth, she'll pass a cloudy mucus, followed by a pinkish or bloody discharge. She may or may not lie down to have her calf. Some cows just strain a few times in between mouthfuls of hay, and out plops the calf. More commonly, though, the cow will lie down and strain for half an hour to an hour before calving.

It is best if she can calve out in the fresh air, in a clean pasture. If not, have a maternity stall ready, and put her in it a few days before she is due to give birth. A box stall about 12 × 12 feet is fine for most cows; make it about 14 × 14 feet for Holsteins and other large breeds. If there is a cement floor, haul in 8 inches of sand or 4 inches of sand and 4 of sawdust. Don't skimp on the bedding!

One of the main reasons I advise having an enclosed area, such as a maternity stall or a grassy pen, is that it's much easier to check on the cow several times a day and at night, if necessary. If she is in a large wooded pasture, sometimes it's hard to locate her, especially after dark. And when cows know they're about to calve, quite often they instinctively go off somewhere secluded to give birth. They can really hide! So it's best to have them where you can find and check them often. Most of the really hard calvings and deliveries of dead calves could have been prevented if someone had seen that the cow was having trouble and helped her or called the veterinarian if it was too much to handle.

A maternity stall is much better than a cement-floored stanchion for a dairy cow to calve in. If she is a little weak in the hindquarters after calving, she won't slip and slide around in a bedded stall. I'd say that 70 percent of the cows that become downers (are unable to rise after calving) suffer from ligament, muscle, and bone injuries caused by sliding around and ending up spread-eagled on the cement.

Normal Calving

In a normal birth, the calf may be delivered in either a front or a rear presentation.

Front Presentation

Most cows deliver their calves front end first; so after your cow has strained hard several times, the first thing you usually see is a dark, round bulge, which is the amniotic sac, or water bag. This is usually followed very soon by the tip of one of the calf's hooves and then the tip of the other.

The calf's hooves should be toes down, so that you see the fronts of its hooves when standing behind the cow, not the bottoms of its feet. These tiny hooves are whitish and soft and have flaky, spongy bottoms. This is normal, so don't worry about the feet being deformed. They are this way to protect the mother from injury at birth. They will soon become hard.

A front presentation calf is born in the position

Labels on figure: Toes down; Note tail arch of mother; Soles pointing up

Normal delivery—front presentation. *Most cows deliver their calves front end first. The first parts that you will see are the soft, whitish hooves with the toes pointing down, followed by the nose of the calf.*

of a diver, with its front legs stretched out and its head between them. The legs will protrude about 1 foot, and then you will begin to see the head, nose first. Quite often the tongue will be out and appear swollen. There will be a momentary pause; then the cow will bear down hard, and the whole head will come out. This is soon followed by the shoulders, and then the calf slides out onto the straw. Usually the afterbirth (placenta) comes along, too, but if it doesn't, don't worry. Most cows lose the afterbirth within a few hours after calving. After calving let the cow clean off her calf, and let her relax.

Rear Presentation

Less frequent, but still considered "normal," is the rear presentation. The first hint of this kind of birth is that the hooves will appear upside down. Instead of seeing the toes, you will see the undersides and soles of the hooves. As the cow strains, the tail and hocks of the calf's hind legs will become visible.

A backward delivery, in many ways, is easier for the cow because there is no bulk at the shoulders to block things. However, there are two problems you may have with this type of birth. Sometimes the umbilical cord breaks while the calf's head is still in the birth passage. When the cord breaks, it is natural for the calf to start to breathe. But, unfortunately, in this position its head is still covered by afterbirth and mucus. As soon as the calf gets halfway out, you should

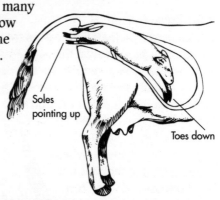

Normal delivery—rear presentation.
The rear presentation is less common but still considered normal. With this presentation you'll first see the undersides of the hooves, followed by the tail and hocks.

take hold of its legs and quickly get it the rest of the way out. Also, be careful that its head doesn't drop to the ground, especially if the floor is cement or the cow is standing. I've seen several calves with severe concussions because of this.

As soon as the calf slides free, quickly clean out any mucus from its throat and nose. If it isn't breathing or isn't breathing strongly, whack it *hard* on the side with the flat of your hand. If there seems to be a lot of mucus in the throat and nose, hoist the calf up by the hind legs to drain it. This will aid in letting the calf breathe. Sometimes poking your finger up its nose or poking it in the eye will make it gasp and start it breathing. Again, when all is well, let the mother clean off her baby, and let them rest.

Abnormal Calving

There are three groups of abnormal deliveries: First, there are the deliveries that can be assisted by the owner, with a little knowledge and common sense. Second are the births that need to be helped along by the veterinarian. Third, and most uncommon, are births that require a cesarean section.

Helping with the Delivery

When you suspect an abnormal delivery, the best thing to do is to scrub up. Wash your hands thoroughly, and trim long finger-nails. Lubricate your hands with ordinary liquid dish detergent, insert one hand into the vulva, and feel around to determine the calf's position. If you find the head and one front leg, loop a piece of binder twine or thin rope around the head through the mouth. (An obstetrical chain works better, but a one-cow homesteader can't afford to purchase a veterinary obstetrics kit merely for one cow who just might have trouble someday.) Keep tension on the rope so you don't lose the head, and push the head and leg back far enough to be able to work the retained leg—usually doubled back, butting up against the pelvis—out through the cervix. While you are bringing the stubborn leg up into position, try to keep a hand over the hoof so it won't poke a hole in the wall of the uterus. Once the leg is into position, the cow should pop the calf out with no more trouble.

If you find two front legs and no head, you're in for a little more work. Try to push the legs back. This in itself is quite a chore as the cow can really bear down, just about crushing your arm at times. However, if you can shove the legs back enough to make a little room to feel around, you'll have an easier time finding the head. Probably the easiest way to track down the head is to feel up one leg to the chest, then around the bulge of the neck and up to the nose. Sometimes you may be able to force the head around into the cor-rect position by just pulling on the nose. Other times you have to grasp the eye sockets with your thumb and finger in order to have enough traction to pop the head around right. (This will not injure the calf's eyes.) Once the head is through the cervix, you can easily place it between the legs, and the delivery can proceed.

If you find the head but no legs, place the rope through the mouth and behind the ears. Keep this tight enough that the head doesn't drop out of reach in the uterus. Shove back on the head. You will have to force it back far enough to be able to bring up both front legs. Again, this is a tiring job, but it *can* be done. Keep a hand between the hooves and the wall of the uterus to guard against tearing.

If the calf is coming backward but only the tail is showing (no legs), you will have to shove the hindquarters in as far as possible. Then you will be able to bend the legs into the correct position, doing each leg separately, for a rear presentation birth.

If the head and front legs are in position but the calf is large or the birth canal is narrow, you can help by fastening ropes to the legs. Here again, obstetrical chains are better since they do not shut off circulation. Be sure they are above the first joint of the foot (the fetlock joint); if they aren't, sometimes the leg will break or the hoof will pull off.

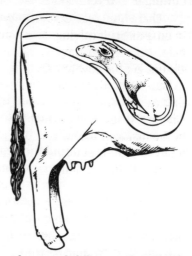

Abnormal delivery—legs back. *If you see the nose first, the calf's legs have caught on the brim of the pelvis and doubled under. You'll need to push the calf back into the uterus so you can bring the front legs into the correct position.*

As the cow strains, pull down on the ropes. Don't jerk, but keep a steady pull as the cow strains, and hold the calf where she pushes it. Sometimes a pole or a pitchfork can be used as a lever. Brace the end or tines against the floor, and put the handle through the ropes and pry down. Don't use a fence stretcher or vehicle to "help" pull the calf. These just pull the cow around and pull at the wrong angle, only jamming the calf worse and often damaging both cow and calf. A better alternative is to use a calf puller, or "calf jack," which is a long pipe with a jacking device on it. A metal britching is set against the cow's rump, just above her bag, and the obstetrical chains are hooked to the jack; with the puller pushing against the cow, it slowly pulls the calf as the mother strains. This puller may be pried down toward the cow's feet, further helping work the "stuck" calf loose. Adding a little liquid dish soap to the birth canal will often help slip the calf free. If you don't have a calf puller, use the soap, and call the veterinarian at once.

Calling the Veterinarian

There are some instances when you should call a veterinarian in on a difficult calving. If you are inexperienced and feel unable to help, call. If you have tried any of the above methods and still cannot get the cow to expel the calf, don't work on her until she is exhausted. Call. The veterinarian has special obstetrical equipment that can greatly speed up the safe delivery of a difficult calf, often saving the calf and the cow. He has the experience and knowledge of the inside of a cow, coupled with tricks of the trade learned from many hundreds of difficult births. Knowing just when to pull, which way to push, how hard to pull, and when to pry comes with much practice.

If the cow quits straining on the calf and just lies there, it's definitely time to call the vet. He can give her an injection that will start uterine contractions again. Even with a calf puller, the veterinarian can have a hard time pulling the calf if the cow doesn't help.

If you check the cow and find a foot, or two feet, tightly encircled by something that feels like a tough bag twisted shut, call. It may be a torsion of the uterus. Here the uterus twists on itself, thus preventing the birth of the calf. The veterinarian can use a torsion rod inserted between the legs to rotate the calf, something like a barbecue spit. It's quite tricky and can be a real job.

If the calf is dead and the cow can't deliver, call the vet. He may have to cut it apart with an embryotomy knife as dead fetuses tend to absorb fluid and swell up. Thus, the calf must be delivered in pieces to save the cow. The embryotomy knife is a special curved knife with a small blade, made to cut the skin of a dead fetus and still protect the wall of the uterus.

Cesarean Section

Once in a while, a cow may need a cesarean section to deliver a calf. The usual cause of this is a heifer that has been bred before she is big enough. No matter how hard you push and pull, you can't get a 29-inch sofa through a 24-inch door. The same applies to cattle.

Many times a cesarean is a poor risk since quite often the veterinarian is called as a last resort and the cow (or heifer) is just too tired and stressed to be a decent surgical risk. Any major operation performed on a sick animal, such as an exhausted cow or a cow with a foul, dead fetus in her, is risky, to say the least. But if you discover the need for a cesarean soon enough and alert the veterinarian right away, the chances for a successful operation are greatly increased.

(For other problems related to calving, see "Eversion of the Uterus" on page 52, "Ketosis" on page 58, "Milk Fever" on page 65, and "Retained Placenta" on page 73.)

Caring for Calves

Ideally, you should allow a newborn calf to stay with its mother or at least let it nurse from its mother three times daily to get the colostrum milk. (Colostrum is the first milk secreted by the cow after calving. It is necessary to the calf to provide antibodies for resistance to many diseases. It is generally discarded for human use.) After the first three days, if you need the cow's milk, you can switch the calf to goat milk or allow it to suck its mother after she has been milked lightly. This strips the cow's milk, saving you from doing it, and also provides nourishment for the calf.

If possible, the calf should be raised on milk, not powdered milk replacer. I do not like medicated feed, especially for very young calves, and most milk replacer contains antibiotics. There is not enough antibiotic in a day's ration of milk replacer to prevent scours or other diseases, and feeding an antibiotic daily can damage enough of the natural and necessary bacteria in the gut to cause scours. If you must use a powdered milk replacer, buy the best one available—usually the most expensive one. Cheaper milk replacers are often insoluble and settle to the bottom in a layer of silt, which causes digestive upsets and scours when the calf eats it. Cheap replacers are also usually low in nutrition. All white powder is not milk; read the label carefully. Do not use human powdered milk: It is low in fat, and calves need the fat to grow and thrive. Remember, Mama's milk is often 5 percent fat or more. But this fat must be digestible in order to prevent scours.

Use a calf bottle to feed milk or milk replacer. When fed from a pail, calves tend to gulp great mouthfuls of milk, which can form large curds in the stomach while being digested. These large curds can easily upset the delicate digestion of a young calf. A nipple pail is somewhat better as the calf sucks and gets less at a time than drinking directly from a pail. The nipple pail does have disadvantages, though. First of all, it is hard to clean thoroughly. Also, an overzealous calf can fling dust, manure, or hay into the open pail and swallow these contaminants with the milk. A calf bottle is best: It allows natural sucking, it is enclosed, and the nipple is easily removed for cleaning.

After the calf is well started on milk, I like to get it on unmedicated calf pellets. Be careful here, too, for many are medicated, and some are of poor quality. Buy the best, and start your calves right. You'll avoid a lot of problems and have much better adults. When a calf consumes a full pound of pellets daily, along with a fair amount of good hay or pasture and sweet feed or calf feed, it can be weaned (taken off milk for good).

Castration

Unless you plan to keep a male calf for breeding, you'll want to castrate it. There are several methods to choose from, though they aren't all equally good.

Clamping, or "Pinching"

The method that I recommend as best by far is clamping. There is no blood, very little shock or setback, and no chance of infection or tetanus. It is quick and very easy to do, even on large bulls. The one disadvantage is the cost of the clamps. The only type of emasculatome, or clamp, that is consistently good or worth using, in my opinion, is that made by Burdizzo. There are many imitations; but if you look closely at the place where the jaws meet to crush the cord, you will see a tiny crack of daylight in the other brands. This is what causes so-called slips, or animals that were thought to have been castrated and found to have one or both testicles still in operation.

If you have only an occasional bull calf to clamp, it is usually very inexpensive to have your veterinarian do it when he is doing something else at your place.

The purpose of clamping is to crush the cords, thus causing the testicles to atrophy and shrink up. They do not drop off, nor is there ever any wound, in contrast to the rubber band method.

Using an Elastrator, or "Banding"

Banding involves using a special, inexpensive tool to slip a heavy, round band over the scrotum and testicles. The band is rolled off the holding pegs of the tool and the band tightens, shutting off circulation to the area. After several weeks, the whole scrotum dies, dries up, and falls off. It is relatively painless, inexpensive, and easy to learn.

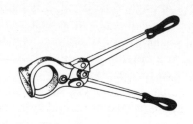

Emasculatome. *Castrating with an emasculatome pinches and crushes the cords but does not cut them, so there's no blood, very little shock or setback, and no chance of infection or tetanus.*

The young bull calf can easily be banded while standing, especially if two people are working with it. One can hold the tool while the other kneels down and works the testicles down into the scrotum. Push the tool up quite high against the body so that you ensure that both testicles are below the band and release the band. As there is a slight wound around the band site, as the scrotum dries, readying to fall away, it is a good idea when banding to also give the calf an injection of tetanus toxoid (or a "tetanus shot"). Without the preventative injection, it is possible for the calf to develop tetanus, for which there is very little help. Do NOT "help" the scrotum fall off by pulling on it or you may cause bleeding.

When preparing to clamp a bull calf, your first task is to restrain the animal. This will make the job quicker and safer for the operator. With a calf up to about 600 pounds, fasten the head by tying it or by securing it in a stanchion or head gate. Have a helper stand alongside the animal, grasp the tail at the base, and raise the tail straight up over the animal's back. This will make it nearly impossible for the calf to kick. The helper should also press one knee under the animal's belly, just in front of the hind leg. This prevents the calf from moving around or sitting down. The same method is used to secure a larger bull, but a couple more assistants and a squeeze chute are always helpful.

Feel the scrotum and testicles with your left hand (if you are right-handed), and identify the cord leading to each testicle. Open the clamp's jaws, and position them across the cord leading to one testicle, well above the testicle itself. This avoids any possibility of mashing the testicle, which would cause shock and swelling. With the cord safely between the jaws, press the handles together all the way. While the jaws of the clamps are still together, check to see that the cord did not slip out of the way when the jaws were being closed. Release the handles, and move on to the next testicle. Do one cord at a time. I always do the right one first, then the left—for the simple reason that, in this way, I never forget which one was not yet done. You'd be surprised at how many people clamp the same side twice! *Never clamp across the center section of the scrotum.* There is a septum separating the two testicles, and you can have serious trouble if this is crushed.

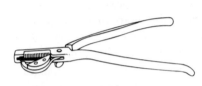

Emasculator. *This is the tool of choice for surgical castration. The emasculator cuts as well as crushes the cords so there is no chance of slips.*

Surgical Castration

Surgical castration is a little more difficult, but it's the surest method. As I tell many cattle raisers, when you see the testicles lying on the ground, you can be sure there were no slips. This procedure requires the use of an emasculator (an instrument that crushes and cuts the cord and blood vessels at the same time), which greatly minimizes bleeding. You also need a sharp knife or scalpel.

Using the same method of restraint described in "Clamping, or 'Pinching'" on page 37 or with the animal tied on the ground, clean the scrotum well with soap and water, and then dry it with a clean towel. Stand behind the animal, grasp the scrotum with one hand, and turn the lateral surface of the scrotum back toward you. Make an incision along the side to the bottom of the scrotum. The incision should be long enough to easily expose the testicle and provide adequate drainage of the wound. (For help in making a proper cut, see the illustration "Surgical Castration" on page 106.) When the cord and testicle are exposed, apply the emasculator. Cut the cord as high as possible. Be sure the crushing part of the emasculator is toward the animal's body, or it won't do any good. Close the emasculator firmly, and count to 10 to make sure the crushing is complete.

There is a layer of tough tissue covering the testicle, called the tunic; remove this along with the testicle. Cutting high, along with removing the tunic, prevents the animal from ending up with a scirrhous cord. This is a buildup of scar tissue that must be peeled out by hand—and is one finger-cramping condition to correct!

Repeat the procedure with the second testicle. Apply a mild antiseptic to the area after you've removed both testicles. Use a fly repellent spray on the hind legs and belly if the flies are bad; just don't spray the incisions.

Dehorning

Horns look nice on some cattle, and dehorning does involve some work for you and some stress on your animals. But, all things considered, it is a necessary job. It's easy for cattle with horns to hurt you whenever you try to work around them; they can also injure each other and themselves. I've seen cattle that died after their horns got tangled in fences, twine, and ropes. I firmly believe that you should dehorn all cattle—with the exception of those breeds whose horns are a special trait, such as the Texas Longhorn.

The best time to dehorn cattle is when they are young calves. It is easier on all concerned, does not require a veterinarian, and shortens healing time. Your options for dehorning calves include caustic ointments, electric dehorning irons, gougers, and elastrators.

Caustic Ointment

This treatment works on calves that are several days old. Before applying caustic ointment, clip the hair around each tiny horn bud. Also, rub a wide ring of petroleum jelly around each eye to protect them in case the ointment runs. Then apply the ointment on the horn bud and around the base to kill the horn cells so no horn grows. Be sure you follow the directions on the container because there can be differences in products.

Always remember that caustic ointment can burn more than horn cells, so apply it carefully. And don't use caustic ointment if it is raining (the ointment will run and burn the face) or if several calves run together (they'll burn each other). Also, avoid the ointment if the calf and mother (or nurse cow) are together, even just at meals; the calf may burn the cow while nursing. And never use caustic ointment if small children are around the calf. If the children touch the caustic ointment, they may receive burns.

Electric Dehorning Iron

This method also burns, killing the horn cells, but has many advantages over ointment treatments. It is safer all around. There is no caustic material on the head, so there's no danger of face burns or burns to children or other animals. It is also less stressful on the animal as it is over and done with in a few minutes and does not cause pain for days. One disadvantage is that a dehorning iron costs more than caustic ointment; so if you have only one calf and can't borrow an iron, the ointment is more economical.

The one problem many people have with an electric dehorning iron is that they do not leave the iron on long enough. The result is a scur (deformed horn). This may turn into the head, pressing right into the skull, or it may get knocked off and cause bleeding. Be sure to follow the directions with your dehorning iron and leave it on the full time, even if the calf bawls bloody murder. Better to dehorn once than to have to repeat the process later. When the bud is properly burned, there will be a copper-colored, indented ring completely around the bud. In the winter or with an exceptionally hairy calf, I clip the hair around the horn first as the hair can insulate the skin and prevent the thorough burn you need to kill the horn cells.

Gouger

This simple instrument has two round, wooden handles with sharp, cup-shaped blades that fit down over a horn or horn button. You just pull the handles apart quickly and snip out the horn. This is the method I prefer for calves up to six to eight months old; it also works on older animals if their horns are small. Gougers are easy to operate and quite effective. There's seldom a problem with scurs growing back, unless you are too timid and cut the button off instead of gouging it out.

I try to dehorn early in the spring, during the winter, or after fly season in the fall. Not only is there less trouble with flies bothering the wound, but there is also less bleeding in cold weather.

As soon as both horns are off, sprinkle blood-stopping powder on the wounds liberally. The bleeding will usually stop in five minutes or so. It may spray in a fine squirt for a minute, so don't be alarmed. It will stop shortly. If it doesn't, place a clean cotton pad on each side, and wrap gauze snugly around the head to put pressure on the wounds. This is seldom necessary, but it is effective when you need to stop excessive bleeding. Remove the pads and wrapping in one day, or they may cause infection. (Remember, any type of bandaged wound invites infection.)

Keep freshly dehorned calves indoors for a few days if flies are around. To control flies, use a repellent wipe on the face or apply fly repellent antiseptic, such as scarlet oil, to the wounds.

Elastrator (Rubber Band Method)

This method starts with clipping the base of the horn. Then the elastrator is slipped tight against the head, placing a rubber band between the head and base of the horn, as close to the head as possible. When you release the band, it cuts off circulation to the horn. Basically, the horn dies and eventually falls off.

Painless? I really doubt it. Wrap a tight rubber band around your finger and see. I must confess that I'm not in favor of this method of dehorning, so if I sound prejudiced—I am! Improper use can result in scurs or other problems. If a band breaks, that horn will develop while the other one doesn't. There is no blood or fly problem, but once in a while, an infection strikes when a horn is partway off. I've also seen several calves with tetanus following dehorning with the rubber band method.

Dehorning Adult Cattle

Unless you are quite experienced, it's best to leave this to your veterinarian. You will need to restrain the animal, ideally in a chute. You could use a stanchion, but you may have problems if the head is not completely immobilized. Veterinarians will usually inject the nerve around the base of each horn with an anesthetic if they plan to manually saw off the horns. If they will use an electric dehorning saw or a large, guillotine-action, manual cutting dehorner, most veterinarians will not use an anesthetic. (The procedure is over so fast that there is little more than afterpain, and cattle seem to suffer more from the injection of the anesthetic than from the dehorning itself.) The dehorner is pushed up close to the head, and the horn is quickly cut off.

After the horn is cut, there is often a stream of blood, about the size of a small pencil, spraying out of the wound. If the cut is close enough to the head, the bleeding arteries are near the surface, and the veterinarian can pick them up and clamp them with heavy forceps. In cold weather the bleeding will stop by itself in a few minutes. If the bleeding continues longer, you may tie a piece of strong twine tightly around the base of both horn stumps; then tie the ends together over the top of the head, further tightening the twine. This stops the

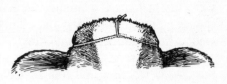

Minimizing bleeding after dehorning. *Tying a piece of binder twine around the horn stumps and leaving it on for an hour or so will help to reduce bleeding when dehorning adult cattle.*

bleeding or at least slows it down considerably. Dust some coagulant powder liberally on the wounds. In an hour cut the top twine. If there is no bleeding, cut the twine off altogether. Do not leave the twine in place longer than absolutely necessary for stopping excessive bleeding, because it cuts off proper circulation and could cause gangrene.

To remove a large-based horn, such as those on bulls or on older cows of some breeds, an electric dehorning saw or a manual saw is better than blade dehorners. Blade dehorners can crack the horn or the skull.

Trimming Feet

The hooves of most cattle tend to grow quickly, especially when the animals are pastured on grass and don't get much exercise. If left untrimmed, the toes often either cross or curl up like elf shoes. This puts a strain on the tendons and can make a cow lame. Any stress of this sort soon lowers milk production of dairy cows and

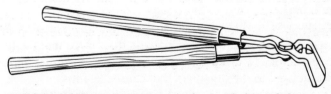

Cattle hoof trimmer. *Trimming the feet regularly can help prevent lameness. Place one side between the toes and the other on the outside of the hoof to trim excess growth.*

causes weight loss in beef cattle. Fortunately, this is easy to prevent. In most cases trimming the feet is a fast and simple job. It causes no pain or bleeding and often extends the life of the cow as well as her productive capabilities.

There are special hoof trimmers for cattle, which you use while the cow is standing, all four feet on the ground. Place one side between the toes of the hoof and the other on the outside of the hoof. A few snips, and those long toes are sound again. If you see pink tissue when you make a cut, stop; the next cut may bring blood. If you do cut too close and bleeding starts, dust the wound with dehorning coagulant powder.

If the toe has curled around and is covering the bottom of the hoof, you may have to lift the foot and snip off that part. This will let the cow walk on the sole of the foot, not on the abnormally grown horn wall of the toe.

DISEASES AND OTHER PROBLEMS

With all cattle there are occasional diseases, common health problems, and parasites. Knowing how to recognize, treat, and prevent them is an important aspect of cattle husbandry. When you recognize a problem quickly, you're more likely to choose an effective course of action. Some problems you'll be able to treat yourself; others will require immediate veterinary assistance. Knowing the difference can save the life of your animal. It's also important to know the normal temperature of your cow so you can check for fever or other abnormalities. The normal body temperature of a cow is 101° to 101.5°F (38.3° to 38.6°C).

Blackleg

Blackleg is a disease that strikes in many parts of North America, causing severe losses in cattle from three months to two years of age. It is caused by the bacterium *Clostridium chauvoei*, which is related to the organism that causes tetanus.

Blackleg organisms live in the soil for years, which explains why some places can be bothered by blackleg year after year until the young stock are vaccinated. Blackleg organisms enter the body

Example of Vaccination Schedule for Cattle

There are many vaccines available today that vaccinate effectively against several diseases at one time, making it convenient and easier on the animal than giving several injections. Your veterinarian can advise you what combination(s) are helpful in your area.

	DISEASE	WHEN TO VACCINATE
HEIFERS	Bovine Virus diarrhea (BVD)	Before weaning and before breeding
	Brucellosis	Calfhood
	Infectious bovine rhinotraceitis (IBR)	Before weaning and before breeding
	Leptospirosis	Before breeding
COWS	BVD	Booster early, before breeding
	IBR	Booster early, before breeding
	Leptospirosis	Every year, before breeding
STEERS	BVD	Yearly
	IBR	Yearly
	Leptospirosis	Yearly

through the digestive tract or through small puncture wounds. They don't grow when exposed to the air; but after they enter the body, the organisms grow in the absence of oxygen and produce a toxin that, when strong enough, kills the animal. Blackleg disease appears suddenly. An infected animal may be okay at night or just a little lame on one leg—and when morning comes, it's dead.

Blackleg is usually quite easy to diagnose. On a living animal, there is often a crackling sound and feel when you touch an affected leg. On skinning out the leg of a dead animal, it usually appears purple, as if it were bruised badly, thus the name blackleg. If you don't see these symptoms in the legs, check around the neck.

If you find yourself in an area where blackleg is a problem—your veterinarian or local cattle raisers can tell you—arrange to have your young animals vaccinated. It costs only a few cents a head and takes only a little while to do a whole herd. It is certainly worth the preventive steps because there is no sure treatment after the animal contracts the disease.

Bloat

The usual cause of bloat in cattle is overeating. This often occurs when cattle are suddenly turned out into lush pasture with clover or other legumes. It's also common to see bloat after cattle break into cornfields or grainfields and overload. Overeating on these types of pasture produces what is called frothy, or foamy, bloat. An abnormal amount of gas forms in numerous small bubbles that the animal is not able to belch up; thus, the gas continues to form, and the animal becomes bloated. If not treated, the animal will stagger, have difficulty breathing, pant, and finally collapse in a heap. Unless you treat the animal immediately, death is usually not far away.

In nearly all cases, the animal will recover promptly if you administer a defoaming agent. It is a good idea to buy a commercial bloat medication from your veterinarian, just to have on hand for emergencies. Lacking that, you can often get good results with corn, peanut, soybean, or safflower oil. Cream or mineral oil can also be effective. Four to 8 ounces of a defoaming agent is usually sufficient for a calf; 1 pint is about right for adult animals. Give the oil by the mouth, knead the sides of the animal well, and then call your veterinarian. Tying a round piece of wood in the cow's mouth, like a horse bit, will often help her belch up some of the gas.

Everyone who has cattle should have a trochar for treating bloated cattle in an emergency (when an animal is weak and close

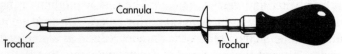

Trochar and cannula. *The trochar is a pointed instrument like an awl, only heavier. The cannula is a small pipe-shaped piece that fits snugly over the trochar. These two pieces are used together to relieve bloat.*

to death). A trochar is a pointed instrument like an awl, only heavier. A small pipe-shaped accompanying piece, called the cannula, fits snugly over the trochar. Insert the trochar and cannula at the highest point of the bloat, on the animal's left side, just in front of the hip bone. (You may need to first make an incision through the tough hide with a sharp knife.) Withdraw the trochar. The cannula stays in to let gas escape without contaminating the peritoneal cavity with debris from the stomach. It will take only a few minutes for

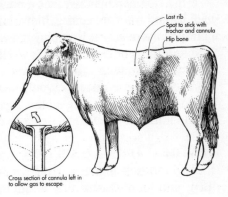

Last rib
Spot to stick with trochar and cannula
Hip bone

Cross section of cannula left in to allow gas to escape

Relieving bloat in cattle. Insert the trochar and cannula at the highest point of the bloat, on the animal's left side, just in front of the hip bone; then withdraw the trochar. The cannula stays in to let gas escape without contaminating the peritoneal cavity with debris from the stomach.

the bloat to reduce, much as if you had popped a full balloon; then the cannula can be removed.

Sometimes a cow will overload on dry feed and develop bloat. This often happens when the cow breaks into the feed room or discovers full feed sacks within reach. In this case the gas is usually in larger pockets, compared with the tiny bubbles of frothy bloat. Here the quickest way to relieve the bloat is to pass a stomach tube and manipulate it to relieve each pocket, one at a time. Caution: Use only a stomach tube, not a garden hose. This can tear the throat or poke a hole in the stomach. I know a lot of cattle owners use them, but I've seen several cases where they caused the death of a cow.

You can get a stomach tube from any veterinarian or order one from a farm veterinary supply catalog. The cost is minimal. It is a good idea to buy one to have on hand for emergencies. A mouth speculum (a pipe-shaped tube with rounded edges) is also a good investment. You put the speculum in the animal's mouth and then insert the tube through the speculum. This prevents the cow from biting the tube.

If the stomach tube releases a pocket of gas (you can hear and smell it) and no more comes, blow down the tube while moving it slightly to make sure it isn't plugged with feed. Watch out, though, because if the tube clears, there is often an eruption of very foul gas and stomach contents. You don't want it in your face!

After the gas is released, you'll see the animal's sides go down dramatically. You may give a bloat medicine to prevent further gas buildup until the animal has had a chance to digest the grain.

Bovine Virus Diarrhea

Bovine virus diarrhea (BVD), or infectious bovine diarrhea (IBD), is a viral disease that is quite common in cattle. It is not always a severe disease; it's more of a chronic infection.

Affected animals will have a higher than normal temperature for several days. They lose their appetites and have diarrhea. Drooling or foaming at the mouth is often a symptom of the disease. You may also notice sores around the mouth, eyes, and nose.

Treatment is often difficult, so consult your veterinarian. Fortunately, it's possible to vaccinate your animals to protect them from this disease.

Breaks

In cattle most broken bones occur in the legs and pelvis. This excludes the broken tails given by people twisting them, trying to get cows to go somewhere they don't want to go.

Broken Legs

Culverts or bridges with holes in them, woods with many downed trees, and stock trailers with rotten floors all rank high in causing broken legs in cattle. To reduce the chance of problems, keep bridges and floors sound and even, and remove excessive debris from pastures. An ounce of prevention is worth a pound of cure!

Even under the best conditions, however, breaks can still happen. If you notice a sudden, severe lameness in a leg, especially if the leg appears floppy or dangling, break is a prime suspect. Do not move the animal unless it is in a really bad place, such as a swamp or scrubby area. If you must move the animal, do it a few steps at a time. Keep the cow quiet, and call the veterinarian at once. If the bone has not come through the skin, there is a good chance the animal can be saved without costing you a fortune. That old idea of "Shoot a cow with a broken leg" is okay for movies, but it's rather costly and foolish in reality.

A plaster cast or a cast-brace combined works quite well in many cattle. The weight a cow carries, along with the animal's disposition, has a lot to do with the success of the treatment. Good aftercare from you is also important. Some animals are quite clumsy with a cast on and need help to get up after lying down. Keep the animal clean and dry, as wet bedding or barnyard muck will soften the plaster and make the cast worthless. Slipping an inner tube over the bottom helps, but you'll need to change it often as it wears out. I've had better luck using Easy Boots, made for horses, on the bottom of plaster casts.

Many legs may also be pinned successfully. Your veterinarian will decide whether a cast or pinning is better for the case.

The healing time varies, but a calf's broken leg usually heals in a month and a cow's in twice that time. With a severe break in an adult cow or a break where the bone tears out through the skin, it is sometimes necessary to have the leg amputated. I once worked on a large Holstein cow whose leg needed amputation. She calved normally and went on to milk 80 pounds of milk a day. It was very difficult to pick her out of the herd as they grazed. It's surprising how well an animal amputee can get around and how unnoticeable the missing limb is to the animal and its owner.

Fractured Pelvises

Most fractured pelvises in cattle occur as the result of a difficult birth or a bad fall. If your cow is having a hard time calving, call your vet. Many times the calf is dead and can be cut apart with a special embryotomy knife; this allows it to be delivered with little risk to the cow. Using a tractor or fence stretcher to pull out a too-big calf can also fracture a pelvis. On a slippery cement floor, a weak or clumsy cow can easily end up in a spread-eagled fall that may fracture the pelvis. In any case, the usual result is a cow that cannot get to her feet, even with help.

Here again, you'll have to give the animal time and some effort to save her. Many of these downer cows will lie for a month or more before rising. As long as they are eating and appear bright and alert, they have a good chance of eventually getting to their feet. There are cow lifters, which fit over the hips and are used to lift downer cows; but a cow with a broken pelvis should not be hauled up. This will only aggravate the problem and make the healing take longer.

Keep downer cows bedded and on their briskets, not lying flat out or spread-eagled. Use bales of hay or straw to prop them up if they tend to lie flat. Turn them twice a day to keep up circulation in their legs and prevent pressure sores. If they are outdoors, provide shade from the sun. Offer plenty of fresh water and fresh feed. A happy cow will get better quicker than a miserable one!

Brucellosis

Cattle brucellosis, also known as Bang's disease, is caused by the bacterium *Brucellus abortus*. It is less common today than it was 50 years ago, owing to stringent testing programs. But it is still too prevalent. It is also a big concern to human health as well as bovine health because it causes undulant fever in humans. Undulant fever often results from drinking raw milk from an infected cow or herd.

In cattle the first symptoms of brucellosis are often abortions and retained placentas. Prevention is the key here; there is no treatment. Vaccinate calves routinely. And when you bring new cattle into your herd, make sure they have been tested and are free of brucellosis. If your herd tests free of brucellosis for at least two years and they don't have contact with untested cattle, you can usually feel safe that your animals don't have the disease. Even if you have only one milk cow on your homestead, test her for brucellosis yearly. It is cheap insurance for your family.

Caked Bag

Caked bag, or udder edema, is a condition you'll find usually just prior to, or soon after, freshening. The bag becomes swollen and feels "doughy" to the touch. If you press your fingers into the bag, fingerprints or dents will remain when you take your hand away. Caked bag is caused by increased blood circulation to the udder, leading to swelling. The blood is carried into the udder faster than it can be carried away, and some of the fluid settles into the tissue, causing the edema. Left untreated, caked bag can cause udder attachments to break down and result in a pendulous udder, which in turn leads to other udder problems. It can also lead to gangrene mastitis if the blood supply becomes completely shut off.

I have had very good luck in reducing caked bag by injecting a diuretic, followed by giving oral diuretics until the bag becomes normal. Diuretics cause the animal to urinate more often, drawing fluid from the body and from the congested udder. Hot compresses and warm udder ointment or udder liniment can help to increase proper circulation and carry away the edema. *Do not limit the cow's water intake.*

Cuts

If your animal gets cut, consult your veterinarian soon after the injury to see whether he thinks sutures are necessary. Most often the cut will not need stitches. In fact, it is a waste of time and money to try suturing certain wounds because of either the placement of the wound site or the type of wound. For instance, it is best not to sew up a gash in areas that are heavily muscled or in "stretch areas." Either the stitches will just tear out in a few days, or they will scar the tissue. A three-cornered tear, with skin hanging, can either be sewn up or have the flap snipped off. (The hole left where the flap was removed will fill in, leaving little or no scarring.) There are some cuts that heal better if sewn up, but many times Mother Nature, plus your good nursing, will heal a cut faster and better than stitches will.

The most important aspect of wound care is cleanliness, followed by fly control. Clip all the hair away from the edges of the wound because it can irritate the cut as well as attract dirt. Leaving hair in or near a wound will double the healing time along with the chances of infection. Other keys to speeding healing include keeping the cut clean (using soap and water) and dry and applying an antiseptic that is also a fly repellent, such as scarlet oil. A 6-inch gash will often heal completely in three weeks with good care.

During the healing process, it's important to keep flies away from the wound for several reasons. Besides irritating the wound, they carry bacteria that cause infection. They also deposit eggs that hatch into maggots. Maggots, in moderation, are not a bad thing, as they eat dead tissue, cleaning out a wound nicely. But when they run out of dead tissue, they go on further and can literally eat an animal alive. So it's wise to keep them away.

Eversion of the Uterus

An eversion (turning inside out) of the uterus is an emergency matter and needs immediate attention. Don't confuse it with a retained placenta, which also occurs after calving and shows as reddened, fleshy tissue protruding from the vulva. While the placenta is stringy and thin, the uterus is heavy and bulky, and the caruncles, or "buttons," stand out plainly. The visible uterus may be from the size of a basketball to the size of a bushel basket.

There is much shock to the cow when this problem occurs, so call your veterinarian immediately. Tell him your cow has thrown her uterus. I've had cattle owners that were too embarrassed to say this; they said only that their cows needed me. It helps a veterinarian if he knows exactly what the problem is, especially in an emergency situation!

While you are waiting for the veterinarian, keep warm, wet towels on the uterus, and do not let it swing and flop around or get in the manure. (Set a bale or two behind the cow, drape it in clean sheets or towels, and place the uterus on that to support it.) If at all possible, get the cow's hind end up a foot or two higher than her front. An old door or sheet of plywood propped up on cement blocks or hay works nicely. This not only makes replacing the uterus easier for the veterinarian but also helps keep the cow from straining and throwing more of the uterus out. Taking this extra trouble may save her life. Also, keep her calm; don't run or excite her. She is in shock, and her heart cannot stand exertion.

When your veterinarian gets there, have a few clean pails of warm water and several towels nearby. If there are a couple of helpers, it will greatly speed up things and may also help save the cow. The veterinarian will administer a spinal anesthetic to reduce the cow's straining. Even with an anesthetic, this is, at best, a rough, tiring job. It's like picking up 60 pounds of liver and stuffing it carefully through a crack, while someone on the other side is shoving it back at you! An injection of oxytocin (a hormone) will help shrink the swollen uterus, making the job somewhat easier. (In an emergency, where no veterinarian is available, you can use plain white table sugar, sprinkled liberally on the cleaned uterus, to produce a similar shrinking effect.)

Once the uterus is carefully cleaned of manure and dirt and is shrinking down in size, the veterinarian usually holds the center of the organ with one hand and carefully stuffs it back into the vagina, a little at a time, working first on one side, then on the other. At first, progress is slow; but suddenly a point is reached where the uterus begins to fall back into place, over the brim of the pelvis, aided by gravity.

The veterinarian carefully inspects the uterus, making sure it is completely turned right side around again, and then inserts uterine boluses to guard against infection. It is usually necessary to lace the lips of the vulva to help keep the cow from throwing the uterus back out, although nothing will absolutely prevent it from coming out again if she strains hard. Thus, the veterinarian may give another spinal anesthetic a few hours after replacing the uterus to keep her from straining until the swelling is gone.

For a day or so after the uterus is in place, it is a good idea to keep the back of the stall built up with hay or straw or to keep the door or plywood platform under the cow's hind end. If she lies down, this will prevent the weight of her bowels from pressing against the uterus, causing irritation or shoving it toward the vulva.

Flies

The most common trouble flies cause is plain irritation, both to animals and to people. Cows bothered severely by flies will produce less milk and lose weight, just from fidgeting and swishing their tails at the pests.

Keeping the barn spotless, both inside and out, will aid greatly in keeping flies down. So will completely eliminating a manure pile outside the barn as well as cleaning up the barnyard. Many farmers who have gone from an outside manure pile to daily manure removal have cut their fly population by over 95 percent. Even if you have only one cow, you'll still get good results by removing manure daily and spreading it on a hay field or an empty part of your garden instead of piling it. Spreading dries the manure, so it won't attract flies; on the other hand, a pile of any size will stay wet in spots, providing ideal sites for flies to lay their eggs. I have had good luck using cleanliness coupled with fly predators, available in many organic supply catalogs, and fly traps set in strategic locations in and near the barn. Those horrible-looking (but effective) sticky, spiral fly catchers also help in milking areas.

Spraying the barn in the morning and at night, when the animals are outside, or spraying the cows themselves should be a last resort. Many of the sprays on the market can do more harm than good because of the dangerous chemicals they contain; so check all of the warnings on the label, as well as the contents of the spray, and always use good judgment when deciding when and where to spray.

If you have a severe problem with flies on beef cattle, ear tags impregnated with insecticide can be a reliable solution. But with all such articles, the total safety is a bit debatable. I prefer to use dust bags hung at the entrance to a watering or salt-and-mineral lick and filled with a somewhat less toxic compound, such as pyrethrins.

Foot Rot

The first sign of foot rot is usually a sudden lameness, often in just one foot. On checking the foot, you may find it swollen, possibly with pus oozing from between the toes. If left untreated, the swelling will increase, and the continual pain will cause the cow to produce less milk. There is a good chance the animal will pick up a bacterial infection, and it may eventually die.

Foot rot is caused by bacteria that live in the soil and enter through cracks in the feet. In winter months cracks may result from cattle stepping on mud that's been cut up by cattle tracks and then frozen, making very bad walking conditions. The flesh between the toes chaps, splits, and is further irritated. In the summer, when cattle congregate in swampy areas or the wet, muddy areas around water tanks, the alternating wet and dry conditions chap the feet, and cracks form.

Keeping cattle away from muddy places in the summer (cementing an "apron" around water tanks often helps) and rough places in the winter will help keep down foot rot. Also, feeding an iodine supplement in the feed or salt will be beneficial in some herds. Making dairy cows walk through a 3 percent formalin or 5 percent copper sulfate foot bath daily will help, especially when one or more animals in the herd have come down with foot rot.

Common treatment often involves a broad-spectrum antibiotic or, in stubborn cases, an intravenous treatment with a sulfa solution administered by the veterinarian. It's also important to keep the foot clean and dry, so don't let the cow walk through mud or manure. A drying powder containing an antibiotic will help, as will a drying liquid like Kopertox.

When the foot rot has progressed too far, it may be necessary to remove the infected portion. Try drawing a rough hay rope through the crack between the toes several times so the friction burns away the dead tissue. Don't be gentle, or you won't accomplish anything. If this is not successful, one claw can be surgically removed. It is much better, of course, to notice the lameness at its start and begin systemic treatment at once. There is a vaccination for foot rot, which can be a help in problem areas; ask your veterinarian about it.

Do not confuse foot rot with a condition known as corns. This quite often occurs in heavy cattle. It is not a swollen, pus-oozing foot but an extra chunk of tissue that extends farther than normal between the toes. Check the other three feet to see the difference. These corns can be very painful, and it's often best to have the veterinarian remove them surgically.

Grubs

Grubs, often called back grubs, are parasitic fly larvae. The parent flies lay eggs on the legs and lower belly of cattle. When they hatch, the tiny maggots burrow directly into the flesh. They migrate and end up just under the skin in the back. Each grub makes a breathing hole and remains there, growing in size, until it drops out of the hole to the ground and starts the cycle over again. These grubs are unappetizing on butchering, and they ruin the animal's hide.

There are many sprays and powders on the market for grubs. Where grubs become a severe problem, cattle owners often resort to using a pour-on insecticide before the grubs become large. A measured amount of insecticide is poured along the back, where it is absorbed and kills the infant maggots in the system. It is often used in the fall and then also gives protection against lice during the winter. If you choose to use an insecticide, make sure you follow the directions to protect yourself, the animal, and the environment.

In mildly affected animals, it is usually best just to leave the grubs alone. Pinching or squashing them on the back can cause an anaphylactic shock; so if you must get rid of one or two grubs, have your veterinarian surgically remove them.

Hardware Disease

Hardware disease, as the name implies, is caused by an animal swallowing nails, pieces of wire, bottle caps, tin cans, or whatever else a cow can swallow. Why bovines like the taste of steel and tin, I'll never know; but I've seen a cow happily munching down 16-penny spikes as her owner patched a barn wall.

These metal objects accumulate in the cow's reticulum. As the stomach churns feed, the sharp pieces of metal penetrate the wall of the reticulum, often traveling into the thoracic cavity and the pericardium of the heart. A nail or wire may migrate to other organs, such as the liver or spleen.

Hardware disease can produce a wide variety of symptoms, depending on where the offending object is in the body. The animal may go off its feed, produce less milk, lose weight, stand with its left elbow cocked out, move slowly, grunt when it breathes out, or have an above-normal temperature. On the other hand, an animal can swallow metal and never show any of the above symptoms.

If you suspect that your cow has hardware disease, call your veterinarian in to thoroughly check over the animal. In early cases the vet can feed a magnet to the cow. It's shaped like a bolus so that the animal can swallow it easily. The magnet gathers the loose metallic trash in the reticulum and keeps it from traveling about and causing harm. If you pasture your animals where they have easy access to metal hardware, it may be wise to give a magnet to all adult cattle as a preventive. Potential problem sites include areas where old buildings have been burned, leaving the nails, and old dump sites, where there are rusted cans or old, rusted baling wire or fence wire. Of course, it is much better to pick up such articles or to cover them with a couple of feet of soil. But if this is not possible, a magnet is a second option.

If a piece of wire has pierced the reticulum, causing peritonitis, antibiotics will often calm the infection. Sometimes a rumenotomy can save a valuable cow that would have to be shipped (sold for meat) without the operation.

To prevent hardware disease, keep cattle away from junk, places where buildings have been torn down or burned, old wire fences, and nails. Do not chop the wire on hay bales with an ax to open them (little pieces of wire break off and are swallowed with the hay); use wire cutters instead. One farmer I knew swept out his cement manger daily with a steel broom, trying to keep a very clean barn. What he didn't realize was that the broom shed bristles in the manger and his cows ate them, giving them hardware disease!

Infectious Bovine Rhinotracheitis

Infectious bovine rhinotracheitis (IBR) is caused by a virus (bovine herpesvirus) and affects cattle of all ages. Symptoms include respiratory distress, abortion, red and swollen eyes, weakness, lack of appetite, and very inflamed mucous membranes of the nose (hence the common name of red nose for the disease). A high temperature, up to 108°F (42.2°C), is also a symptom. A cow with a genital infection may show a raised tail head, increased urination, a swollen vulva, ulcers of the vulva, a vaginal discharge, or pustules on the vulva.

As IBR is caused by a virus, there is no treatment other than good general care and the use of antibiotics to knock out secondary bacterial infections, which are common. Affected animals will usually recover in about two weeks, but they remain a source of infection for other animals.

There are very effective vaccines available for IBR at a low cost. Talk to your veterinarian about the type of vaccination program he would recommend for your area.

Johne's Disease

Johne's (pronounced YO-nes) disease is caused by the bacterium *Mycobacterium paratuberculosis*. It spreads through the manure of affected animals, often contaminating the pasture, water, and feed. A calf can even pick up the infection after nursing its dam's dirty udder.

Symptoms include diarrhea, usually becoming chronic, with a foul odor; this is commonly followed by weight loss and a drop in production. There is no fever in most cases. The animals weaken and eventually die. There is no treatment.

Johne's disease affects primarily cattle, but it can also harm sheep and goats. If this disease breaks out in your herd, you should test any new animals that you have brought to the place. Also, test any animals that have chronic diarrhea. Culling affected animals, coupled with testing and strict sanitation, is the only means of reducing an infection in a herd.

Ketosis

Ketosis, or acetonemia, is a metabolic imbalance occurring mainly in higher-producing milking cows after calving. It most often happens when you are feeding the cattle hay and dry feed while keeping them in a barn or barn lot.

There is primary ketosis, which happens by itself, and secondary ketosis, which happens along with or because of a problem such as mastitis or a displaced abomasum. The cow will usually stop eating, produce less milk, and act generally depressed. These symptoms, by themselves, could be caused by any number of ailments. But if the cow is in the barn, has just recently freshened, and is a fairly good producer, it would pay to check her for ketosis. Do not wait. It's important to treat ketosis right away, or the animal may die.

It's very easy to check a cow's milk for this problem with ketosis test powder, also known as acetone test powder. (This is available at many rural drugstores, from your veterinarian, or from a veterinary supply catalog.) The only problem is that the powder does not combine well with colostrum (a cow's first milk after giving birth, usually two days' worth) to give an accurate reading. In such cases you may have to test her urine instead. This involves standing around behind her (seemingly forever!) with your little sterile jar, ready and waiting for her to urinate. Then just try to catch a jarful without getting drowned. (One hint: Cows usually urinate soon after they rise, after lying down for a while.) If a urine test is too inconvenient, have your veterinarian test the cow's blood.

When a test indicates a positive result for ketosis, there are several treatments to choose from, depending on the severity of the illness. For instance, some cows respond to drenching with 1 or 2 pints of molasses. If you're using this treatment, mix the molasses with the same amount of warm water, or else it could be quite a mess getting it in the cow. Usually, one dose will provide relief; if not, try a second dose in an hour or two. If the cow doesn't perk up soon after a second dose, call your veterinarian because there may be another cause of the ketosis, such as a displaced abomasum.

Cortisone injections, according to a veterinarian's recommendation, are another option. (This treatment is based on the theory that the adrenal cortex becomes exhausted and quits producing enough glucocorticoids.) Drenching the cow with propylene glycol or giving an intravenous injection of 500 to 1,000 cc of 40 percent dextrose daily will also work in most cases. All of these treatments are usually given only once, but you may need to repeat them in a day or so if the cow doesn't improve or if she has a relapse. Some cows respond to one approach but not to any of the others; so, if possible, get your veterinarian out to look at your cow and choose the treatment. If you must administer a treatment without a veterinarian's guidance, be sure to read and follow the directions on the product label.

Be aware that cattle sometimes also exhibit a craziness with ketosis. The animal may run in place with her head up against the barn wall or in her stanchion, circle to one side, or try to attack a person. Keeping in mind that these also could be symptoms of rabies—so don't get her slobber on you—carefully work the cow into a well-bedded stall or a chute where she can't do much damage to herself or hurt someone. Call the veterinarian at once. Luckily, ketosis is usually a much less dramatic problem. If you check your herd at least twice a day, you can easily catch the disease in its early stages and treat the problem successfully. Sometimes a heavy concentration of molasses in the grain ration before and for a few weeks after calving will prevent ketosis, and it surely won't hurt anything.

Leptospirosis

Leptospirosis is a contagious bacterial disease in cattle as well as in many other animals, including humans. It usually spreads through contact with streams, ponds, or surface water contaminated with the feces or urine of affected animals.

Symptoms include fever, weakness, anemia, abortion, lowered milk production, and the production of abnormal milk. The urine may contain blood, turning it a red or wine color.

If you suspect leptospirosis in your herd, call your veterinarian at once. With prompt testing and treatment, you can usually stop this disease. Treatment typically includes antibiotics, blood transfusions for anemic animals, and good nursing. It's highly recommended that you isolate affected animals to protect the rest of your herd. You'll also want to vaccinate the animals that are not showing signs of the disease.

Prevention includes routine vaccinations as well as fencing to keep animals away from contaminated ponds and streams. Keep cattle feed free of rodent contamination. Buy replacement animals from herds that are vaccinated yearly and that have no leptospirosis in any of the cattle.

Lice

Lice can appear on any cattle at any time of the year, but they are most often a problem during the winter months. They do not like sunlight and exposure, so they wait until long hair and dark days come along. Unless you are specifically looking for lice, the first sign that your cattle are lousy is the rubbing that suddenly begins. The affected animals, usually all of the herd, will begin to rub and scratch their necks on fences, the stanchion, the brush, or anything handy—including you! Pretty soon, the hair will wear away, especially on the neck, making the animals look moth-eaten. They may also look as if they have dandruff. When you part the remaining hair and peer around at the skin, you will see little gray bugs that are smaller than a grain of rice. They are oval shaped, with a head at one end that often appears to be red. Suddenly you feel crawly. Don't worry: Lice prefer cows to people and very seldom stay on a human to dine.

Lice may be small, but if there are sufficient numbers on a cow, their feeding can cause anemia and literally bleed the animal to death. Get rid of the pests as soon as possible. There are many louse powders on the market, carried by your veterinarian or a veterinary supply catalog. Caution: Be sure you use a powder formulated for dairy cattle because some powders can get into the milk and cause toxicity.

Mange

Several types of mange can occur in cattle. All true mange is caused by tiny mites that burrow into the skin. These cause itching, a moth-eaten appearance, scales, crusty spots, pustules, and thickened skin. If you suspect an animal has mange, have your veterinarian test it and recommend a treatment. Many cases of suspected mange turn out to be something else. A mange remedy will not help an allergy, a vitamin deficiency, or urine scald!

Complete isolation is a must for an animal with mange. It is bad enough to treat a single animal with it, without having to treat 10 or 20. Lime-sulfur dips, given weekly for at least six weeks, are effective in treating chorioptic mange, the most common mange found in cattle. For beef cattle or nonlactating dairy animals, topical application of ivermectin is the quickest, surest treatment. Other remedies include various sprays and local treatments. Lindane was used in the past, but it is toxic and is not permitted to be used or sold in some areas.

Mastitis

Mastitis is an inflammation of the mammary gland: the udder. Many bacteria can cause mastitis, including streptococci, staphylococci, *Pseudomonas*, *Corynebacterium pyogenes*, and *Escherichia coli*. There may or may not be watery, lumpy, bloody, or otherwise abnormal milk, but there usually is some change in the milk.

The California Mastitis Test (CMT) is the most economical test for mastitis and is also easy to use. You can purchase a test kit at most rural community drug- and feed stores, through a farm-ranch veterinary supply catalog, or from your veterinarian. For best results, use the test routinely—approximately every month—on the entire milking herd. Also, use it in between routine testing if you suspect mastitis in an individual cow. With regular testing you can identify mastitis in its early stages, before it lowers milk production or damages the udder and becomes harder to treat successfully.

Keep in mind that some cows' udders will swell a bit and feel harder than normal to the touch a few days to a week after freshening. If the milk checks normal with the CMT and her temperature is normal, don't worry. In a few days the bag will go back to normal.

Also, it is quite common for some cows to pass a few "plugs" or "strings" in their milk while at the end of their lactation or when first fresh. This also can be normal. There are physiological changes in the milk during freshening, drying up, and even some heat periods that can cause slightly abnormal milk. A cow can and does sometimes freshen with mastitis; but unless her milk stays stringy for a day or she shows signs of sickness, test—don't worry.

There are several types of mastitis, but here I'll try to explain three: acute, gangrene, and chronic.

Acute Mastitis

This type of mastitis develops rapidly. The cow may be all right one night and sick the next day. At first you'll usually notice a marked reduction in milk production, especially in affected quarters of the udder. There may be flecks in the milk or gummy strings or sometimes a watery fluid that in no way resembles milk. The bag is usually hot and swollen in one or more quarters. The sick cow commonly runs a temperature of 103°F (39.4°C) or higher. Quite often she will also go partly or completely off her feed. She looks and acts sick.

If possible, your veterinarian should take milk samples for culture and have sensitivity tests run to identify the causative agent and the correct antibiotic for quick, effective treatment. Where such a test is not possible and you need to start treating a very sick cow, the best thing to use is a broad-spectrum antibiotic or antibiotic combination such as penicillin-streptomycin. Be careful in your choice of antibiotics, and read the directions carefully, especially in regard to the milk-withholding times. (You must withhold the milk from treated animals from market for several days.)

One treatment, known as intermammary infusion, involves injecting an antibiotic compound directly into the teat of a cow with mastitis via a plastic syringe with a flexible tube tip. I do not often use this approach, as systemic treatment usually seems to clear up the infection quickly. I believe that in many cases, using mastitis tubes actually prolongs mastitis or even makes it worse by irritating the teat canal. No matter how careful you are to wash the teats and disinfect the tube tip, there are still bacteria in the barn, just waiting to catch a ride on the tube into the teat canal. It is nearly impossible to totally disinfect skin—merely rubbing alcohol on doesn't immediately kill off all bacteria—and a cow's teats are far from surgically clean!

Along with drug treatments, massaging the udder with warm cloths, applying a warming udder ointment, and milking the animal several times a day will all help to quickly relieve most cases of acute mastitis. Milking the cow by hand (which is more gentle than a machine) every two hours or so is like draining an abscess. It helps flush out the causative bacteria, thinning their numbers and making the drugs work faster. Never milk a mastitis cow with the milker you use on your other cows. You can't disinfect it thoroughly enough in between cows, or even in between milkings, to be sure you won't spread the infection to other cows. If you normally milk by hand, milk the mastitis cow last. Either way, always scrub your hands thoroughly after milking her, until she is well cleared up. A lot of folks don't think of mastitis as an infection, and they treat it too lightly. But besides ruining or even killing one good cow, it can also spread to others in your herd.

Acute mastitis is quite often brought about by stress, such as a bump, bee sting, or cold, which enables the bacteria to multiply and become dangerous. Misuse of the milking machine is one of the main causes of mastitis in cows. Do not leave a milker on a cow for over three minutes. Longer milking times increase the chance of damaging the udder. I have been in barns where one person, working alone, had three milking machines going at one time. This is not physically possible—that is, if the milking is done right. Figuring the time it takes to do a good job washing and drying the bags, putting milker belts on the cows, dumping the milk (assuming that the milker is not milking cows on a pipeline milker, of course), dipping the teats after milking, plus walking back and forth, nobody can use more than two milkers at once without help.

Gangrene Mastitis

This type of mastitis can follow acute mastitis or appear suddenly by itself. When the udder feels hard and hot, worry and call the vet. When it feels hard and cold, panic and call the vet. Once the bag, or part of it, becomes cold and has a "dead" feeling, you need to get help soon, or the cow will die. Many times gangrene mastitis is caused when the swelling of acute mastitis shuts off the circulation in one or more quarters of the udder. The part with no blood supply actually dies and will literally rot off, if the animal doesn't die first. If the animal receives poor treatment or no treatment at all, she quickly becomes toxic and then dies.

Proper treatment often consists of intravenous antibiotics, supportive fluids, surgical removal of the affected quarter or quarters, and long-term antibiotic therapy following the surgery, in addition to excellent care until the cow recovers.

Chronic Mastitis

With chronic mastitis the same cow or cows will show repeated periodic flare-ups of mastitis. A cow with chronic mastitis is usually not as sick as a cow with acute mastitis; in fact, she may not appear sick at all. The udder may swell, but usually the first sign of trouble is when her milk will not pass through the strainer. Stripping the four quarters separately into a strip cup *before* every milking for every cow will let you catch the very first symptoms of mastitis. You can begin mastitis treatment sooner and provide the extra cleanliness and isolation needed to prevent its spread to other cows. Not many people use a strip cup, because they feel it's too much trouble. But it's a lot easier to strip-check than to explain to the dairy why you have mastitis milk in today's shipment!

Dry cow treatment (the use of special mastitis infusions while the cow is not milking) can help some chronic mastitis cows if you are exceptionally careful to have the teats clean and keep the tube tips sterile before treatment. Do not, for instance, open all four tubes, lay them in the straw, and then clean the teats; the tubes will become contaminated. To clean the teats thoroughly, scrub them with warm, soapy water. After rinsing and drying them, apply Betadine or rubbing alcohol, and allow it to dry. Also, clean your hands thoroughly. Then, infuse one teat at a time, opening the tube just before infusion.

Once a cow has chronic mastitis, the problem is seldom completely knocked out. Instead, it lies hidden in scar tissue in the udder, and any stress lets it break out again. If you have a cow with chronic mastitis, milk it last in the herd, and if possible, use a separate milker. When culling time comes, it might be best to choose her to ship rather than a cow that doesn't give quite as much milk, perhaps, but is mastitis-free. As long as a chronic mastitis cow is in the herd, she is a source of infection for all the others.

Preventing Mastitis

As with many diseases, mastitis is easier to prevent than treat. Start by eliminating trouble areas, such as a high concrete step into the barn (cows will bang their udders on it). Bed the stalls generously so cows don't hit their udders against the floor when they lie down. If possible, keep cows from lying in muddy areas, where they can chill their udders in cold weather and pick up bacteria from the muck. Keeping the cows from hurrying or running (and consequently banging their udders) will also help. If the person who brings in your cows is impatient, you'll see a lot of mastitis in your herd.

Religiously dipping the teats after milking will greatly cut down the chance of mastitis because it kills many bacteria. Dipping also helps prevent chapping, another stress to the teat.

If you have a cow with a hanging, pendulous udder, it helps to use an udder support, especially when she first freshens. This will keep the udder from banging on her legs as she walks. When you have a chance, cull that cow from your herd.

In the same vein, choose heifers out of cows with great udders. I would rather have a tight-uddered cow than one that milked more but had a pendulous udder. The tight-uddered cow will be with me longer and be much less apt to get mastitis.

Keep the udders clipped, especially in the winter. Hair encourages the clinging of filth and makes it impossible to wash the udder thoroughly. A token splash with water does not count as washing the udder. The proper technique is to wash the entire udder, including the areas between the quarters as well as the teats. This not only makes the udder clean to milk but also stimulates milk letdown, letting the cow's milk out quickly.

Finally, but perhaps most importantly, have someone experienced, such as a maintenance person from your milking equipment dealership, thoroughly go over your milking equipment. Problems such as incorrect vacuum, pulsation rate, liner length, and bore diameter all are frequent causes of mastitis in a herd. Just because a milker gets milk out of the cow and into the tank does not mean it is easy on the cow's udder! Spending a few minutes and a few dollars can lead to great savings in the end.

If your herd has a mastitis problem, discuss the possibility of vaccinating the animals with your veterinarian. But also be very aware that mastitis vaccination is not a replacement for good husbandry and milking practices.

Milk Fever

To begin with, an animal with milk fever has no fever. In fact, it usually has a subnormal temperature! Milk fever occurs in high-producing milk cows, with the greatest incidence in Jerseys. A cow that produces only 20 pounds of milk a day will very seldom come down with it. I have seen only one beef cow with milk fever, and she was part Holstein. Milk fever doesn't occur very often in heifers but rather in cows that have had two or more calves.

Milk fever is caused by low blood calcium. A cow can come down with milk fever several weeks before calving, but it usually happens one or several days after calving. Milk fever causes an ascending paralysis, beginning with the hind limbs and progressing up the body. Keep a close eye on any newly fresh cow that is staggery in its hind limbs or that staggers when trying to rise. If it's milk fever, the condition will get progressively worse until the cow is unable to rise. The next thing you will notice, in most cases, is the characteristic bend, or kink, to the neck. The cow will twist her head to one side and be unable to hold it straight. Not all cows will exhibit this, but many do.

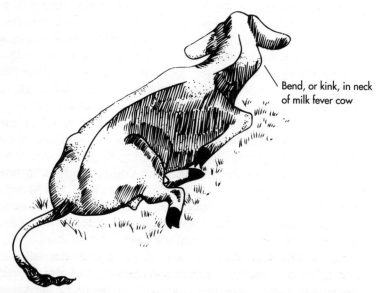

Bend, or kink, in neck of milk fever cow

Cow with milk fever. *A cow with milk fever will gradually develop paralysis in her hind limbs until she can no longer stand. In most cases you will also notice a bend, or kink, in the animal's neck.*

Milk fever is an emergency: If the cow doesn't get prompt treatment, she may well die. It is also one thing that should, if possible, be treated by a veterinarian. There are several reasons for this. First of all, the calcium-phosphorus solution used to treat milk fever must be given intravenously for the quickest results. It can be given intraperitoneally (into the abdominal cavity), but it is absorbed more slowly that way. This may be all right in a mild case, but many times the cow is quite far gone when the problem is discovered. I once treated a little Jersey with irregular, labored breathing and dry, open eyes, as if she were already dead. The intravenous treatment brought prompt relief, and she was standing and chewing her cud in half an hour. She wouldn't have had a chance with intraperitoneal treatment.

Another reason to let your veterinarian treat this problem is that calcium is a powerful stimulant to the heart. A cow with milk fever may already show an abnormal heartbeat. Sometimes an amphetamine injection or other drug can be given to regulate this, for giving calcium to a cow with heart abnormalities can kill her.

Some stubborn cases of milk fever need more than one bottle (500 cc) of calcium. But your veterinarian should make this decision because he has had the experience to make the right call. There is no need to give two bottles if the cow is simply tired from her efforts to get up. Giving too much calcium, or giving it too fast, can kill a cow. Even the veterinarian can be wrong, as nothing is ever sure in medicine; but his chances for a correct decision will be better than those of an inexperienced layperson.

If you do not live fairly near a veterinarian (within 50 miles or so) and you have one or more high-producing milk cows, it would be a good idea to obtain an intravenous outfit and two bottles of calcium to keep on hand. Ask your veterinarian to show you how to use them in an emergency. And I would advise home treatment of milk fever only in an emergency situation. If you must treat an affected animal yourself, work carefully; take your time, and do it right. When starting the intravenous injection, start it slowly, first clearing the tube of air before attaching it to the needle in the vein. Bubbles in the bottle should rise one or two at a time, not in a continuous stream; that is too fast and can kill your cow. Lower the bottle to slow down the rate.

Make sure the needle—I like a 16-gauge, 2-inch needle—is threaded well into the vein, not just sticking into it. Calcium irritates the skin; if some leaks out under the skin, it can make a section of the neck slough off. A veterinarian can't do much to treat this problem, and the damaged area looks ugly for quite a while. (For more information on giving this type of injection properly, see "Intravenous Injection" on page 371.)

After you have given one whole 500-cc bottle, your cow should begin to shake, look brighter, and manure as the paralysis wears off. Don't be in a big rush to get her to her feet, as many cows are hurt trying to get up when they are still too wobbly. Remember, she almost died! She will get up when she is ready. Provide her with good footing and plenty of bedding. Don't let her slip and slide around on cement; throw a bushel or two of sand down under her. Make sure she doesn't have her head in a corner or up against a wall, as cattle have to throw their heads and necks out to balance themselves when getting up. If she is in a stanchion, release her head. When it is time for her to get up, she will have a better chance of making it, especially if you grasp her tail to assist her.

If she still can't get up after several hours, you may have to give her the second bottle. Also, some cattle relapse into milk fever after getting to their feet; so be sure to watch a treated cow for several hours and check in on her regularly for a couple of days.

I don't like to treat a cow for milk fever until she goes down: The treatment is dangerous, and sometimes the cow is just a little wobbly from calving and really doesn't have milk fever at all. It is, however, a good idea to call your veterinarian and let him know you have a cow you think is coming down with milk fever; he will try to stay within phone reach in case you do need him.

Once a cow has had milk fever, she is quite apt to have it each year after (or just before) she calves, as may her daughters since she is probably a good producer and will pass this trait on to them. If you have no problem in getting prompt veterinary help, I wouldn't necessarily advise selling milk fever–prone cows, because they are good producers; but it does mean watching them like a hawk around calving time.

So far, there is nothing that is sure to prevent milk fever. To reduce the chance of a problem, don't milk out a cow completely for three days following freshening. Take just enough milk, from all four quarters, to feed her calf and to take the pressure off the udder somewhat. Also, cut down on her grain for a few days. These steps will not prevent milk fever for certain, but they will help.

Dietary prevention consists of reducing alfalfa in the diet, as alfalfa is a feed high in calcium and potassium. As a dairy cow becomes close to freshening, cutting out the alfalfa and substituting it with a grass-based hay may help prevent milk fever on refreshening. It has recently been found that potassium plays a part in the milk fever complex and alfalfa is also high in potassium.

With high risk cows (cows that have had milk fever in the past or have come from dams prone to milk fever), it can help to give them calcium chloride gel immediately after freshening in order to boost the blood calcium.

Pinkeye

Pinkeye, or infectious keratitis, is most common during the summer months. The first sign of trouble is an eye that is watering or tearing. Soon the eye will begin to squint and appear bloodshot. If left untreated, a cloudy film may appear there. This film will spread and cover the eye, which will become bluish white. The cow will lose sight in that eye. If both eyes are affected, she will go totally blind.

Pinkeye is spread by flies that walk on the tears of the infected eye and then move on to other animals. Sometimes it will clear up untreated, depending on the causative organism, but don't count on it. It can spread quickly not only among your animals but also among animals in nearby herds. If your neighbor's herd has pinkeye, look out for it in your cattle.

There are several eye powders on the market that usually stop pinkeye before it gets past the tearing stage. These antibiotic powders sometimes contain a local anesthetic to cut down the pain and itching. Some also contain a dye so that if you have many cattle, you can easily tell which animals have been treated.

In cases where the eye has clouded over, I have had very good luck using subcutaneous foreign protein injections. (For details on giving this kind of injection, see "Subcutaneous Injection" on page 373.) Antibiotic injections don't usually work very well as the eye has a natural protective barrier that keeps out much of the antibiotic. Injecting foreign protein, however, stimulates the body to produce nonspecific antibodies that are natural to the body and thus can get through this barrier into the eye and attack the infection. I give these injections daily or every two days until improvement is noted. I've found that 90 percent or more of these cloudy-eyed cattle clear up entirely with treatment. If injectable foreign protein is not available, try injecting sterile nonfat canned milk, available from the grocery store. (The fat could cause body reactions, so make sure you use nonfat milk.) A large cow usually requires 10 cc, given once weekly until the eye is clear.

Fly control during the summer will help prevent pinkeye, but there's nothing that will completely stop it. If you have to treat one or more head of beef cattle for pinkeye and the flies are very bad, it is often wise to use treated ear tags to keep the pests away from the infected eyes. This will not only help the affected animals but also prevent the pinkeye from spreading to your whole herd. If pinkeye is a yearly problem in your area, ask your veterinarian about vaccinating your animals.

Pneumonia

This is another disease brought about by stress, such as a change in the weather, shipping, changes in the feed, or confinement in damp quarters. I have found that dampness seems to cause many respiratory problems in the winter months, and the difficulty is not confined to animals stuck in old, rickety, overcrowded, dirty barns—although these aren't the best of conditions for cattle. I have treated pneumonia in animals that were kept in damp barns designed by agricultural engineers and that were cared for by animal husbandry specialists. But the barns were too warm (I don't like a barn warmer than 50°F [10°C] in the winter), and "sweat" dripped constantly from the ceiling. That is too damp. Animals are much more comfortable—and less stressed, less prone to pneumonia—in a cold but dry barn. A moist, warm barn is more "comfy" for you to milk in. But remember, you can leave after a little while and get out in the fresh air. The cattle stay in the dampness and become chilled.

Dry, clean bedding and adequate ventilation do much to help a barn stay dry. So does allowing adequate space for the animals, where they are not packed in too closely. You would be better off to let young stock run in and out of a shed that is cold but dry and draft-free than to put them in a pen in the barn and crowd the cows inside. Here again, I recommend loose, or free, housing, where at all possible. When cattle are free to come and go, they can go outside and stand in the sun, come in out of the wind, or move about if chilled, whereas a confined animal has to take whatever conditions you and the barn provide.

Pneumonia can be caused by many organisms, quite often a *Pasteurella* bacterium as well as viruses and fungi. Usually, the animal is stricken suddenly, with no warning. The first signs are abnormally quick breathing, a drop in milk production, and perhaps a few dry, unproductive coughs. Next the cow begins to puff, often running a temperature of 104° to 106°F (40° to 41.1°C), and goes off its feed. If left untreated, the animal begins to show signs of breathing difficulty: The neck is extended, the nostrils flare, and the cow will grunt heavily on each breath. The animal usually dies shortly after beginning to grunt and foam at the mouth from lack of oxygen.

At the first signs of rough breathing and depression, it is best to isolate the animal as much as possible in a comfortable, draft-free stall. Take the cow's temperature. If the temperature is above 102°F (38.9°C) or the breathing doesn't improve in a few hours, call your vet. It is possible to successfully treat an advanced pneumonia case, but the chances for complete recovery are much better if the animal is diagnosed and treated in the very early stages of the disease. Once the cattle show advanced symptoms, such as stretching their necks out, grunting, and lying down, they may survive with treatment, but there is usually severe damage done to the lungs by this point. Nothing can be done to repair them, and you will end up with animals that are like persons with emphysema. A beef animal will remain thin, using every bit of energy to breathe, and a dairy animal will not milk decently. A young animal won't grow as well as one that breathes normally.

If a veterinarian is not available to make a positive diagnosis, you will have to do a little guesswork and treat the sick animal for pneumonia. But please, do not go ahead and treat a pneumonia cow if you do have a veterinarian handy, since he can sometimes advise other ways to help save the animal. Based on his past experience, he may recommend steaming, a process that involves placing a humidifier or a bucket of boiling hot water under an animal's nose, covering its head with a blanket to create a "tent," and allowing the animal to breathe the steam. Other options include cortisone treatment, injectable expectorants to help clear congested lungs, electrolytes to restore fluid balance following a fever, and other remedies. Whenever possible, let the vet choose the treatment.

A broad-spectrum antibiotic treatment (one that treats a wide variety of bacterial infections), such as penicillin, Tylan, or tetracycline, especially the long-acting formula, seems to work best unless a culture proves otherwise. (Having your veterinarian take a blood test for culture is worth the expense so you'll be able to choose the best antibiotic for the job.) Continue antibiotic treatment as recommended by your veterinarian or in the directions for treatment given on the antibiotic bottle for the full course of treatment. If you stop giving the antibiotic—or, worse yet, give only one shot—the organisms causing the problem may develop a resistance to that antibiotic, and the animal will suffer a relapse. This is much harder to treat than the original pneumonia, and you cannot use the same antibiotic or one that acts against it. (For more information on how antibiotics can work with or against each other, see "Antibiotic Compatibility" on page 375.)

Sulfonamides, oral or injectable, also usually work well in treating pneumonia. Remember, there are *many* sulfa drugs and many more sulfa combinations. Make sure the sulfa you use is for pneumonia! I have had very good luck with triple sulfas, such as sulfadiazine, sulfamerazine, and sulfathiazole combined. When using any sulfa drug, make sure that the cow or calf is consuming plenty of water, because sulfas can be hard on the kidneys if the animal doesn't drink enough.

Puncture Wounds

In many ways a puncture wound is more dangerous to cattle than a wide-open gash. A typical puncture happens when Bessie steps on a nail out in the old shed and comes hobbling home. Most times the nail has come out, leaving a tiny black hole that bleeds only a few drops, if at all. But on its way in, the nail carried bacteria with it, and the warm, moist environment provides perfect conditions for the bacteria to multiply. In addition to blackleg and tetanus organisms, many other bacteria can cause a severe infection, making the prompt treatment of a puncture wound—especially in the foot—very important.

As soon as you notice a wound, tie the cow in a clean place where you can work on it to treat the area and keep it clean. Soak the wound, scrub it well with hot, soapy water, and irrigate it with an antiseptic like Betadine. You can use an old syringe or any number of improvised items (such as a doll bottle with a stiff plastic nipple or an ear syringe) to spray the antiseptic into the wound. The important thing is not what you use but that you get the antiseptic clear down to the bottom of the wound.

After treating the wound, it is a good idea to give the animal a three-day systemic treatment with a broad-spectrum antibiotic as a precaution. Injecting tetanus antitoxin is a good idea, too. Cows do not get tetanus as readily as horses do, but often enough that you should respect the risk. It is also a good idea to soak the injured foot in hot Epsom salts twice a day for three days; keep it out of manure and dirt in between soakings. This not only will reduce the soreness but also will clean the wound and help protect against infection.

Retained Placenta

A cow usually expels her afterbirth within a few hours after calving. If she has not expelled it 48 to 72 hours after giving birth, she is said to have a retained placenta. Have your veterinarian come out to check the cow.

Sometimes it is easy to remove the placenta manually. Inside the cow it is attached to the uterus by means of meshing potato-shaped "buttons" on the placenta (called cotyledons) and matching "buttons" on the uterine surface (known as caruncles). Removing the placenta manually involves reaching into the cow and gently peeling apart the "buttons" by hand, freeing the afterbirth. There are quite a few attachments, so it takes a while to clean each one thoroughly.

In other cases swelling or an infection may make manual cleaning impossible. Also, many veterinarians prefer not to manually clean a cow as it is possible to introduce bacteria into the uterus or damage the organ, no matter how gently they work. Many farmers insist on "having the cow cleaned," and they pull and yank on the placenta until it comes away. This is dangerous because some of the attachments on the uterus can pull off, too, and the cow may not be able to carry another calf. There's also a chance of severe bleeding or infection due to pieces of the placenta being torn and left inside the uterus.

Many times your veterinarian can give the cow an injection to help the uterus cast off the placenta. He can also place boluses or powder in the uterus to prevent infection and help dissolve the afterbirth. It is important to keep as much of the placenta hanging through the cervix as possible. If the cervix closes before all the shreds have passed through, there is considerably more chance of infection, which may either ruin the cow's reproductive ability or kill her. Keeping the placenta hanging through the vagina will help provide gentle traction, which also encourages the uterus to release the placenta naturally.

Ringworm

Ringworm is not a worm, nor is it caused by worms. It is a dermatitis caused by a fungus, typically *Trichophyton verrucosum.* It appears as rough, scaly, round patches of baldness, usually on the face and neck. You'll most often see it during the winter months since, like lice, it thrives in long hair and dark conditions. Small patches of ringworm are not dangerous, but if not treated, they can spread over quite a bit of the body, interfering with normal skin functions. Ringworm is also very contagious, and a herd of cattle or young stock with ringworm will not grow properly or carry normal body weight. The stress can also make the animals more prone to other health problems.

To treat ringworm, remove the thick, scaly dandruff by soaking with warm, soapy water, and apply any one of the antifungal drugs. Tincture of iodine is one of the best treatments, and it is easy to get. Scrub the antifungal drug into the lesion, working from the outside of the affected area to the inside. (Don't scrub from the inside out, as this can spread the lesion.) Use a small brush, and really scrub. Repeat this treatment every day or as often as the directions on your chosen product recommend. Do not get the drug in the animal's eyes. (Rubbing a ring of petroleum jelly around the eyes will help protect them, as will working carefully when you apply the treatment.) Getting your cattle into the sunlight will also help rid them of ringworm.

Scours

Scours is a term used for diarrhea in farm animals. It can affect both young and older animals.

Scours in Calves

Calves in the 3-day to 3-week age group are the usual victims of this problem. The most common causes are stress and overeating—especially milk. Stress refers to any considerable change in the animal's environment, from dramatic changes in the weather, moving, or emotional upset to changes in the feed or the feeding routine. It's no wonder that calves bought at a sale barn often come down with scours! After a calf is older than 3 weeks, it is usually past the calf scour stage, so you can relax some.

When raising calves, it is a very good idea to have a couple of packets of oral electrolyte powder on hand as well as a simple scour medicine, just in case you do need it. Have your veterinarian make his recommendations. I have had very good luck with a kaolin-pectin-bismuth solution containing antibiotics. The kaolin solution soothes the gut and helps dry the stools; the antibiotic works on the destructive bacteria present.

If you notice a loose stool in a calf in the scour age bracket (3 to 21 days of age), give that animal immediate attention. A normal calf stool is yellowish and like gooey putty, with some form to it. You know a calf has trouble when you see puddles of nasty mush in its bedding instead of manure or wet manure stuck to its tail. If you notice the stool is slightly loose, cut the milk feedings in half. If the stool is very loose, stop all feedings of milk. Provide adequate water and dry feed. Do not try to give additional dry feed or pellets to make up for the lack of milk. It will only cause additional stress to the digestive tract. A calf with scours needs less to digest, not more!

I do not recommend giving scour medicine every time a calf passes a loose stool, as many times the animal will return to normal if you just stop feeding milk for a day. To help determine the right treatment, take the calf's temperature. If it is 101.5°F (38.6°C) or below, just replace its milk with electrolytes or barley water. Feeding an electrolyte solution instead of milk will help to get fluid into the animal and restore the electrolyte balance in its body. (For more information on electrolyte therapy, see "Electrolytes in the Body" on page 382.) If you can't get an electrolyte solution, feeding barley water will often help. Make this by simmering ½ pound of barley in 1 gallon of water until the barley is tender. Drain off the liquid for the calf, and save the barley to eat yourself. Feed the barley water, 1 pint at a time, every 2 hours throughout the day in place of milk.

When a calf's temperature is higher than 101.5°F (38.6°C) or when its stools seem to be getting looser and more frequent, begin the scour medication. Please read all directions, and follow them exactly. Scours is nothing to play around with. If the cure doesn't come quickly, the calf will die. It may not seem that a 100-pound calf full of bucks and kicks can die in a couple of days just from diarrhea, but it can.

A calf that acts sick and is running a fever, as well as scouring, usually also benefits from injectable antibiotics. Ask your veterinarian to recommend a suitable treatment, as you want something that will not act against the antibiotic in the scour medication.

If you have any trouble clearing up the scours in two days, call your vet. Sometimes an intravenous electrolyte injection over a 24-hour period is necessary, and a blood transfusion may work miracles. I knew one Angus calf that was so sick it was laid out flat for two days, unable to raise even its head. We had it in the clinic with an intravenous drip for 36 hours straight and under a heat lamp (it was so sick that it was running a subnormal temperature—usually a symptom of imminent death). The only way we knew the calf was still alive was by its shallow breathing. Then at night we heard a bawl from the clinic. The calf's head was up, and its eyes were open and bright. Two hours later it took some oral electrolytes from a bottle, and little sweat beads appeared on its black nose—usually a sure sign that all is well. The calf had stopped scouring and was on its way back to good health. Two days later it nursed by itself from our old nurse cow. Today it weighs 800 pounds, and its owner is glad he gave it a chance and gambled on such a poor risk.

Buying young calves at an auction barn is the surest way to get great experience in doctoring scouring calves. There the calf is subjected to more stress than possibly anywhere else. First there is the emotional trauma of being separated from its mother, often soon after birth. (Possibly it never even received colostrum.) Then comes the strange ride to the yards confined in a trailer or truck or, even worse, jammed into a sack or into a load of other animals. Next it is unloaded and pushed into a strange pen with a large number of calves, where they spend hours swapping germs. Maybe one or more sick calves are in the bunch, scouring badly, dumped by an owner who figured they would probably die. You buy your calf and take it home, changing its diet, schedule, and surroundings again. You sure wouldn't treat a three-day-old human infant that way and think it would be okay!

If you do buy a young calf at the auction barn, be prepared for scours, and start medication as soon as the first loose stool hits the ground. Also, be very stingy with the first three days of meals. If you can, give only 1 quart at a time, but feed every 3 hours; this is better than giving 2 quarts twice a day. There are also many commercial products that you can give to calves to head off scours. Ask your veterinarian to recommend one, and give it to your new calf as soon as you get home. Even if it doesn't prevent scours altogether, it may help reduce the severity of the case.

While calves may get scours even with the best care, it is worth taking precautions to reduce the chance. (For tips on proper calf feeding, see "Caring for Calves" on page 36.)

Diarrhea in Adult Cattle

During the summer months, when cattle are on lush pasture, their stools become quite loose and are sometimes mistaken for scours. If in doubt, bring the animal into the barn or a dry lot, and feed it hay for a day or two. If the looseness was due simply to eating lush green grass, the hay will cause the stools to return to normal. If not, or if the animal is acting depressed (less active, not eating well), take the animal's temperature. Diarrhea is often a symptom of such diseases as Johne's disease and shipping fever. (Keep in mind that an animal does not have to be shipped to come down with shipping fever. For more information on the other symptoms of these two problems, see "Johne's Disease" on page 57 and "Shipping Fever" on page 78.)

If the temperature is normal and the animal acts fine but for the diarrhea, take a stool sample in to your veterinarian. (By stool sample, I mean just a tablespoonful of manure—not a whole bushel basket full, as one farmer once brought in!) The veterinarian can examine the sample under a microscope and tell if the animal has trouble with worms or other intestinal parasites, one of the most common causes of diarrhea in cattle. You will not necessarily see worms in the manure when the animal has parasites, as some dangerous ones are microscopic. If the sample is negative, there is no reason to worm. Wormers are toxic and can kill a sick animal that is not wormy. Don't just assume the cow is wormy and worm it: Be sure.

Many things can cause scours in cattle. An allergy to a certain plant, eating a slightly poisonous plant or a moldy chunk of hay, too much feed, feed changes, heat cycles, and other factors can all cause scouring. Fortunately, it is usually easy to remedy. Your veterinarian may prescribe some astringent antidiarrheal medicine. This comes in various forms: bolus, powder, or liquid. Give the medication according to the directions.

During the winter months, especially when confined in a barn, cattle become susceptible to what is called winter scours, or winter dysentery. This comes on suddenly, with several animals in a herd, or perhaps just one or two, developing serious diarrhea. If there are many animals in the herd, it usually will spread quickly until most, if not all, of the animals are affected. In milking animals there will be a sharp drop in milk production. One farmer whose entire dairy herd came down with it said, "I didn't get any milk this morning. Just manure, and lots of it!" He was sloshing around in a foot of sloppy manure in what had previously been a spotless barn.

Affected cattle can pass mucus and quite large quantities of blood. If you notice the problem quickly—and it's hard to miss—start treating the animals with an astringent antidiarrheal. Try 1 percent copper sulfate solution (75 to 150 ml daily for no more than three days) or catechu (gallotanic acid) along with ferrous sulfate and copper sulfate several times daily. Also, use electrolytes to combat dehydration, if needed. These treatments will usually hold the animals until the "bug" (believed to be a virus) dies out. Winter scours is a nasty condition but seldom kills cattle.

Shipping Fever

Shipping fever, also known as hemorrhagic septicemia, is a pneumonia-enteritis complex. This means it involves pneumonia in the lungs and frequently diarrhea or inflammation of the bowels, as well. It is most often brought on by stress; since shipping is a frequent stress in cattle, the name of shipping fever became common. An animal does not have to be shipped to come down with shipping fever.

An affected animal often has a high temperature, sometimes reaching 105°F (40.6°C). You will notice rapid breathing with a rasping cough. There may be a heavy nasal discharge, and the animal will often have diarrhea. Death can be caused by dehydration or lung consolidation (the scarring and filling of the lung with fluid or pus).

Shipping fever is usually quite contagious, so it's necessary to isolate any sick animal. Sulfas, tetracycline, dihydrostreptomycin, and antiserum have been used to treat the disease. Researchers differ on the use of antiserum: Some say it works well; others say it is worthless. Antidiarrheals, expectorants, electrolytes, and good nursing will all help. Adding 1 percent cobalt chloride to the water (1 ounce per animal) will aid in stimulating the depressed appetite.

When at all possible, involve your veterinarian in the diagnosis and treatment of cattle you suspect have shipping fever. If you get him involved early in the course of the disease, he has the best chance of promptly starting effective treatment and prescribing the right nursing care that will help the animal recover quickly.

To help prevent shipping fever, vaccinate your animals three weeks or more before an anticipated stress, such as shipping or showing. Also, isolate all new animals for at least two weeks after bringing them home, before introducing them to the herd. Other common-sense steps include providing adequate ventilation and keeping your animals and barns clean.

Teat and Udder Injuries

Cows are more prone to udder and teat injuries than any other domestic animal. This is due to their weight and clumsy ways as well as to intentionally inbred "deformities" like huge udders and long teats. What most often happens is that the udders and teats get stepped on or snagged on something. If a cow doesn't manage to step on her own teat, some kind neighboring cow seems willing to do it for her. Sometimes nothing more serious than a bruise results, but many times there is a cut, tear, or mashed teat to contend with.

If you catch a teat injury while the cut is still new or fresh (not dried up and scabbed over), the chances are good that if your veterinarian comes out and sews it up, it will heal rapidly and uneventfully. After a day or so, though, stitches will probably not hold well, and the suturing may seal in bacteria that will cause infection and scarring. With an older cut, it's best to let your veterinarian decide the proper course of treatment.

A cow objects to being milked when she has an injured teat, so the easiest course of action is to use a milk tube inserted in the teat to let the milk run out. Some milk tubes have caps on their ends that can be unscrewed to let the milk out at certain times of the day (normally at the usual milking time). Tubes like these are helpful as it is a bit unsanitary to have a cow leaking milk out all over the barn floor, especially in the summer. The flies might like it, but the injured cow with flies on her sore teat doesn't. Before inserting a milk tube, scrub the teat with warm, soapy water; then rinse, dip in Betadine, and allow to air-dry. Sterilize the tube by immersing it in boiling water for 15 minutes. Scrub your hands well, rinse and dry them, and then insert the cooled tube. All this extra care is worth the effort because otherwise you may introduce bacteria into the teat canal, which could cause mastitis in the already stressed teat.

It's not uncommon for cows with large, low-hanging bags to snag and rip their udders on almost anything handy. Barbed wire fences and old dead brush seem to rank high on the list of causes of cow snags. Most bloody rips can be successfully sewn up, leaving little or no scar, so don't let anyone talk you into shooting your cow. Get your veterinarian out to assess the damage and treat the wound. Udder rips can be quite ugly. Many times they gape widely, bleed profusely, and leak milk. After such an injury, the affected quarter or quarters may not give as much milk as before, but generally it is well worth the money to have your veterinarian treat the damage.

To stop excessive bleeding from a teat or udder injury, pack clean cloths against the injury quite firmly until the blood stops flowing. This may take several minutes. Leave a cloth on the wound, as the blood will clot between the cloth and the injury; if you pull the cloth off, it will often start to bleed again. Don't put anything on the wound before the veterinarian arrives. It is sometimes hard to suture a wound that has been gobbed up with powder or gooey salve. The important things are to call the veterinarian as soon as you see the injury and to keep the area around the animal as clean as possible. No barn surgery is sterile, but it won't help an animal with a gaping wound to lie down in 6 inches of manure and dirt.

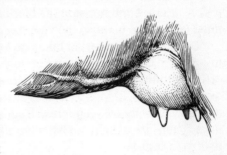

Milk vein. *One milk vein runs along each side of the cow's underside. These large veins are the site of many injuries. Serious injuries will require the attention of your veterinarian.*

Milk Vein Injuries

While we're on this part of the cow, let's move just a little forward to an injury that is fairly common in larger cows. On each side of a cow, viewed from underneath, runs a very large blood vessel known as the milk vein. On a large, high-producing milk cow, this vein is as much as 3 inches across, making it a prime target for injury. Cows sometimes catch the milk vein on a nail, step on it while rising, or hook it with a sharp dewclaw on a front leg. If this vein is cut badly, the cow can bleed to death in less than 15 minutes.

If a cow injures a milk vein, check to see how badly it is bleeding. Remember, a little blood sometimes looks like a lot. If it is dripping, leave it alone, and call your vet. If it is running out in a stream, applying a pressure pack of clean cloths to the area will usually stop it or at least slow it down considerably. Keep the pack on, and have someone else call the vet. Make sure you tell the veterinarian you think the cow cut her milk vein: That classifies the injury as an emergency, and your veterinarian will get there in a hurry.

When a milk vein is cut badly enough that the blood is pouring out in a heavy stream, you need to take steps to reduce the bleeding right away. Get a rope 10 to 12 feet long, or fasten several hay strings together to make a rope. Tightly pull it around the cow's body, in front of the bag, to form a tourniquet, while someone else runs to call the vet. The rope will usually slow down the bleeding to a slow drip but will not stop the bleeding permanently. The wound must be sutured because the vein has probably been severed.

Once your veterinarian takes care of the wound, you will have to keep the cow inside. Keep her very well bedded so she doesn't catch the stitches and rip them loose, starting the whole thing over again. To help speed the healing process, wrap a sheet around her belly to keep straw from poking the injury for a few days. There are usually no bad aftereffects from a properly treated milk vein injury.

Tetanus

Tetanus is caused by *Clostridium tetani*. Although it is more commonly a problem in horses, it does occur quite often in cattle. Tetanus organisms grow in the absence of oxygen, so they are a hazard only in a puncture wound or some other sealed-off wound. I have seen several cases of tetanus in steer calves following castration with elastrators (the rubber band method). I've also seen it following dehorning and surgical castration. When tetanus follows surgical castration, it is almost always due to an incision that's too small. After the castration this tiny incision closes off, making a dandy incubator for tetanus organisms.

A cow or calf with tetanus will usually be reluctant to move. It may stand with its neck stretched out, possibly drool, and be unable to eat or drink. (Use caution when working around an animal like this since these could also be symptoms of rabies.) The membrane in the corner of the eye typically covers nearly half of the eye. The stiffness progresses until death follows. There is no sure treatment for tetanus, although massive doses of tetanus antitoxin or penicillin have worked. If you suspect an animal has tetanus, call your veterinarian immediately to make a definite diagnosis and suggest the proper course of action.

Cattle are usually not vaccinated for tetanus, but there certainly is no reason why they should not or cannot be, especially if the problem has happened before in your herd. If an animal is injured, you can prevent tetanus by giving the antitoxin as soon as possible. This immediately builds up immunity and thus gives quick protection, although the protection doesn't last long. It's a good idea to give the antitoxin after an injury even if the animal has been vaccinated with tetanus toxoid, because no vaccine is 100 percent sure.

Ticks

Ticks are the same type of creature as lice but larger. They are flat and vary in size from the head of a pin to nearly a fat nickel when full of blood. The size also depends on the age and kind of tick. Ticks are usually a darkish brown or black color, although they become grayish when attached to an animal and full of blood. Besides sucking blood and looking ugly, ticks can spread disease as they feed.

In some geographic areas, ticks aren't much of a problem. Cattle in these areas get only an occasional tick, which you can pick off at milking time. (On beef cattle the ticks will fall off when full.) In other areas where ticks are more prevalent, you may need to dip, spray, or powder your cattle periodically. While lice are most numerous in the winter, ticks prefer the warmer summer months and seem to have a "season" when they are the worst. Your veterinarian or county agent can tell you how prevalent ticks are in your area and if they can carry any serious diseases.

To pick off a single tick, simply grasp its body with your fingers, and pull slowly until it releases its hold. If your animals have many ticks, you may choose to dust them with rotenone powder or use one of the many sprays on the market. Where ticks are extremely thick, you may choose to use a pour-on insecticide, which is absorbed into the body and blood stream, repelling and killing ticks as well as lice and flies. If you choose to use this product and are using it on dairy cows, be sure to buy a product labeled for use in lactating dairy cows. Be sure to read labels before buying a tick treatment as many are very toxic and unfriendly to the environment.

Tuberculosis

TB causes a general wasting illness, light fever, weakness, and often a nonproductive cough, followed by death. Once very common, TB has been nearly wiped out in the United States and Canada, owing mainly to very stringent testing programs. It is, however, not completely gone. There are affected herds left, and sources of infection from a wild population or other animals are still there. (Bison, elk, llamas, deer, opossums, and humans all are possible carriers of TB.)

There is no reliable vaccination available for cattle at this time. To protect your cattle, always test all new animals before introducing them to the herd. If TB has recently been found in animals in your area, your veterinarian may also recommend testing your whole herd periodically.

Worms

Volumes can—and have been—written about internal parasites of cattle. There are many families and many individual worms involved. And with cattle moving more, on account of hauling long distances to pasture, sales, feedlots, and shows, previously localized infestations of certain worms are becoming more and more widespread. Some of the worms that are common to cattle include common stomach worm, tapeworm, small stomach worm, hookworm, threadworm, lungworm, and large-mouth bowel worm.

Possible symptoms of worm infestation include weight loss, potbelly, bad hair coat, general weakness, and coughing. If you suspect an animal has worms, take a small fecal sample to your veterinarian for examination. It is not enough that you don't find any sign of worms in the manure with your naked eye; many are microscopic.

Once you know what worms your cattle have, you can treat them with a wormer effective for their specific problem. All wormers do not get all types of worms; thus, it's important to get a diagnosis so you can choose the right treatment. If your cattle don't have worms, you may actually kill the animals by worming them improperly. Cattle that were weak from pneumonia or lice have been killed by well-meaning owners who figured the trouble must be worms. Cattle should be checked for worms more frequently than they are: Many cattle, both beef and dairy, would do much better if they didn't have to feed a belly full of worms!

With the advent of injectable wormers, such as ivermectin, and the use of pour-ons, it is possible to control, if not eliminate, severe worm problems in cattle. I do not like to use systemic wormers, as their safety to human consumers is debatable—but where they are warranted, I do not hesitate.

There are many other steps you can take to help reduce a worm problem. Rotate pastures to give the soil and grass a chance to rest and naturally get rid of worm eggs. Keep fecal contamination out of feed bunks, mangers, and water tanks. Establishing a routine worming program and having your veterinarian periodically check for worms will also help make worm problems a thing of the past.

Liver Fluke

Liver fluke is a serious problem, especially in swampy or lowland areas where snails are prevalent. The snails pass encysted fluke larvae, which adhere to grasses and leaves. When eaten by a grazing cow, the cysts break, and the new liver flukes penetrate the intestine and migrate to the liver. Here they ramble about, destroying liver tissue as they go. An affected bovine may keep its weight and just suddenly die. (On autopsy, you'd wonder how it possibly seemed well for as long as it did.) Or it may begin to act listless and progressively get worse, no matter what you do to help it.

Sometimes it is possible to find the eggs of the liver fluke in a fecal examination. In most cases, though, you will need to wait for an autopsy on the dead animal for a positive diagnosis. Once you know that flukes may be present, you can treat your remaining cattle properly. Treatment for liver fluke is more promising today than in the past, when the treatment was nearly as bad as the problem. There are several new drugs available, which your veterinarian may use to establish a treatment program. Fencing off any lowland snail habitats will also help prevent reinfection.

GOATS

General Care and Management

*G*oats have become the dairy animal of choice for people with a limited amount of space. They are also ideal for those who need only a moderate amount of milk and dairy products. Through the years dairy goats have been improved in milking ability, so it's common to have a doe (not "nanny") that provides a gallon of milk daily. Goats are such clean and pleasant animals, with a nice, intelligent personality, that it is no wonder they are so popular.

Although many folks think of goats as replacements for cows, goats are not just small cows—they belong to an individual species and have their own particular problems along with several ailments shared by many domestic creatures. As with other animals, though, goats can be productive and rewarding if you provide them with a safe, healthy environment and good overall care.

Housing

Goats hate getting wet. A few drops of rain will send a herd stampeding for shelter, screaming as if they were being eaten alive by wolves. So be sure your goats have access to shelter!

Open, or Loose, Housing

Dry and milking does do best if they can wander in and out of their shelter at will. Does that are kept tied or in stanchions are more prone to arthritis, lameness, and leg swellings. Large, draft-free, well-bedded loafing pens, with an outside pasture for exercise and sun, keep does healthy and happy.

It's smart to plan an extra pen for kidding so you can separate a doe when she is ready to kid. A roomy pen sited next to the other goats is ideal. That way, the other goats won't bother her while she's kidding, and they won't be hurt by her if she is an overprotective mother.

Don't forget the buck when allowing room for pens. All too many bucks are shut away from the herd in a small, filthy, dark pen and basically ignored except during breeding season. A buck needs exercise, sunshine, and companionship as much as your does do. A sunny pasture and a companion can go a long way toward preventing nervous habits, such as chewing on wood, beating the wire with his head, or masturbating. Possible companions include another buck, a wether (castrated buck), or a doe that is not being milked, such as a doe raising special doe kids. (If the latter, remove those doelings before late summer, or they will be bred too early.)

Fencing

Unlike sheep and cattle, which are basically grazers, goats tend to be browsers, preferring tender willow tips and other brush. This is the

PARTS OF A GOAT

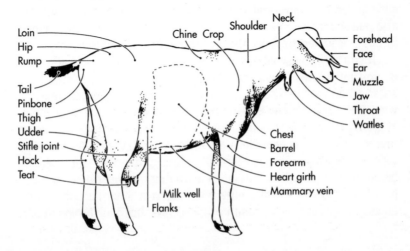

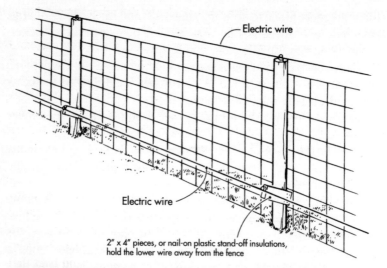

Electric wire

Electric wire

2" x 4" pieces, or nail-on plastic stand-off insulations,
hold the lower wire away from the fence

Goat-proof fence. *Goats are smart and athletic, so it's often hard to
keep them contained. But in my experience, a combination of electric fence
and woven wire stock fence is effective.*

most important reason for having a goat-proof fence to contain them.
Apple and other fruit trees rank high on a goat's goody list, as do
flowers and ornamental shrubbery. As a rule, goats are hard to contain because of their intelligence and athletic abilities. Barbed wire
won't do anything but rip udders, and the animals will quickly destroy
plain woven wire stock fence by climbing and pushing on it. It's possible to contain some goats with a two-strand electric fence, but I've
also had some determined caprines that gritted their teeth and dashed
through or under the fence in spite of the shock they received.

If you plan to use electric fences, you must train your goats. That
is, you must teach them that those flimsy-looking wires will "bite
back" when touched, so the goats will be afraid to even go near the
wire. Training is simple: Put one goat in the fenced area, and set a pan
of grain just outside to tempt it over to the fence. Then walk away so
that when the goat gets shocked, it doesn't think you did the dirty
trick! If you don't do this "formal" training, the goat will probably
break the wire, tangle it, and never learn that the wire caused the jolt.
It's also important to train only one goat at a time. Putting several
goats in together to train ensures that you will be fixing broken fence.

When one goat receives a shock and bleats, the others often charge about, hitting the fence and getting loose.

I've found on my farm that a combination of electric fence and woven wire stock fence or heavy gauge 16-foot-long "stock panels" will contain anything placed inside. This is more formidable than just the electric wire, and yet the electric wire is there to keep animals away from the woven wire. (It seems that one of the goats always has to graze on the other side of the fence, smashing the wire down if it's unprotected by the electric fence!)

Confined Housing

A heated barn for goats is not necessary, even in the coldest climates, and really does more harm than good. A warm barn is quite often a damp one, and a close, damp barn causes pneumonia and other respiratory problems. If you must have a cozy place to milk, build a small milking parlor in one corner of the barn, and heat that slightly. The goats won't be in it long enough to have trouble from it, and you won't have cold hands.

Overcrowding can also lead to many problems, so make sure you have enough room for your animals. A single pen cannot support as many goats as a setup with a loafing barn and free pasture access. In any group of goats, there is a "pecking order," with the toughest goat being boss. The stronger goats will hog the hay rack, grain trough, and even sometimes the water pail or salt block. When one of the meeker animals tries to eat or drink, the bossier ones butt it away, keeping it in its place. Sometimes severe injuries and even death can result. If necessary, you can keep a small group of goats in a large stall, but be sure to provide a long manger and keep it stocked with hay at all times to reduce fighting. Also, keep confined goats separated when you give them their grain.

Staking

If you have only one or two goats, you may choose to keep them staked out. But be aware that there are many problems with staking. A dog can worry and even kill a goat since a tied goat doesn't have much defense and can't run away. Sunstroke is also a problem. When you tie out the animal, make sure the site has at least some shade all day. Where there is shade in the morning, there may be none for the

First Aid Kit for Goats

Here are some basic ingredients that belong in a caprine first aid kit. All of the items below are necessary if you keep a herd of goats. If you have only one or two goats, at least keep those items that are marked with an asterisk. Of course, there are many other things you can keep in your kit, but this is a good start. Ask your veterinarian for his advice for your situation. He may also be able to supply items that you can't find at your local farm supply store or in a farm veterinary supply catalog.

Balling gun (calf-sized)*

Betadine*

Bloat medicine

Blood stopper

California Mastitis Test

Electric disbudding iron

Emasculatome

Forceps/needle holder

Heat lamp

Hoof nippers*

Intravenous outfit

Kid feeding tubes*

Mouth speculum

Rectal veterinary thermometer*

Roll of cotton

Scarlet oil*

16- to 10-gauge, 3-inch needle (for bloat)*

Stomach tube

Teat dip*

Three or four 18-gauge, 1½-inch needles*

12-cc syringe*

Two rolls of 3-inch gauze*

Veterinarian's phone number*

hot afternoon. If this goes unnoticed, there may be a dead goat in the evening.

It is challenging—but necessary—to provide water for staked-out animals. It seems they always tip the pail over 10 minutes after being watered. Or they manure in the bucket, and goats will never touch fouled water. Check the water supply several times a day to make sure your goat has clean water to drink.

Another problem with staking is finding the right length of rope. A goat on a short rope won't get much exercise, and it'll get tangled up on a long rope. Goats often break legs after wrapping them up in a chain or rope and then panicking and thrashing about. Be sure to check on staked animals often and untangle them if you see a problem.

Feeding

Goats, like dairy cattle, must have good food to produce a decent amount of milk and maintain their weight and health. Speaking of weight, a dairy goat, to many people, looks thin. It is perfectly normal for a milking doe to have a "bony topside." So many new goat people are shocked at the "underfed" appearance of their new goat and swear the previous owner starved her. They immediately begin to fatten her up. In six months the previously healthy goat looks like a fat beef steer and is having breeding or kidding problems. A high-producing milk doe many times puts her all into the milk pail and loses much fat. She is not skinny but trim, like a race horse.

A goat that is naturally chubby quite often does not milk well. She is what is called a meat goat, with the bloodlines that produce meat-type animals, not dairy animals. This is not to say that a skinny goat is in good shape. A goat with her backbone sticking out and no flesh on her ribs at all certainly needs weight. She cannot produce milk if she is emaciated! If you are unsure of the proper weight for your goat, ask your veterinarian or an experienced goat breeder in your area.

Pasture and Hay

Ideally, dairy goats should have access to a pasture, preferably seeded with a legume-grass mixture. There may be small brush for them to browse, although once in a while, goats may eat brush that gives an off-flavor to the milk. I prefer a pasture that's divided into sections so the grazing can be rotated. Move your animals to the next area when their current pasture is showing signs of stress, such as bald spots or trampled areas. When you move your goats from one section to another, mow the grazed section to control weeds and rank grass; then let it rest. In this way, your pasture will always be fresh and palatable, and you will greatly reduce any parasite problems.

In their shelter keep a rack of fresh hay for your goats to munch on when they come in for protection from the sun, rain, or cold wind. Change the hay daily, giving the "leftovers" to cattle or horses. Goats are very fussy eaters and often refuse hay that has been nibbled on—or even breathed on! While this hay is perfectly good, they may let it stay in the manger until it becomes moldy or dusty, which causes health problems. If you clean out those feeders every day, your goats will eat more hay, and they'll be healthier and produce more milk.

Grain

A young, dry doe on good pasture requires little, if any, grain. Good lush pasture or legume hay will usually keep the dry doe in good flesh but not overly fat. As the doe becomes heavy with kids, it is usually wise to increase her grain steadily: It is during the last month or so that the kids begin to grow large enough to become a drain on her. Just before kidding, cutting back slightly on the amount of grain you feed may help prevent milk fever in high-producing does. Do not reduce the amount greatly or cut it out altogether, or you may bring on a problem called ketosis. After freshening you may again gradually increase the amount of grain, bringing the doe to full milk production.

There is no hard and fast rule about the exact amount of grain that goats need. Every animal is an individual, and you must feed it as such. Also, there is a great variety of feeds available. You can talk to your county Cooperative Extension Agent (usually located in your county seat) about the feeds available in your area, stressing that you are feeding dairy goats. If you can't get any other advice, you won't go too wrong feeding the following amounts of a good, high-protein, mixed-grain-with-molasses ration, often called sweet feed:

- Kids, birth to four or five months: free-choice, fed in a creep feeder
- Older kids to dry yearlings: 1 to 2 pounds daily
- Bred does, dry: 2 pounds daily or less, depending on other feeds available, such as lush legume pasture or hay
- Does heavy with kid: 2 to 4 pounds daily
- Milking does: ½ to 2 pounds for every 2 pounds of milk given daily
- Bucks with heavy service: 3 to 6 pounds daily

Split the daily grain ration into two feedings per day, and increase or decrease it as the animals' condition indicates. The amounts may be changed to suit the needs of individual goats.

Do not feed goats urea or feed containing urea! Much mixed dairy ration today contains urea, a cheap protein supplement. Read the label on the bag, or ask the feed store operator—whatever it takes to make sure. It's easy to poison goats by feeding urea. Feed meant for cattle often contains urea, but goats can't handle it without disaster.

Salt and Minerals

Keeping a constant supply of trace mineral–iodized salt available may help prevent a variety of health problems. Or you may choose to supply these minerals in a feed supplement. Many areas of the country are lacking in one or more minerals; other areas have an overabundance of certain minerals. Before feeding a mineral supplement, contact your county agent.

Water

It's best if your goats have free access to water at all times. Otherwise, water them at least three times daily, and allow them to drink as much as they want. Always provide the water before giving grain; watering after feeding grain may lead to bloat. In the summer the water should be cool, and the winter water should have the chill taken off. The more water the goats drink, the more milk they will produce and the healthier they will be.

If you leave a pail of water for your goats, make sure they are drinking it, especially during the summer. Goats will very seldom drink unclean water, even if they are very thirsty. Manure, a dead mouse, or other unsavory material falling in the water will usually keep the goats away. And drinking less water will mean a drop in milk production.

Supplying Feed and Water

The best way to keep your goats' feed and water clean is to use "keyhole" mangers and access points to water tanks. These are easy to make from a sheet of ⅝-inch plywood. Make the head holes about 8 inches in diameter, and cut the slots below the holes about 4 inches wide. (Measure your largest goat's head at the eyes and neck to be sure the keyholes are wide enough for it; this way, it won't bang or rub its head entering the keyhole.) The head holes for mangers should be higher than the goat can reach by standing on the floor. On the lower face of the plywood, screw a sturdy 2 × 4 to make a step. The goats will quickly learn to step up on the 2 × 4 to enter the keyhole. This prevents them from wasting any hay or grain. (Be sure the bottom of the keyhole slot goes down far enough that they are com-

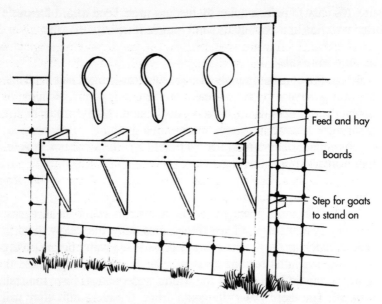

Keyhole manger. *Keyhole-shaped access points to mangers will prevent your goats from wasting their feed and hay. Make the opening higher than the goats can reach from the ground, and give them a step.*

fortable while eating.) The keyhole for the watering tank does not need a step up as nothing will be pulled out and wasted.

Since there is one keyhole per goat and the animals are contained while eating, keyhole mangers will prevent many injuries caused by fighting over feed. They also keep the feed cleaner as none is contaminated by manure or dirt; so your goats will waste less feed while eating more. Likewise, their water is always pure, encouraging them to drink more. The time and effort you'll be saved in changing feed and water are an additional bonus!

Restraint

The first step to restraining a goat is catching it. If your goats are used to being handled, this should be easy, especially if they have collars. To catch a difficult goat that does not have a collar, get as close as possible, reach out quickly, and grab the beard. With a beardless goat, put a hand under the chin, and tip the head up; then push it against the side of the pen. This will keep it off balance and easy to hold.

The goat, being smaller than a cow and somewhat of a pet, is easier to restrain. Usually the only restraint needed is a stanchion. A milking stanchion works well because it is raised, giving the goat less area to dance back and forth on. Another alternative is to tie the goat with a halter or collar to a solid object. Goats, distracted by a measure of grain, easily learn that routine hoof trimming or hair clipping does not hurt and soon ignore it. They will also quickly learn to tolerate other minor examinations and procedures.

Working on an injured teat or teaching a young doe to stand for milking calls for a bit more patience on your part. You'll have to press your arm against her leg to guard against kicks and to keep her from dancing around so much. It usually does no good to simply hold one of her legs, especially when teaching a doe to stand for milking: You can't milk her the rest of her life by holding her hind leg up! With a very nervous doe, it is sometimes necessary to slip a figure eight of light hay string or rope around her hocks. Have a helper hold the string or rope. Do not tie it, because if she should fall or panic, she could break a leg.

Another way to restrain a jumpy goat is to press your head firmly into her flank and hold her against a solid wall while her head is secured in a stanchion or tied. Don't quit or give up if she does jump around a bit. She may just be testing you to see if she can make you quit. If she can't dissuade you by dancing about, she may give up.

The easiest way to drench a goat or give it a bolus is by straddling the neck, facing forward, tipping the chin up, and giving the dose. When giving a drench, pour slowly so the animal doesn't choke or get any of the fluid in its lungs. (This may cause aspiration pneumonia, which quite often kills the goat.) When giving a bolus (pronounced bowl-us), coat it with corn oil first to make it go down easier. If you must give a large bolus, it is usually best to break it in half or thirds to prevent choking. Many boluses are made with cattle in mind and are a little too big for a goat to swallow with ease.

When taking a goat's temperature, it is usually easiest to crowd the animal against a solid wall with your knee and then slip the lubricated thermometer into the rectum. Goats do not like their tails pulled or even touched; so it is easier to get them to stand still while having their temperature taken if you don't handle their tails.

To restrain a small kid, you may hold it between your knees while seated or have an assistant hold it while you drench, dehorn, give pills, or provide other treatment. When you need more restraint, use a kid box or bag. The box can be heavy cardboard with a head hole in it, with the cover tied with heavy twine. It should be just big enough for the kid to fit into but not roomy enough for it to squirm around in. A kid bag should be made of heavy canvas with either a reinforced hole for the head or a drawstring, making the bag snug around the neck to prevent the front feet from coming through. You can use a box or bag for dehorning, descenting bucklings, or treating facial lacerations. If you need to give an injection or treat some other part of the animal, cut a small hole in the side. If you have many kids, it is a good idea to make a kid box out of wood, with a hinged lid and sturdy latch. The wooden box will outlast the cardboard box and provide a lot more security because it will not come apart.

Breeding

Breeding is one of the most important aspects of goat ownership. When a doe doesn't produce kids, you lose time, milk, meat, and money, as there are no products for you to sell or use at home. Understanding the breeding cycle and trying to get the timing right so your doe is efficiently bred to a very good buck will do much to ensure routine breeding and economic gain.

The Heat Cycle

The doe normally comes into heat every 21 days, more or less, mainly in the late summer through the winter. If they are not bred, many continue coming into heat until spring or early summer, so it is not impossible to have does kid every month of the year. Bear in mind that it is generally easier to get a doe bred in the fall than in the spring, though. The doe will be in heat from 1 to 3 days. Remember that each doe is an individual: She may differ from the "norm" and still be normal.

If you have a buck running with your does, it will be easy to detect when a doe is in heat. The buck will show extreme interest in that doe. He will paw at her, sticking his tongue out, or nibble along her body, making guttural grunts. She will respond by wagging her tail, urinating, squatting, and bleating.

If the buck is not running with the does, the doe in heat may suddenly start hanging around as near to the buck pen as possible. She may bleat, run back and forth, wag her tail, ride other does, or be ridden by them. Her vulva may be red and swollen. She may have strings of mucus on her tail or sides. When stroked across the back, she may wag her tail. When she is taken to the buck, he will show extreme interest in her. (There are some bucks that show extreme interest in any doe, whether or not she is in heat; so know the buck!) If the doe is in heat, she will allow the buck to mount her.

If you have only one doe and no buck, it can be difficult to tell when she is in heat and ready to breed. There are many cases where a doe is sold as sterile, simply because her owners didn't manage to get her to a buck when she was in heat! Sometimes you may notice a drop in milk production or a change in personality. She may get bossy, nervous, or very friendly when in heat.

If possible, it is best to take her to the buck you plan on using (make reservations first, in advance of the heat) and leave her there for a month. If he breeds her the first day you take her there, fine. But it is possible to be just a tiny bit late or early; to make sure, it is wisest to leave her there until she is a few days late with her next scheduled heat period. It may cost a few dollars for boarding fees; but if you're a novice one-goat owner, you'll save in the long run by not having to feed a doe you thought was bred, missing out on all that milk in the spring and following months.

Providing 20 hours of light per day (including artificial light, as needed) for two months of the winter, then returning to the normally available daylight, will often cause does to come into heat as a group. There are other heat-synchronizing techniques available. If you have interest in this, contact your veterinarian.

The Pregnancy

After your doe has been bred, let her settle down to her routine life. If you are very anxious to know if she is pregnant, your veterinarian can use an ultrasound scanner. This method is very accurate and easy for a skilled operator, but it can be costly for you. If you have many purebred goats, there are now inexpensive ultrasound devices that are effective, and with many does, it becomes economically sound to buy one and learn to use it. A less expensive method is the estrone sulfate test performed on urine or milk.

Do not try to get a pregnant doe fat by dramatically increasing her grain ration. Just continue feeding on the basis of how much milk she gives and her general condition. Be sure she gets daily exercise, especially during the winter. A doe that gets little exercise will have poor muscle tone when kidding time arrives; she will have a harder time kidding and will have weaker kids. I'm not talking about strenuous exercise like climbing and jumping but gentle movement such as walking around for hay, salt, and water, which have been placed to encourage her to move about frequently.

Normal Kidding

A doe will kid approximately five months from breeding. Just prior to kidding, she may or may not lose interest in her feed, paw, appear restless, grunt, or lie down and get up repeatedly. When she passes strings of bloody mucus, you'll know she's beginning labor in earnest.

There are two presentations of the fetus that are normal. The most common is the front presentation.

Front Presentation

With the front presentation, the first thing you'll usually see is a dark, round bulge (the amniotic sac, or water bag). This is closely followed by two feet and a tiny nose. The average doe (if there is one!) usually works 15 to 45 minutes to deliver the first kid. The kid is born in three stages: first the head and front feet, then the shoulders, and finally the hips and back legs. If all appears well, leave the doe alone. Too much "help" can upset her and cause trouble.

A first-freshening doe usually has a single kid, whereas older does quite often have twins or triplets. Soon after the birth of the first kid, the doe will usually repeat the process until all her kids have been delivered. Clean each kid's nose and mouth of afterbirth and mucus to prevent suffocation or inhalation of fluids. If the kids are born in very cold weather and it is below freezing in the

Normal presentation of twins. It's not unusual for older does to have twins. Usually the second twin will work its way into a front presentation position before it is delivered.

barn, dry them immediately, and provide a heat lamp. Ears and feet freeze very easily, and frozen parts will become gangrenous and fall off in time.

Rear Presentation

The other normal birth position is the rear, or posterior, presentation. Here the water bag is followed by two feet but no head. The toes will point up instead of down, as seen in the front presentation. It is generally easier for the doe to give birth to a kid when it is in this position because there is not the abrupt bulge of the head and shoulders to deal with. (Think of a triangle, point first, in this delivery.)

The only problem encountered with the rear presentation is that as soon as the umbilical cord breaks, the kid begins to breathe. If the head is still in the birth canal, the kid can suffocate or inhale fluids and die. For this reason, it is best to help a doe having a "backward" kid as soon as the kid is out about halfway. Don't yank, but apply firm pressure downward as the doe pushes. When the head emerges, clean out the mouth and nose thoroughly. If the kid is not breathing well, hold it upside down by the hind legs, and smack its side with the flat of your hand. Any mucus and fluid are generally forced out, allowing normal breathing. This is what doctors do with human babies: The shock of that slap causes the kid (human or caprine!) to draw a deep breath, after holding it by the hind legs has let the fluid drain out.

If the kid is still not breathing, dry the mouth and nose again; then cover the mouth and nose with your mouth, and gently blow into the airway. Do not blow hard, as the kid is small and you could injure the lungs. A little firm puff is generally all that is needed.

After the kid is breathing well and is dried off, apply an antiseptic, such as iodine, to the navel. This will help prevent navel infection, scours (diarrhea), and some crippling joint infec-

Normal delivery—rear presentation.
In this type of delivery, you'll first see two feet with the toes pointing upward. As soon as the kid is out about halfway, it's best to assist with the delivery to get the kid out and breathing properly.

tions later on in life. A wide-mouthed half-pint jar nearly full of iodine is good: Just hold it tight to the belly, and slosh it around well to completely drench the whole umbilical cord. Daubing a little on is not enough for thorough coverage.

Abnormal Kidding

There are more possible abnormal positions in goats than in other animals, due to multiple births and legginess of the kids. This is not to say there are more problems with goats but a wider variety of possible problems.

Front Presentation—Head Back

If your doe has been in labor for some time and has produced only two front legs and no head, you can strongly suspect that the head has deflected off the brim of the pelvis and is turned back. *Do not pull on the legs.* It will only make matters much worse.

Scrub up with a mild dish soap, and lubricate your hand and bare arm with it. Carefully slip your hand into the doe to check the position of the kid. Work down one front leg to the chest. Make sure both legs belong to the same kid (remember, there may be more than one kid!). Then follow up the neck, and locate the head. Usually you can cup the head in your hand and draw it back into position in the birth canal. If needed, you can also get a grip in the eye sockets (this will not hurt the kid) or in the lower jaw. You may have to push the forelegs back to get enough room to slip the head into the birth canal. Once the kid's head is in between its legs, gentle, firm traction will aid the tired doe in moving it on its way into the world.

Front Presentation—One or Both Legs Back

If the doe labors for a while and produces nothing but the water bag or perhaps

Abnormal delivery—head back. *If the doe strains for a while and produces only two front legs, the head may be turned back. You'll need to push the kid partway back into the uterus so you can bring the head around.*

just the tip of the nose, suspect that the front legs are folded back, preventing the birth. (If only one leg is back, you will see one hoof and maybe the nose.)

Again, scrub up, lubricate your hand and arm, and go in to investigate. Follow the neck down to the chest and then to one leg. Be sure it belongs to the kid whose head is in the birth canal! It can be easy to grab the twin's leg—and two kids can't be born at once! You may have to shove the kid's head back to get space to slip the legs up. I like to put a rope or chain around the head to prevent losing it, as you'd be surprised at how complicated things can feel in that crowded uterus. Shield the uterus from the hoof by cupping your hand over it; then gently pull the hoof and the leg over the brim of the pelvis and through the cervix. Get the head into place, and then reach for the other leg, also easing it through. When everything is in position, applying a little traction (remember, pull down as she pushes) will help the doe finish the job, as she may be tired.

Breech Presentation—Both Legs Back

With this birth position, the doe will strain for some time but may not work as hard as usual, and nothing but the water bag is produced. When you examine her, you will run into a round, firm ball: the kid's rump. Work your hand down to find the stifle of one leg and then the hock. Gently shove forward, just above the hock, and at the same time, try to slip the leg back over the brim of the pelvis. Work carefully, and keep the hoof covered as soon as you can grab it: A torn uterus can mean a dead doe. When one leg is up, you can grasp it and shove the kid back; this will make it easier to bring up the other leg. Once the legs are in the proper position, treat this delivery as a normal rear presentation. Be sure to clean out the nose and throat well.

Mixed Delivery—Tangled Twins

Here there can be a wide variety of possibilities. You'll often see a leg of one twin and the head and leg of the other. If a doe labors over half an hour without giving birth, it is advisable to go in and feel around to find out what's happening. If all seems okay, withdraw and give her a bit longer. Some does are just slow or may require only a bit of gentle traction to help. If there are tangled twins, you'll have to untangle them.

When trying to untangle twins, work carefully and slowly. Shove back one twin (usually the one without its head in the birth canal) to make room, so you can position the other twin correctly and move it farther into the birth canal. It may take some doing; but once the twins are untangled, the delivery should proceed fairly easily. You may need to apply a little traction to slide the first kid far enough out that the second kid will not interfere with the first birth.

Calling the Veterinarian

You should examine any doe that is in hard labor for over 45 minutes without producing a kid. If the problem is just an abnormal position, you'll usually be able to deliver the kids by yourself, as described earlier in this section. If you do not feel confident doing this or if you work with the doe for longer than 15 minutes without results, it is best to call your veterinarian. Sometimes a really difficult birth needs a veterinarian's added experience. Too much trauma is a huge stress, which can easily put a doe into shock. Such a doe is a poor risk, and no veterinarian likes to work on a half-dead doe.

If the kid is just too large to pass through the birth canal, the veterinarian may perform a cesarean delivery. This generally has very good results, provided the doe is not exhausted when the surgery is performed.

Occasionally a doe experiences a torsion, or twisting, of the uterus. This most often happens in older does with twins or triplets heavy in the uterus. The uterus gets twisted, making delivery impossible until the torsion is corrected. This can be quite a job, as it is hard to figure out which way the uterus has turned. A torsion rod is often a great help. This is fastened to the kid's legs, making turning the uterus easier. The only problem is space. If the uterus was twisted tight before any part of the kid entered the birth canal, there is no way to get hold of the legs or work the rod in. In cases like this, rolling the doe over will often flop the uterus over into appropriate position. This is tricky, even with experience, because if you roll her the wrong way, there is the possibility of making the uterus twist tighter instead of going into the proper position. Sometimes a cesarean is the only course of action.

Occasionally a kid dies before birth. When this happens, the fetus may absorb fluids and swell up. If it becomes too large, it sometimes is necessary for a veterinarian to remove a leg and shoulder in order to gain room for the rest of the fetus to pass. This is done with a special hooked knife called an embryotomy knife, which has a small blade that can be shielded by the hand to protect the uterus from accidental cuts.

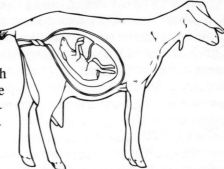

(For other problems related to pregnancy and kidding, see "Eversion of the Uterus" on page 125,

Torsion of the uterus. *If the uterus gets twisted, you will need veterinary assistance to correct the problem and allow the kid to be born.*

"Freezing" on page 127, "Infertility" on page 129, "Ketosis" on page 133, "Milk Fever" on page 138, "Retained Placenta" on page 142, and "White Muscle Disease" on page 147.)

Caring for Kids

Most kids are fed twice daily. But where it is possible, feeding young kids smaller amounts in four daily feedings, until they are eating hay and grain well, will help them to avoid digestion problems. If it's not feasible to leave the kids with their mother, nurse does work well because the kids can "snack" at will. Some goats will accept several kids; the number, of course, depends on the doe's milking ability and patience! If a nurse doe is not available, you can, of course, bottle feed your kids. They can be fed either, preferably, goat milk, or reconstituted milk replacer. If you are going to use a powdered milk replacer, either buy lamb, or better still, kid milk replacer. Feeding "people" instant, non-fat dry milk or dry calf milk replacer does not raise healthy kids. The formulas are not right for kid goats and they will often fail to thrive or develop scours (severe diarrhea).

The amount of milk each kid needs depends on its size and vigor. It can vary from half a cup to a pint to start with. Big-boned, strong, vigorous kids can handle a larger amount than kids that are smaller and somewhat "backward."

Chilled, tiny, or premature kids may not have much nursing instinct. But you can save them and keep them free of scours by tube-feeding them until their sucking instinct becomes stronger. Use a plastic tube (a French tube or catheter) and a 12-cc or larger syringe. Feed the milk (actually, it's colostrum for the first three days) at body temperature or just a little warmer. Simply stick the tube into the milk, draw up a full load, and then insert the tube slowly but firmly into the kid's mouth and down the throat. Wait until the kid begins to swallow, and then slowly shove the tube down. It is possible to mistakenly get the tube into the lung, but this is rare; if you watch for the swallowing, you should do fine. If the kid coughs when the tube is all the way or partly down, withdraw it and try again. The tube is inserted far enough to just reach the end of the esophagus (the tube in the throat that delivers food and fluids to the stomach); eyeball it by the length of the neck. When injecting the milk, push the plunger of the syringe in slowly, or the milk may churn around, making the kid squirm. This is a safe, easy method to use, and the entire process—feeding and washing up the tube and syringe afterward—can be done in five minutes. Kids fed by a stomach tube (until they are stronger and can suck normally) will do better than kids that have milk poured into them. The latter kids usually develop diarrhea and are susceptible to aspiration pneumonia, as well.

When a kid begins to munch hay and graze, I like to get it eating Calf Manna, or another nonmedicated pelleted milk replacer, and grain as soon as possible. This avoids many digestive upsets and gets the stomach working well early in life. I do *not* like to use medicated pellets of any kind as a routine, daily feed. Animals can develop resistant bacteria, and the antibiotics can kill normal, necessary gut bacteria, resulting in a host of problems.

Castration

Only the best of bucklings should be left as bucks. Selling a buck born from an inferior doe or using a buck born from an unplanned breeding as a breeding animal will only injure the reputation of dairy goats in general. And keeping such a buck "because he's pretty" or some such reason will only degrade your own stock. Surplus bucklings should be castrated, even when they are sold for meat, used for meat at home, or sold for pets. (It takes a real goat lover to have a *buck* for a pet!)

Clamping, or "Pinching"

This is my choice in castrating. First of all, it is bloodless. There is no open sore at any time to become infected or pick up tetanus organisms. And it is easy to do or very inexpensive if your veterinarian does it. The cords and blood vessels are simply crushed, and the testicles slowly atrophy and shrink up. They do not die and drop off, as with the use of the elastrator. There is little pain, and it is over in a few seconds.

To use this method, beg, borrow, or buy a Burdizzo emasculatome. (I've seen too many slips from imitations to recommend the "economy" tool modeled after the Burdizzo.) There are different sizes, ranging from those used for bulls and stallions to smaller ones intended for use on kids and lambs. The smaller lamb model is the best choice because it is less clumsy for an inexperienced person to use than the larger sizes. This method may be used on all bucks, regardless of size or age, although younger kids are easier to do and require less restraint (and a smaller Burdizzo).

To use the emasculatome, first have an assistant hold the kid. (If you have an older buck, tie it with a short rope, and have the helper hold the animal against a wall or partition.) Grasp the scrotum, and identify one testicle; then feel upward to identify the cord. Place the jaws of the emasculatome across the cord. Make sure that the center division between the testicles is not in the way. Clamping this division can lead to serious problems, such as shock, pain, and swelling. When you're sure the jaws are in the right position, close the handles of the clamps, and hold them closed for a few seconds. Then repeat the procedure on the second testicle.

Surgical Castration

This is a sure and quite safe operation for the animal. I would advise giving a tetanus antitoxin injection following this procedure, just to be safe. But I've never known a goat to get tetanus when operated on in a clean manner, as long as the incisions were large enough. Once in a while, bleeding is a problem, but you can generally avoid this by working carefully.

Very young kids are easiest to do, and the operation is safer for them at this time. Kids over one week old but less than six weeks are quickly castrated with little shock, pain, or bleeding. Have an assistant hold the kid across his or her lap while you wash its scrotum with warm, soapy water. Hold the testicle between your thumb and forefinger, bulging it toward the bottom of the scrotum. Using a scalpel, single-edged razor blade, or sharp knife, make an incision across the entire bottom, at least an inch long. Then pull the testicle and tunic (the white membrane covering the testicle) through the incision.

If the buckling is quite young and small, the cord will be thin, requiring no tying or crushing; just pull until the cord snaps. There is little, if any, bleeding this way. If the kid is larger, you can use a knife; but don't make a sharp cut—just scrape the cord until it breaks. This will lessen the chances of bleeding. Make sure you draw the cord and tunic well out of the scrotum before scraping because if any tissue hangs out, the healing will be incomplete. This can result in a buildup of scar tissue known as a scirrhous cord. And it is a mess to repair.

When castrating large bucks by surgery, it is advisable to use an emasculator to crush the blood vessels and cords while cutting at the same time. Make the incisions, and draw out one testicle. Apply the emasculator to that testicle, keeping the crushing portion toward the body. I usually hold the emasculator in place after the testicle has been cut free to make sure the cord and blood vessels are well crushed. Then repeat the procedure with the second testicle. If you use a scalpel or knife, instead of an emasculator, to cut the cords, you can tie off the stumps with catgut (available through your veterinarian). But

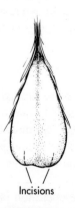

Incisions

Surgical castration. *This method is easiest on very young goats. Restrain the kid, and wash the scrotum with warm, soapy water. Then make an incision at least 1 inch long across the bottom of the scrotum below each testicle.*

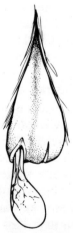

Removing the testicle. *After making the incision, pull out the testicle and the tunic (the white membrane covering the testicle). Pull until the cord snaps, or scrape the cord with a knife to break it with minimal bleeding.*

crushing is usually safer since these ligatures sometimes slip off.

When you are done, it's a good idea to dust an antibiotic powder on the incisions. Also, keep the flies away. Under these conditions healing is very rapid. (This is why I prefer to castrate surgically during the seasons flies are not present.)

Using the Elastrator, or "Banding"

Banding involves using an inexpensive elastrator, which is used to slip a special, heavy rubber band over the scrotum and testicles. The band is slipped off the holding pegs of the instrument above the testicles, shutting off circulation to the area. After several weeks, the whole scrotum dies, dries up, and falls off. It is quite painless, inexpensive, and easy to learn.

The young buckling is easiest held by an assistant, cradled upside down on their lap. The elastrator is squeezed open and slipped over the testicles. The operator carefully inspects them to ensure that both testicles are outside the elastrator band, with the elastrator being held as close to the body as possible. The band is then rolled off the pegs and the elastrator removed. There is a slight wound around the band site as the scrotum dries, readying to fall away. Therefore, it is a good idea to give the buckling an injection of tetanus toxoid at banding time, just to be safe, as tetanus is always possible with any wound. Do NOT "help" the scrotum fall off by pulling on it or you may cause bleeding and pain.

Dehorning

Generally speaking, horns cause trouble when left on goats. Even the most gentle doe can accidentally swing her head around and catch a person in the face or eye. Children are often injured in this way: They cannot grasp the fact that their beloved pet could hurt them, even though she loves them dearly.

Goats can also injure each other with their horns. I lost a registered Nubian doe when her stall mate—a nice, gentle, but horned doe—got angry when they were competing for feed and hooked the Nubian's belly, rupturing her spleen.

Horns on bucks are a particular danger. True, not many bucks are mean, but horns are an invitation to trouble. All bucks play to show their good spirits and virility. This play can sometimes get a little out of hand, especially if a buck has a 4-foot rack of horns! I know of several people, as well as other goats, injured this way. One man had his leg ripped open and required 18 stitches. And once a buck finds use for his horns, he often gets a little "pushy" or belligerent with the discovery of his newfound strength, and he really becomes a problem to handle.

Horns can harm the wearer, too. Goats like to shove their heads through woven wire fencing to nibble on grass on the other side. Some horns can be squeezed through the fence, but then the goat cannot back out and can hang itself if not spotted in time. Likewise, horned goats often tangle themselves in hay strings, mangers, tether ropes, and even each other's collars, with fatal results.

Dehorning Kids

The best age to dehorn dairy goats is when they are young kids. When done at this age, very little shock and less work are involved. The easiest method, and the best by far, is the electric disbudding iron. The electric iron is inexpensive as well as safe and sure when used properly. The procedure is as follows:

1. Restrain the kid in a kid box or bag, or have an assistant hold it firmly.
2. Clip the hair away from the horn buds.
3. Heat the iron well—it should scorch wood quickly.
4. Firmly apply the iron to the first horn bud for about 10 seconds.
5. Rotate the iron, pushing it firmly to the head. Do not stop if the kid bleats. Disbudding may well save its life later on or save a person from injury.
6. Move to the next bud, and repeat the process.

When you are finished, examine both buds. There should be a copper-colored, indented ring around each one, with no breaks in the ring. If all is well, release the kid, and give it a feeding. You will be forgiven at once.

In a few days, the scab will come off and the head will be smooth permanently, unless you worked too quickly or missed a spot by not rotating the iron. In this case scurs (misshapen horns) may appear. Remove these with the iron while they are still small. Just be sure you do a more thorough job!

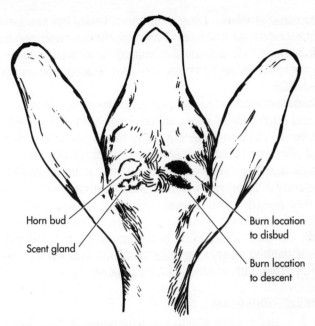

Horn bud

Scent gland

Burn location
to disbud

Burn location
to descent

Dehorning and descenting. *Dehorning is easiest when goat kids are young. It's best to use an electric disbudding iron. If the kid is a buck, you can descent it at the same time by also burning the scent gland with the dehorner.*

Gougers, or scoops, which are made for calves, work well on kids. They leave unsightly holes in the head for some time, but the holes heal nice and smooth. The gougers have a sharp mouth that fits over the horn bud. You must have them down close to the head so there is hair taken out with the horn bud. When the blades are in position, force the handles apart quickly to neatly clip out the bud. Control the bleeding with an electric disbudding iron. Not only will it stop any bleeding but it will kill any horn cells around the base of the horn, which if left unburned may well grow horns or scurs. One note: The wound can look like a hole "into the brain," as you may notice bubbling in the cavity when the animal breathes. In this case the hole is possibly into a sinus (not the brain) and will not cause a problem, so don't worry.

I won't go into the use of caustic ointments or elastrators (rubber bands), as I don't like either method, especially on goats. There are just too many problems. Caustic ointment works, but you have to be very cautious about it causing burns by running over the animal's skin or being rubbed onto another animal. Goats are more active than calves, and the chances of a burn from caustic dehorning ointment are much greater.

Elastrators are hard to place on goats due to the wide base of the horn, and often owners wait until the horn is an inch or two long to help keep the band in place. But goats have horn cells farther down into the skin than do cattle; if you don't kill or remove this skin, scur formation is nearly a certainty. Also, rubber bands can break and fall off, resulting in horn regrowth. When the horns are partially off, they are easily snagged and broken, resulting in pain and bleeding. Infections and tetanus are also a problem. And if all that weren't enough, this method is painful to the animal. Ask people who have used this method on milking does, and most will tell you that their does dropped in milk production for a long period.

Dehorning Adult Goats

In dehorning adult goats, you'll need more experience, more equipment, and more complicated techniques. It's common to use a tranquilizer along with a local anesthetic around the horn bases. I have had excellent results with an anesthetic put out for cats: ketamine hydrochloride. It is a short-acting anesthetic and quite safe for goats. An adult buck will require from 5 to 7 cc (100 mg/ml). Smaller doelings and bucklings generally take 1 to 2 cc. Give this anesthetic with an intramuscular injection.

The usual tool for dehorning an adult goat is a hacksaw or wire saw. Take care to cut deep enough into the head, not flat across the horn. A proper cut will remove a band of skin and hair with the horn, leaving an unsightly bloody hole. The holes will be larger in a mature buck than in a doe, owing to the size of the horn bases. Do not be alarmed when blood runs in droplets from the nose or mouth. This is normal in many cases as the blood trickles down the sinus cavities into the nose and mouth. Likewise, the holes left by the dehorning may bubble with each breath. You have not cut into the brain, only the sinus. It will heal up nice and smooth in a few weeks.

In fly season daub the fresh wounds with scarlet oil to prevent maggots. (I prefer to dehorn surgically when flies are not present to avoid this problem.) If your goat bleeds quite a bit, place a cotton pad over each horn wound, and wrap gauze snugly around the head like a bonnet. Be sure to remove the pads and gauze after 24 hours.

Keep the area around the cuts clean and free from hay, manure, and feed. It helps to feed hay from a box on the ground until the head is healed. Otherwise, feeding from mangers may cause hay chaff to get into the incisions, preventing healing and often causing infections.

Descenting Bucks

One drawback to owning a buck is the odoriferous musky smell he emits during the breeding season. Contrary to old wives' tales, the odor is not connected to the buck's virility; does are just as attracted to a descented buck as to his "stinky" brother. A castrated buck does not have an odor, because the glands remain inactive when there is no longer hormonal stimulus to produce the musk. Likewise, a doe has no odor since she does not have scent glands.

In bucks the major scent glands are on the head behind the horn base. Other glands are found on the legs and near the tail, although these are small compared with those on the head. You can feel and, in many instances, see the scent gland bumps on a clipped head. (Smell your hand afterward!)

A simple and effective way to descent a buck kid is to burn the glands at disbudding time with the electric dehorner. This leaves a double ring burned into each side of the head: one for the horn bud and the other for the scent. It looks unsightly for a few days and takes a few more days to heal, but it is definitely worth it because you'll have years of relatively "scent-free" buck ownership.

Older bucks can be descented surgically. Using a tranquilizer and local anesthetic or Ketaset, your veterinarian can quite easily remove the gland, leaving a fairly neat-looking head. He will shave the skin, paint it with antiseptic, make the incisions, and lift the skin to expose the bumpy glands underneath. By using blunt dissection, he'll peel them away, leaving a clean and smooth (although somewhat scalped-looking) head. After the procedure control the bleeding with a cotton pressure pack, and sprinkle the area with antibiotic powder. Just to be on the safe side, also give a tetanus booster or antitoxin and four days' treatment with a broad-spectrum antibiotic.

Even a descented buck will have some odor at breeding time as part of the breeding ritual involves urinating on his chin and forelegs. To help keep this odor to a minimum, keep him clipped at breeding time, and sponge his forelegs with Massengil douche when he gets too rank. Keep in mind, though, that does are attracted to this scent, and a clean, sweet-smelling guy may not stimulate a doe that is not in a strong heat.

Handling Goats

Goats are naturally friendly animals that like plenty of attention and handling. Treating them kindly and gently will make dairy animals that are easy to milk from the start. They love to have their necks scratched, shoulders rubbed, and sides petted. But they *hate* having their ears pulled! I have Nubians, and it seems that visitors simply must pull their long, floppy ears; so be on the alert with your company, or your goats may become timid.

Pulling or wrestling with a goat's horns is a sure way to invite trouble. The most mild-mannered goat can become nasty with its horns if taught to do so by its owners. I know of a little horned buck that was teased this way—that is, until he finally put his owner in the hospital with 18 stitches in his leg.

Trimming Feet

Goats need their feet trimmed regularly. This is relatively easy to do yourself, and it is definitely worth your time. Untrimmed feet can lead to many problems with goats, from lameness to completely crippled legs due to contracted tendons. Some goats with long-neglected feet can be brought back close to normality by careful and repeated correct trimming, but many are forever crippled.

There is no set formula for how often you should trim the feet. Different types of ground, the natural hardness of the hooves, the amount of exercise, and the type of feed can all influence hoof growth and wear. Just check the feet regularly, and trim them when they begin to look a bit sloppy. If you handle your goats often, they will allow you to pick up their feet with little struggle. A distraction of grain can also help. While one person can easily manage to trim feet, it is helpful to have an assistant, especially if you have more than one animal to do.

There are several instruments available for trimming goat feet, ranging from a sharp jackknife to special hoof nippers. All will work fine if you use them properly. The main thing is to trim the wall of the toes so it is level with the cushion, or frog, on the underside of the foot.

DISEASES AND OTHER PROBLEMS

No matter how well you care for your goats, there's always a chance that an accident or illness will pop up in your herd. Being aware of signs and symptoms of common problems will help you catch and treat them before they take the health or life of your animal. Many times you can treat the problem yourself; other times you'll need to call your veterinarian at once. Making the right decision requires

Suggested Vaccination Schedule for Goats

Here are some guidelines to show which vaccinations to consider and when to give them. But because different problems are common in different areas, you should check with your veterinarian to work out a specific schedule for your particular situation and location.

	DISEASE	WHEN TO VACCINATE
KIDS	Enterotoxemia (*Clostridium perfringens* Types C and D)	8 to 10 weeks if dams not protected, 12 weeks otherwise; repeat in 21 days
	Tetanus (toxoid)	8 weeks
DOES	Enterotoxemia (*C. perfringens* Types C and D)	Two doses, 2 to 3 weeks apart, the 1st year as adults; if doe is pregnant, give second dose in last third of pregnancy
	Tetanus (toxoid)	Yearly
BUCKS	Enterotoxemia (*C. perfringens* Types C and D)	Yearly
	Tetanus (toxoid)	Yearly

knowledge as well as experience. When in doubt, call your veterinarian for advice. It's also important to know the normal temperature of your goat so you can check for fever or other abnormalities. The normal body temperature of a goat is 102° to 103°F (38.9° to 39.4°C).

Abscesses

Abscesses are fairly common in goats. They can pop up anywhere, seemingly overnight. In most instances they either break and drain themselves or just quietly disappear. But they can cause trouble, especially if there are abscesses in the udder or internal organs or if they start affecting several members of your herd.

Corynebacteria are a common cause of abscesses in goats, as are staphylococci, streptococci, *Escherichia coli,* and many lesser-known organisms. Therefore, no one treatment or preventive will work in all cases or in all herds.

If a goat or a herd is bothered by abscesses, the best course of action is to have your vet take a sample for culture and sensitivity tests. This will tell not only just which specific organism is causing the trouble but also what antibiotic will work on it. A broad-spectrum antibiotic, such as oxytetracycline or a sulfa combination, will usually work; results can be disappointing, though, since abscesses are walled off from the body and have little blood circulation to carry systemic antibiotics. Occasionally you may need to treat an abscess problem with an autogenous vaccine made from the specific organisms causing the infection. Check with your veterinarian to see what is available.

When working with an open abscess, be sure to wear plastic or rubber gloves as some of the bacteria present may cause problems for you. Also, don't allow children to play with a goat with an abscess, and don't use the milk from a doe with an udder abscess.

It is easy, although not especially pleasant, to treat a simple, once-in-a-while abscess. First, isolate the animal because an abscess that breaks and drains is spreading millions of potential abscess-producing bacteria. Trim the hair around the abscess lump, and try systemic treatment: injectable antibiotics for four days. This may or may not help the abscess you see; however, it may be effective on internal abscesses you do not see but that can cause trouble just the same. Remember to read the label on the antibiotics, and withhold milk from sale for the length of time required. Milk with antibiotic residue does not make good cheese or yogurt, and it should not be used by a person sensitive to that antibiotic. It is fine to give the milk to calves or kids (goat kids, that is!).

Keep an eye on the abscess as you continue the antibiotics. If it does not reduce in size after the four days of treatment, you may think about lancing it. It is a good idea to draw some fluid out of the suspected abscess with a sterile needle and syringe before lancing it. Once in a while, the swelling is not an abscess (which contains yellowish or whitish pus) but a hematoma (blood-filled sac). If an inexperienced person lances a hematoma, the animal could bleed to death. When the abscess is on the udder or in the throat area, call your veterinarian to handle the treatment; it's easy to cut the blood vessels there by mistake and kill the animal.

To lance the abscess, scrub its surface well with warm, soapy water, and pat it dry with a clean paper towel. Paint the surface with Betadine, allowing it to dry. While wearing plastic or rubber gloves, make a quick incision at the bottom of the lump, at least 1½ inches long. (Many people make an incision at the top or center of the lump; but this will not allow adequate drainage, and there will always be a pocket of pus left.) Clip a strip of skin off along the incision to widen the hole and ensure that the inside heals. Clean out the pocket of the abscess with a sterile gauze pad. Flush out the pocket with warm, soapy water, rinse, and then let dry. Fill the pocket with iodine, Betadine, or an antibiotic.

Caseous Lymphadenitis

Caseous lymphadenitis is a term that describes a serious abscess problem in goats. Here the lymph glands become infected with *Corynebacterium pseudotuberculosis,* and then they abscess. As with other lymph gland diseases, it spreads easily throughout the body, and it's

Cleaning the abscess. a. Using plastic gloves, clean out the pocket of the abscess with a sterile gauze pad. b. Be sure to clean out all debris from the farthest reaches.

often unnoticed by an owner. Sometimes the first sign is a well-fed goat that just keeps getting thinner and thinner until it finally dies. Other times you may notice abscesses near the skin surface. To treat them, clip the hair, and apply heat (hot packs and hot liniment or ointment) to draw them to a head. Open and drain them as described on page 114; then pack them with an antibiotic.

The trouble with caseous lymphadenitis is that often internal abscesses form in addition to the external ones. The internal abscesses may involve body organs and kill the animal. Antibiotic therapy doesn't often help this condition. Because it is a serious problem, it's best to cull (or permanently isolate) an affected animal.

There are a few steps you can take to prevent caseous lymphadenitis. Avoid raising kids on the milk of animals that have abscesses, and keep the kids totally away from the adults. Isolate or cull any adults with abscesses. Do not buy a doe with a history of abscesses or one that comes from a herd with an abscess problem. Strict sanitation will also help keep problems to a minimum.

Arthritis

Arthritis is a crippling of the joints. It is commonly found in goats that have not had their feet trimmed regularly. As the toes grow long and twisted, the deformation puts excessive strain and pressure on the joints, often causing arthritis if not taken care of promptly.

Arthritis can also be related to abscess troubles. As opposed to the arthritis found in older animals, this kind of arthritis can strike goats of any age, even young kids. There is no single organism responsible for all arthritis in goats, but it can be caused by *C. pseudotuberculosis* (which may also produce abscesses) or by the virus that causes caprine arthritis and encephalitis (CAE). (For more information on this problem, see "Caprine Arthritis and Encephalitis" on page 122.) *E. coli*, staphylococci, and many other organisms also have caused arthritis in goats, often entering a kid's body shortly after birth.

With arthritis there is commonly puffiness at the joints and pain. If you catch the problem early, a veterinarian can draw off fluid from the joint for culture. Antibiotic therapy can sometimes reverse this disease, depending on its cause, but many times results are discouraging. Once the animal is severely crippled (if the joints have been damaged and the bone deformed), nothing can help.

If the joint infection is stopped early, there may still be trouble from bent knees caused by contracted tendons due to disuse of the legs. This will force the goat to remain in an abnormal kneeling position or a crouched, half-kneeling stance. You may be able to correct this by working with the affected legs daily. Draw each leg into as normal a position as possible, without causing severe pain. Release; then stretch it again. Repeat the process 15 to 20 times a day, and do it every day until the animal can stand normally.

If the stretching does not help and your veterinarian feels the only problem is contracted tendons, he may be able to put on light casts. This will work only if the legs can be brought into proper position without a lot of pain. The casts should go from fetlock to elbow. Leave them on for two weeks, remove them to check the progress and look for pressure sores, and then replace them, if necessary. Another option for correcting contracted tendons is a tendonotomy. This is a relatively simple operation that can be performed at your veterinarian's clinic, under a local anesthetic. Bear in mind that if the legs are permanently damaged or the infection and inflammation are still active in the joint, there's nothing you can do to restore the usefulness of the legs.

There are a few steps you can take to minimize the chance of arthritis affecting your animals. First, choose sound, good-boned breeding stock from herds that are free of arthritis. Keep your goats in dry, well-bedded stalls—not on bare cement floors—and trim their feet regularly. And disinfect the navels of all newly born kids with iodine. If one of your goats does show signs of arthritis, cull it, or isolate it and have it tested for CAE.

Bloat and Indigestion

Most goats bloat owing to improper feeding, whether by accident or from ignorance. There are two types of bloat: frothy bloat and dry bloat. In frothy bloat the gas forms in numerous tiny bubbles, which are nearly impossible to belch up. This usually follows overeating on lush legume pastures. Dry bloat is generally caused by indigestion, eating too much grain, or eating large amounts of grain and then drinking equally large amounts of water. Here the gas forms in pockets and is trapped. More and more of it forms, and the animal is unable to belch, thus bloating.

Frothy bloat is more dangerous because it occurs suddenly and is many times fatal. To minimize the chance of problems, never turn a herd of goats out into lush pasture, especially alfalfa or clover, unless they are used to it. Otherwise, they will overload and may well bloat. If your animals are used to being in the barn lot and eating dry feed, help them adjust by cutting and feeding a few armloads from the pasture daily. Increase the amount you bring in each day until you see that the goats are leaving some uneaten. Then turn the animals out in the afternoon of a dry day. (Wet legumes bloat animals more than dry pastures do.)

Even with this extra care, it's important to watch your animals closely for the first few days you turn them out. If you notice signs of bloat, call your veterinarian immediately. If he is not available, you may be able to relieve the bloat yourself by drenching with ½ pint of corn, peanut, or mineral oil. Adding 1 to 2 teaspoons of turpentine (*not* paint thinner or anything else!) to the oil and mixing well before drenching is helpful. Kneading the bloated area after drenching will also help break up the gas. It is wise to have a bottle of bloat remedy on hand for just such an emergency. Ask your veterinarian what he recommends.

Sometimes it is necessary to pass a stomach tube to relieve the pressure. *Do not use a garden hose or anything but a stomach tube.* Any other tube can slit the esophagus and kill the goat. It's usually best to have your veterinarian do this unless you happen to have a calf-sized stomach tube on hand. (For details on using the tube, see "Bloat" on page 46.)

In an emergency, when you don't discover a goat until she is very full of gas (like a balloon) and in severe distress from the pressure, it may be necessary to use a trochar and cannula to relieve the gas at once. The trochar is an awl-shaped instrument with a tube (the cannula) fitting over it. (See "Trochar and Cannula" on page 46 for an illustration of these instruments.) Your veterinarian is the best person to decide if the case calls for this tool.

Use a pocketknife only to save an animal that has totally collapsed and appears near death. Unlike the trochar and cannula, the knife makes an incision only, and nothing carries the gas and stomach contents through the peritoneum and out of the body. With the knife all this boils into the peritoneal cavity, later to cause infection and sometimes death. A 3-inch-long, 16- to 10-gauge intra-

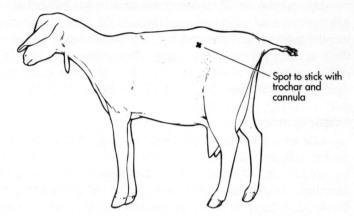

Spot to stick with
trochar and
cannula

Tapping a bloated goat. In an emergency you may need to use a long, heavy-gauge hypodermic needle or a trochar and cannula to relieve the gas. Stick the goat at the highest point of the bloat on the left side.

venous needle is better than a knife as it acts as both trochar and cannula. If you live quite a distance from the veterinarian, it's a good idea to invest in one, just in case you need it; the cost is minimal.

If you must stick a goat, push the needle through the wall of the rumen at the highest point of bloat on the left side, just in front of the hip. This is an emergency measure only, as some animals never really recover after being relieved in this way—possibly because some of the stomach contents leak into the peritoneal cavity or adhesions form.

Indigestion

Many goats will get indigestion, rather than bloat, from overeating grain or greens. They will at first appear colicky, stamping their hind feet, grunting, and biting or nosing their sides. The goats may then lie down, act generally sick, and not want to get up (but can if you make them). Diarrhea usually follows in a few hours. A classic example was my old Nubian doe. She was used to eating grass, hay, and garden greens. One day I took her along for a walk in the woods. I looked at the beautiful spring wildflowers—she ate them. That evening she was in misery with a good old bellyache!

In most cases a dose or two of Kaopectate will completely clear up the problem. But in cases where the goat is in pain from gas, your veterinarian can give it a shot to quiet the stomach cramps. Also, giving oil orally (as you would for bloat) will stop the gas buildup as well as help move the offending material through the goat. If your goats get into the grain bin and overload, it's a good idea to get a dose of oil into them at once, before trouble starts. (Remember, corn, peanut, vegetable, or mineral oil—not car oil!) This will help move the feed through faster and usually prevents acute gastritis or bloat.

Simple Diarrhea

Kids are a prime target for digestive upsets. This is because they are fed milk, and milk can easily cause problems if fed wrong. If kids are not running with their mother, they need a feeding of colostrum four times daily for the first three days. The colostrum acts as a laxative to move the first bowel movements through naturally and also provides the kids with protective antibodies. Otherwise, the hard fecal material can irritate the bowel, often causing scours.

When kids are on milk, they sometimes overeat (usually your fault) or eat wrong (their fault). Gulping milk can lead to indigestion and diarrhea. While this often occurs when hungry kids suck a bottle, it can happen when they nurse on their mother, as well. At the first sign of loose bowels, cut the milk given at the next feeding in half. (If the kid is nursing on its dam, simply milk her out when you notice the diarrhea.) In most cases this will quickly remedy the problem.

Where the diarrhea continues, you'd better check with your veterinarian. He may want to examine the kid or check it for coccidiosis, which is quite common in kids. (See "Coccidiosis" on page 122 for details on this problem.) Your veterinarian can also provide an antidiarrheal medication. There are two basic types: astringents and kaolin-pectin preparations. Antibiotics may be added to kill harmful bacteria, preventing irreversible scours. Give the medicine regularly and carefully, exactly as directed. If you give it haphazardly or only when you think of it, the medicine won't do the job, and you may lose a kid.

Breaks

In goats most broken bones occur in the legs. Common causes include car accidents, dog bites, getting a tie-out chain or rope wrapped around a leg, and catching a leg in a fence, stall divider, or brush. You can strongly suspect a broken leg if a sound goat suddenly becomes severely lame. Most broken limbs dangle, and the goat will not walk on the affected leg. Sometimes you are able to see the bone sticking up against the skin or even through the skin. In any of these cases, call the veterinarian immediately.

A broken leg or even two on a goat doesn't mean an automatic death sentence. Proper care before and after the leg is set is important. When you discover a goat with a suspected broken leg, keep the animal quiet to prevent further damage. Leave it where it is unless it is in a dangerous or very inconvenient place. If you must move the animal, do it very slowly so that you don't further injure the leg. Sometimes the bone gets pushed through the skin if the animal thrashes around. This makes it easy for infections to start, and it may also make it more difficult to set the break. If the animal is in serious shock, from either the accident or the pain, your veterinarian may choose to immobilize the leg with a temporary splint until the shock has been taken care of.

If the bone is not through the skin, a plaster cast or a Thomas splint reinforced with plaster works well in most cases. Some breaks, especially those of kids, are easy to repair with intramedullary pins as there is very little encumbrance after the bone is set with pins, compared with a cast or splint.

When the leg has been set with a cast or splint, you must check it at least twice daily. Check above the cast (and below, if the cast doesn't include the foot) for swelling, dampness, and odor. These indicate potential problems such as a too-tight cast, sores under the cast, or infection. When possible, feel the foot to make sure it is warm—an indication of normal circulation. If it suddenly becomes cold and loses feeling (pinch or prick the skin between the claws to check), call your vet immediately: This indicates loss of circulation. If you don't correct the problem, it could turn into gangrene.

While the leg is healing, it's critical to keep the cast dry. Wet bedding, mud, rain, or swamps mean disaster for a plaster cast or plaster-reinforced splint. If you turn out the goat in a pasture where there is mud or damp grass, slide a section of inner tube over the cast, and tape it in place. A little car-starting fluid (ether) sprayed on the sticky side of duct tape will make it really stick. Do not leave the tube on all the time, though, as the cast and the leg must "breathe." It is best to limit the goat's time in the pasture while wearing the cast.

Most casts or splints must remain on two to three weeks for kids and four to six weeks for large adults. They may need to be replaced if left on over three weeks; your veterinarian will advise you.

Caprine Arthritis and Encephalitis

The CAE virus is a common cause of arthritis in goats. It also causes mastitis, in which the udder is quite swollen, firm to the touch, and producing little milk. Another related problem is encephalitis, often in kids less than five months old, causing lameness, paralysis, and seizures. Death usually follows the encephalitis.

Unfortunately, CAE is all too common today. There is no treatment, only strict preventive measures. When buying new goats, make sure they come from a CAE-free herd. Test your existing herd regularly, and cull any affected animals. Raise kids from a suspect animal on pasteurized milk (including pasteurized colostrum)or powdered goat kid milk replacer from the time they are born; never allow them to suck their dam. Also, raise kids in strict isolation from affected or possibly affected goats. The CAE virus is plentiful in the milk. If infected soon after birth, kids can carry the infection for life and may develop symptoms (arthritis or mastitis) at a much later date after seeming perfectly healthy.

Coccidiosis

Coccidiosis is a very important problem in dairy goats, which results in reduced milk production, unthrifty animals, diarrhea (especially in younger animals), and kids that fail to mature properly. It is caused by protozoa (coccidia) that invade the intestines. Coccidiosis is passed from adults to kids, usually through fecal contamination of the feed and water. Adults seem to build some immunity to coccidiosis, but they continue to shed oocysts in their manure; these protozoa are then picked up by nonimmune kids. Symptoms can progress from diarrhea, weight loss, and fever to emaciation and death. Fortunately, it is possible to control this problem.

Have your veterinarian check any young goat that develops a diarrhea of unknown origin that either continues or comes and goes. A simple fecal examination will tell if coccidiosis is present. When it is, your veterinarian will prescribe a cocciodiostat, which you can often put in the drinking water or milk.

Where coccidiosis has become a herd problem—and it often does—using a coccidiostat routinely often helps. In addition, strict sanitation is a must. Keep kids away from older animals, and give them clean, very dry quarters. Do not allow kids to run through their feed troughs and mangers; use kid-sized keyhole mangers to keep the hay, grain, and drinking water clean. Talk to your veterinarian for other suggestions in developing a coccidia elimination plan for your herd.

Cuts and Miscellaneous Injuries

The key to treating an injury successfully is being calm enough to assess the situation. Don't panic. If you think the injury is bad enough, call your vet immediately, and describe the situation to him *exactly*. I had some folks call me one day, saying their doe had broken a window and had a piece of glass in her nose. I asked how badly it was bleeding; they replied that it bled a little, but the bleeding had stopped. Could I come and get the glass out for them?

I saw in my mind a sliver of glass perhaps ½ inch long. No hurry, right? Luckily, I was able to go right out—that glass was 2 feet long! In fact, I don't know how she kept from breaking it when she moved. It entered one nostril and came out the other. The doe looked like a cannibal with a bone in her nose. But it looked worse than it was, and there was no trouble after the "piece" of glass was removed.

Most cuts on animals heal very well with no suturing. Many times people argue in favor of stitches because their own doctors sewed up a half-inch cut on their hands. But there is often quicker healing with less scarring if a cut is not sewn up. Of course, there are some cuts that do need suturing, but let your veterinarian decide. And let him make the decision while the cut is still fresh. After a day or two, there may be swelling, contamination, or stiffness in the skin, and even a cut that might have been better sewn up can't be.

A puncture wound is something to take very seriously. Clean it well to the bottom of the wound, and flush Betadine through it thoroughly. Tetanus is always a possibility with a puncture wound or any wound that is not open to the air. Therefore, an injection of tetanus antitoxin is advisable, just in case—especially with animals that have not been routinely immunized.

A clean wound, whether sutured or not, is generally a healthy wound. Try to keep it that way. Clip all the hair away from the wound. Hair is irritating at best and only retards healing—if it doesn't cause more serious trouble. Also, keep dirt and manure washed out of the wound with plain warm, soapy water.

Very few wounds should be bandaged. Animals heal quicker with the wound exposed to the air. A bandage often just slows down healing and can hold or attract bacteria, causing an infection.

Keeping flies away from a wound is a must. Flies lay eggs on the wound and on surrounding hair. In a very short time, these eggs become maggots and enter the cut; there they begin to clean up the dead tissue. Great. But when that's gone, they begin eating live, healthy tissue. This will continue until the poor goat is hosting a seething mass of maggots. Scarlet oil or other healing maggot control daubed in and around the wound will keep the flies out.

Other miscellaneous injuries that afflict goats are generally the same types of problems people incur, including bruises, strains, sprains, burns, and heatstroke. When in doubt, treat the injured goat as you would a human with the same problem. If you can't get in touch with your veterinarian, try a first aid manual for treatment advice.

Enterotoxemia

Enterotoxemia is commonly known as overeating disease. Like tetanus, this disease is caused by a *Clostridium* bacterium, in this case, *Clostridium perfringens.* Although this problem is usually confined to young goats that are overfed, especially on grain, it can break out in any herd. Show kids being pushed for size and growth, meat animals being fattened for slaughter, and herds owned by a person who routinely overfeeds are all prime targets for enterotoxemia. However, overfeeding is not always the cause; in some herds it "just happens." The deaths are sudden, with little or no warning. Diarrhea, circling, convulsions, incoordination, and weakness are all symptoms.

As with tetanus, treatment for enterotoxemia is quite disappointing once you notice the symptoms. Luckily, vaccination is very effective, and many people routinely vaccinate all kids and all adults every 6 to 12 months. Does should receive two injections of vaccine, two to three weeks apart, during the last third of pregnancy and one booster yearly thereafter. Follow your veterinarian's recommendations.

Eversion of the Uterus

The uterus, in essence, is a fleshy pouch to contain the kids before birth. It is very muscular and well supplied with blood. Once in a while, the doe may continue straining after the kids are born, turn this pouch inside out, and force it out of the body.

Eversion of the uterus can be a hereditary problem, so never knowingly buy a doeling out of a doe that has had this trouble or a doe who, herself, has thrown out her uterus. Once a doe does this, there's an 80 percent or better chance she'll do it again and again, possibly dying from it.

If a doe kids and continues to strain, you can sometimes prevent her from throwing her uterus by standing her on a piece of plywood raised 5 to 12 inches in the back. This will take the weight and pressure of her stomach and intestines off her uterus. If this doesn't work, call your vet. He can check to make sure there isn't a problem such as a retained mummified fetus. Then he will give her a spinal anesthetic, which will usually last until the uterus shrinks back to a smaller size. Without the bulk of a large uterus, as it is just after kidding, the doe usually stops straining.

If a doe does throw her uterus, you will recognize it as a fleshy red bag protruding from the vagina, covered with caruncles ("buttons"), which are the size of a hardball or smaller. The uterus looks like a bumpy pouch with veins. It is the size of a grocery bag when fully out. Do not confuse this with a retained placenta, which is stringy, thin, and lightweight. (For details on this latter problem, see "Retained Placenta" on page 142.)

Eversion of the uterus is definitely an emergency situation, so call your veterinarian immediately. There is a tremendous amount of shock involved, and some does die within 10 to 15 minutes after the uterus is entirely out. Most can survive longer; but the sooner it is put back, the better chance the doe will have. (Although you will not want to use her for breeding again, she can milk well for a full lactation period and be used for meat when she dries up.)

After calling for help, elevate the doe's rear end, and keep her quiet. Running around will increase her shock and the possibility of tearing the uterus on a nail, wire, or other sharp object. A tear can mean her death. Keep a warm, moist towel on the uterus. This not only keeps it clean but also greatly cuts down the shock involved.

Resting the uterus on a bale of hay that's been draped with clean towels will help when the veterinarian arrives. The uterus is heavy and sloppy, making it hard to handle, so the extra support is a help. In place of a bale of hay or straw, two people, one on each side, can support the uterus in a towel, like a hammock. This makes it much easier to put it back into the body.

Many veterinarians use a spinal anesthetic to stop the straining, both during the replacement and afterward, which will prevent the doe from throwing it out again. It is also often a help to give the doe an injection of oxytocin (a hormone) to help shrink the uterus before attempting to put it back.

Afterward it is sometimes necessary to close the lips of the vulva, which can help to keep the newly replaced uterus from being pushed out again. But this alone will not keep the uterus in if the doe really gets to straining hard. So have her rear end elevated to cut down pressure, keep her occupied with feed or her kids, and *watch* her. If she begins to strain, call your vet. Don't wait to see if she will throw it out again, because she may. Usually a second spinal is all that is needed. By that time, if all is normal, the uterus is shrinking down well, and the urge to push is gone. Remember that this tendency is hereditary, so do not keep kids from this doe to use for breeding—not even that pretty buckling.

Foot Rot

Foot rot in goats is an infection seen in the feet, usually after the animals have been confined to pens with damp bedding. Lameness is usually the first sign of trouble. On examination you'll often notice a foul odor, and the foot may be swollen; sometimes you can see pus between the claws. If left untreated, the entire shell of the toe may slough off.

Keep in mind that other problems, such as a stone or thorn lodged in a toe or poorly trimmed hooves, can also cause severe lameness. So if you see an animal having trouble walking, wash and inspect the feet thoroughly.

Systemic treatment with antibiotics for a week usually helps to heal foot rot. You must also keep the feet thoroughly clean. Soak the affected foot or feet in a warm solution of Epsom salts daily, allow to dry, and then treat with a drying foot rot solution, such as Kopertox. If several goats in your herd are affected, force the animals to walk through a foot bath of 5 percent formalin or copper sulfate mixture (450 grams to 1 gallon of water); repeat this two or three times a week.

Remember, foot rot is most common in damp conditions; so prevention consists of keeping the stalls and running pens clean and dry. Also, trim the hooves regularly to help prevent manure from building up in the feet. Feeding an iodine supplement may help prohibit foot rot in some herds—a block of iodized white salt is seldom enough. Consult with your veterinarian if your animals are frequently bothered by foot rot.

Freezing

The natural breeding season of goats is August to January, so many give birth in very cold weather. It always seems that it's the night when it's -35°F (-1.7°C) and the wind is howling that a doe decides to kid. Being damp from amniotic fluid and afterbirth, the newborn kids—especially their ears and feet—are prime targets for frostbite and freezing. The doe can sometimes manage to dry off and warm a single vigorous kid born on a cold night, at least enough to keep it from freezing; but a doe who has twins or triplets can seldom handle all of them.

In mild cases of freezing or frostbite, the ears or feet will be swollen, tender, and hot to the touch. Stiff ears or unyielding feet and legs are signs of serious freezing. If left untreated, the damaged parts will become gangrenous due to insufficient circulation, and they'll eventually dry up and fall off. With ears, it is unsightly; with legs and feet, this leaves the goat with a severe handicap. A goat can survive the loss of one leg or two feet but will hardly do as well as a goat that is sound.

Preventive measures are the best way to "treat" this problem. If you live where subzero winters or low windchills are common and you don't have enough animals in your barn to keep the temperature above freezing, try to have an individual pen available for each doe due to freshen. A heat lamp or two will usually generate enough warmth for the newborn kids. Make sure you protect the heat lamp with a cage to prevent accidents—and *please*, double-secure it: A few extra minutes could save a lot of heartache. A fire in a barn is a terror. You don't want to keep the doe too warm; but the temperature in the stall needs to be above freezing, and there should be no drafts. After she kids, wait a day until the kids are all active and dry, and then slowly withdraw the heat.

If you discover a doe that has kidded during the night and has a kid suffering from freezing, carry the kid to the house, fill your bathtub with warm water (just a bit cooler than you like your bath), and stand the kid in it. If the ears are frozen or frosted, soak them well. Continue soaking the feet and ears for 15 minutes, warming the water as needed. Have someone warm several towels by throwing them in the dryer or hanging them by the oven or furnace. As soon as you are done soaking the kid, throw the warm towels on your lap, place the kid on them, and rub it dry, gently. *Do not scrub those frozen parts!* You may damage them. A hand-held blow dryer also works well for drying, and you don't have to touch the affected parts.

When the kid is thoroughly dry, place it in a box with some warm cloths near a source of warmth, such as a heat register or wood stove. Or place a heating pad on the floor, invert a cookie pan over it, and place the box on the pan. Be sure to supervise the heat source closely to prevent accidents! Then fix Junior a nice warm bottle. It may help to give intramuscular cortisone injections for four days, which raises the blood pressure, increases circulation, and reduces swelling and pain. If you don't catch the ears before they are damaged, wait until they begin to shrivel up; then give a week's treatment with antibiotics to prevent infection. Obviously, the best prevention is to keep the buch away from does in August through early November in cold climates to avoid kidding during freezing weather.

Fungal Infection

To the untrained eye, there isn't much difference between a fungal infection of the skin and mange, which is caused by mites. Even a veterinarian with experience must often take a skin scraping to make sure. So don't assume every bald or irritated-looking area on the skin is mange until it has been diagnosed by a veterinarian—not by a neighbor! Few mange remedies will work on a fungus, which can spread wildly while being incorrectly treated.

A general fungal infection of the skin is usually easy to treat. First, clip the affected area. Examine all the skin well for other lesions, and clip away additional hair, as needed. (Afterward be sure to soak the clipper blades in a fungicide.) During the warmer months, scrubbing the skin with a shampoo containing a medication works well. Be sure to follow directions carefully. In the winter treat the areas with a medication supplied by your veterinarian.

Infertility

Much of the "infertility" in does, especially with a first-goat owner, is due to poor timing and misinformation on the owner's part. Although does can and sometimes do come into heat and conceive in the spring, the months between August and January are their natural breeding time. Even when does show a summer heat, many do not conceive, so it's not fair to label them sterile.

Unless you keep a buck at your place, you should plan to leave a doe with the buck owner for at least a month. This is the safest, surest, and cheapest way to ensure pregnancy. Many does are brought to the buck a day or even a few hours late. Even if the doe stands for service, she may not conceive. Some does, especially young ones, are a bit timid; when hauled to an aggressive buck, they are afraid of his advances and seem to go out of heat quickly. Also, some does experience what is called a silent heat. There are no outward signs of heat, but many times the buck will know, resulting in a successful breeding that might otherwise have been missed.

Abortion

If a doe that you thought was bred suddenly comes into heat, it is quite possible that she aborted the fetus. Many people do not realize how small a fetus is before the last month or two before it is born. At 74 days the fetus is about the size of a baby mouse, and at 94 days, about the size of a hamster. So it's no wonder that many does abort and no one ever knows about it.

Many things can cause an abortion. Injury, natural causes (such as the doe's body rejecting an abnormal fetus), poor nutrition, fatigue, bacterial infections, viruses, poisons, and so forth—all have caused does to abort. (I have listed them in what I feel is the order of common occurrence.) To minimize the chance of problems, do not allow does heavy with kid to jump up on things or climb, and keep them separated from rough goats. The does need adequate exercise but not strenuous activity. Also, feed them carefully to keep them in good shape.

A single abortion in a herd is usually nothing to worry about. But if it is repeated or there seems to be an associated problem, call your veterinarian.

Cystic Ovaries

Once in a while, you may see a doe that is continually in heat. Instead of the regular 3-week cycle, she appears in heat every week or every few days. She will ride other does and accept service from the buck. Often such a doe has cystic ovaries. Positive diagnosis is difficult in many does without doing a laparotomy (surgical examination). Some does have a rectum large enough to allow a veterinarian to perform a rectal examination of the ovaries, but unfortunately, these are in a minority.

Often a veterinarian can be fairly certain, after observing a doe and hearing a complete history, that she does have cystic ovaries, and he can treat her accordingly. Injections of chorionic gonadotropin or progesterone will often help, and you can breed the doe on her first *regular* heat. In some cases surgery is necessary; in others nothing can be done to help. Fortunately, this condition is fairly uncommon.

Pyometra and Metritis

Pyometra and metritis are similar conditions that prevent conception and often interfere with normal heat cycles. Both terms basically refer to an infected uterus. With pyometra there is more pus in the uterus. Metritis means an inflamed uterus, but often there is a considerable amount of pus and exudate present. These conditions are commonly due to incomplete expulsion of the afterbirth or the death of one or more fetuses.

There may or may not be drainage from these conditions. When there is drainage, it is good in some ways. It lets you know there is serious trouble present; indicates the cervix is open a little, which facilitates drainage and treatments; and lets you begin treatment sooner because you become aware of the problem sooner. Otherwise, you may notice only that a recently kidded doe seems "off" or is running a fever. When you suspect a uterine infection, it's smart to have your veterinarian examine the doe.

Hormone injections, which force the uterus to contract and thus expel the pus and exudate, will often help treat these conditions. Infusions of antiseptics and antibiotics may be useful, as well. If the doe is running a fever or acting sick, you'll also usually have to start systemic treatment with antibiotics.

Retained Corpus Luteum

Once in a while, a doe will not come back into heat after having kidded. She may have a retained corpus luteum (yellow body). The corpus luteum is a glandular mass in the ovary, formed by an ovarian follicle that has matured and discharged its ovum. If the ovum is impregnated, the corpus luteum increases in size and remains for several months. If the corpus luteum does not rupture or degenerate after the birth of the kids, it "tells" the body that the doe is still pregnant, and she will not come into heat.

Of course, there are other conditions that will prevent a doe from having heat cycles, but a retained corpus luteum is quite common. It is generally easier to correct than many sterility problems, and one or two injections of estrogen (a female hormone) will often start normal heat cycles.

Vaginitis

Vaginitis, in itself, is not a serious condition. It can have simple causes, such as irritation due to kidding or breeding; but it can also result from a bacterial or viral infection, and metritis can follow. Vaginitis can be spread by a buck, by first breeding an infected doe and then a healthy doe. A doe with vaginitis will usually come into heat regularly but just fail to conceive. This is because the pH of the vagina is changed, which can kill the sperm.

The doe is seldom sick; but in severe, untreated cases, she may run a fever and act depressed. To see the condition, you'll need to part the lips of the vagina or use a vaginal speculum. Along with a reddening of the vaginal walls, there may be pustules and perhaps a foul odor. If you see any of these symptoms, have your veterinarian examine the doe to determine the extent and cause of her vaginitis.

When the vaginitis is caused by simple irritation, it will often remedy itself if you avoid breeding the doe for several weeks or if you use artificial insemination instead. If the condition is due to a bacterial infection, your veterinarian can suggest a successful treatment. He may recommend a mild douche with an iodine solution or infusion with a soothing antibiotic.

Fertility of the Buck

So far, I've neglected the buck in the discussion of infertility. This is only because it's more common to see does with sterility problems, simply owing to the fact that there are more does than breeding bucks.

Overuse is a common factor affecting the fertility of some bucks, especially well-bred bucks in heavy demand. Although many bucks can and do serve four or five does in a day, it is much safer to stagger breeding dates to cut that number in half.

The buck should be in very good physical shape at the approach of breeding season. This includes an examination and treatment, if necessary, for internal parasites and lice. Vitamin deficiencies can sometimes cut down on fertility, as can hormone imbalances. Also, the testicles of a buck should be full and oblong. They should be even, too. Shrunken, hard, or knotted testicles indicate past injury, inflammation of the testicle, or infection.

Most aggressive bucks in heavy service lose some weight during the breeding season, so it is a good idea to make sure yours is at his maximum *healthy* weight at its onset. However, remember that a buck that is quite a bit overweight will tend to have fewer successful breedings than a buck in top shape. The potency and sperm motility are greatly reduced in an obese buck. To stay healthy, a buck needs daily exercise. He should have an outside yard with toys, such as an old tire hanging from a tree, or another buck or a wether to play with. This play can be quite rough at times, but it is what builds muscle in a buck instead of flab from standing around inactive all day.

Hermaphroditism

Hermaphroditism occurs fairly often in goats—often enough to discuss, at any rate. The hermaphrodite doe will generally have an enlarged clitoris and sometimes a swollen or elongated vulva. She may look more bucklike than is normal. Her neck and shoulders will be heavier, and horns, if she has them, will be larger at the base than usual. Her heat periods will not be normal, or they will be completely absent. Obviously, if she does not have ovaries, she will not come into heat. The hermaphrodite buck may appear normal but either will not breed or will be sterile when bred.

The most frequent occurrence of hermaphroditism is in goats originating from the mating of two naturally polled (hornless) parents. When a horned (even if disbudded) goat is mated to a naturally polled goat, the kids will nearly always be normal. But when naturally polled animals are mated, a very high percentage of the offspring are hermaphrodites. Unfortunately, it is almost impossible to tell if a goat has been disbudded at an early age or is naturally polled. Some owners have intentionally bred two polled animals in an attempt to "breed out" horns, as was done with Polled Hereford cattle. With cattle this works, but not with goats.

Of course, hermaphrodites can occur from the mating of two horned animals, as well. But this appears to be simply an occasional happening, as it is with other species of animals.

Ketosis

If you notice a doe acting strangely several weeks before freshening, you should suspect ketosis. She may act a little "dumpy" or "slow," or she may stand in a corner with her head down. Later, coordination becomes poor, usually followed by weakness and staggering. The doe finally is unable to get to her feet. The entire course of this disease, or metabolic disturbance, often takes only several days from first signs to death.

Ketosis generally shows up in underfed does—not a starved doe necessarily but often a doe that's not receiving enough grain and legume hay to provide adequate carbohydrates for herself and her fetuses. Ketosis often shows in does carrying multiple fetuses.

Consult your veterinarian early if you suspect ketosis. Testing is quick, inexpensive, and simple. If you begin treatment when you notice the first symptoms, the animal will usually respond successfully. If she is still eating, boosting her carbohydrate level by increasing her feed with a palatable sweet feed can aid in relieving the ketosis. In some cases feeding glucose intravenously or giving propylene glycol orally with 40 units of insulin (intramuscularly) helps. Some does benefit from molasses drenches; dilute 4 ounces of molasses with water, and give the dose twice daily. It is difficult to successfully treat does with advanced cases of ketosis with drugs. If a doe is near kidding and comes down with ketosis, delivering the kids via cesarean section usually saves the doe and the kids.

Lice

Lice can be a real problem with goats, especially during the winter months. The long hair and shorter daylight hours encourage the intense breeding of lice, and they bother smaller animals, such as goats and calves, quicker than they do adult cows or horses. Aside from the itching and irritation, lice can cause severe anemia and death. They suck the blood, and if enough are on an animal, they can actually bleed it to death. Lice lower an animal's resistance and stamina, often causing it to look thin even if you are feeding it well. An infested animal will also be weakened, making it easy prey for intestinal parasites, disease, and metabolic problems. Milk production and growth rates also suffer.

It pays to check several animals in your herd, at random, each week during the winter because lice can multiply rapidly. Dandruff and patchy bald spots, accompanied by itching and rubbing, are signs of lice. The lice themselves look like tiny, oval-shaped, gray flecks, the size of a grain of rice or smaller. They usually don't move around; they attach themselves to the goat and stay put. A magnifying glass can help you spot them in parted sections of hair on the neck, throat, or body.

If you find lice or strongly suspect they are present, get a good dairy louse powder, and follow the directions on the package. Dust all of your goats, whether or not you've seen lice on all of them. Treat them weekly for three weeks. This will kill lice as they hatch, before they can breed and lay more eggs.

Mange

Mange is caused by mites and comes in two varieties: demo-dectic and sarcoptic. It can be a serious problem and is difficult to diagnose without having your veterinarian take skin scrapings. Mange can resemble many other skin problems, such as fungal, staph, and viral infections as well as allergic dermatosis. On goats most mange shows as baldness with small nodules like pimples, followed by scabs and crusty areas. The skin is either itchy or extra- sensitive to the touch; it may get thick and "stiff."

A small area of mange is very much easier to treat than an extensive area; so when in doubt, call your veterinarian out, or run your goat to the clinic for a check. Mange can spread on one goat like wildfire or spread through a herd equally quickly. Always keep a suspected animal isolated.

Treatment is sometimes difficult and depends on a correct diagnosis, followed by good nursing, a good mange remedy, and good luck. Many dips, sprays, powders, and rub-ons are effective against mange. Some work fine on limited areas but are toxic if used on the whole body. Others, such as liquid treatments, are better used in the summer as the animal will be wet. Your veterinarian will make the correct treatment choice for your particular situation; follow his advice and instructions.

Clip all hair away from a mange lesion, or clip the whole goat if the problem is widespread. Bathing the area with hot, soapy water before each treatment will help by removing any dandruff or loose scabs. It will also soften the skin, making it easier for the mange remedy to get to the mites, which burrow into the skin.

Mastitis

Mastitis means inflammation of the udder, usually caused by bacterial infection in a stressed udder. It is very common in goats. But with knowledge and good general care, you can prevent it or quickly detect and treat it, so it does not become a chronic condition.

Acute Mastitis

With acute mastitis the doe will act sick, running a temperature of 103° to 107°F (39.4° to 41.7°C). (Goats can differ in "normal" temperature, so it's a good idea to record what is normal for your individual goats when they are healthy.) The udder on one or both sides is usually hot, swollen, and hard. Mastitis means inflammation of the mammary gland, but most people think in terms of the abnormal milk that is usually present: It may be thick, chunky, bloody, watery, or puslike and smelly.

Acute mastitis is caused by a stress on the udder, which allows bacteria to multiply and cause trouble. This stress can be anything from a bump or bang to a bee sting or a cut teat. Does with low, pendulous bags are very prone to mastitis from knocking them about. A doe who tangles her teats in her legs while walking is a prime target—all the more reason to breed does for good udder attachments.

If you use a milking machine, it's important to watch it closely. If left unattended, it can creep up on the bag, causing stress that can lead to mastitis. Many does let their milk down all at once and are completely milked out in a minute. This leaves no time for you to go off and feed kids, water the buck, or do other tasks.

Most goats milked by machine are run through a milking parlor, where there is a short vacuum line. However, if you use a long line with several cocks, be sure the vacuum is the same at both ends. Improper vacuum, as well as improper inflation sizes or pulsation rates, can stress the udder and can cause bad mastitis flare-ups.

As for treatment, the very best thing is to have your veterinarian take a sample of the milk for culture. This way, you'll find out just what bacteria are causing the trouble. Most cases of acute mastitis respond to combination sulfas or a broad-spectrum antibiotic given systemically. Many veterinarians no longer use intramammary infusion (mastitis tubes), as there is a great risk of introducing other bacteria into an already-stressed udder. You can't sterilize skin, and 99 percent of the tube tips that enter the teat are not sterile, even if you do dab them with alcohol. Systemic treatment is better because it goes to work in the body all through the tissues, not just on the surface of the interior of the udder. Remember, the inside of the udder looks like a sponge, not an open, hollow ball full of milk. Getting an antibiotic forced through the teat and massaged into all those little pockets where there is active infection is darned near impossible.

Another part of treating acute mastitis is reducing the swelling in the udder. Cortisone injections can help, but don't use them if a doe is pregnant, owing to the danger of abortion. Another option is to massage warm udder liniment or ointment into the udder twice daily. Milking the infected side of the udder dry several times a day will hasten recovery time and also often help keep milk production from failing. Flushing out those bacteria (which are present in the milk) in this way is like draining an abscess, making healing easier and faster than if they were left inside. Always use good sanitation when working around a goat with mastitis to reduce the chance of spreading it to other does. Milk the affected doe last, and milk her by hand, not with a machine. It's also a good idea to dip the teats in a teat dip solution after each milking; dip the good teat first if the mastitis is only on one side. And scrub your hands well before handling other goats.

Chronic Mastitis

Once a doe has had acute mastitis, she is more prone to chronic mastitis. If you didn't treat the acute mastitis completely—perhaps you didn't give the antibiotics for the prescribed length of time, you switched antibiotics, or you used udder infusions improperly—tiny pockets of bacteria could remain. These bacteria are walled off by scar tissue in the udder, just waiting for an excuse (stress) to start trouble.

With chronic mastitis the doe usually isn't visibly sick, but she gives chunky or abnormal milk for a day or so, which then seems to clear up. The udder may swell but not with the hard, hot swelling of acute mastitis. There are often hard lumps, fibrous scar tissue, in the udder. She may flare up, on occasion, with acute mastitis. I seriously doubt that a doe with chronic mastitis is ever really cleared of it. As long as she is with your other does, she will be a potential source of infection.

Do not allow a mastitis doe to run with your other milkers, because it is possible for her to drip milk that another doe might lie in. Always milk the mastitis doe last, and milk her by hand if you use a machine on the others. Then scrub your hands immediately. The spray of milk that hits your hand contains millions of bacteria, which can be transferred to other does if you forget to wash up and you handle their bags. These steps might seem excessive, but they're really not when you consider the possibility of cutting six or seven years off a doe's production due to mastitis. That means a great loss in both milk and finances.

As you may guess, it is a lot easier to prevent mastitis than to "cure" it. Dipping the teats after milking will help keep mastitis down. The dip not only seals the teat canal from infection, but it also helps keep the teats from chapping and heals small cuts, all of which are stresses. Use fresh dip for each doe, however, as bacteria can live in teat dip long enough to be transferred from one doe or teat to another. But dipping teats will not help if the mastitis is caused by poor management practices, such as improper milking or having high doorsills that does can bang their udders on.

If your herd often has mastitis problems or if you just want to be on the safe side, you can test your does routinely for the presence of mastitis. Use the California Mastitis Test, available through your veterinarian or farm veterinary catalog. Test monthly or whenever you notice a goat producing suspicious or abnormal milk.

Gangrene Mastitis

Gangrene mastitis is a serious problem that can follow udder edema or other kinds of mastitis. It is many times caused by a combination of coliform bacteria and impaired circulation, as can be found with a caked bag or injury (usually a bang or bruise). If you ever notice that a doe's whole bag, or even just one side of it, feels cold like a piece of meat from the refrigerator instead of warm and alive, get help *immediately!* A doe can absorb enough toxin from a gangrenous udder to die in a day or two.

If you spot gangrene mastitis quickly enough, your veterinarian may be able to stop it, but that has a lot to do with luck. The bag may be fine and milk normally at night and be in a bad condition the next morning. Treatment consists of systemic antibiotics, cortisone, and heat applied to the bag to stimulate circulation.

In severe cases of gangrene mastitis, the affected part of the bag may have to be surgically removed to save the doe. If only one half is removed, you can still use her as a milker in the future since the remaining half will usually compensate. Of course, she will never give as much milk as she did before she lost half of her bag, but she *can* raise kids. If the entire udder is lost, she is usually fattened for the freezer unless she is a pet or produces great kids. Of course, her kids will have to be fed by another doe or raised by hand.

Milk Fever

Milk fever is a misnamed condition as there is no fever but instead a subnormal temperature. It can occur just prior to kidding, but usually it occurs one to four days after. It is generally found only in high-producing does. Likewise, it's seldom seen in a first freshener unless she is an extremely good milker.

The first signs will be unsteadiness in the rear quarters since milk fever causes an ascending paralysis. The doe will stagger, bleat, and go down. She will sometimes assume a froglike position as she tries to rise, dragging the rear legs backward. She will finally quit trying to rise and remain down. Her eyes will look glazed. She will seem not to know what is going on around her. If she is not treated, she will lapse into a coma and die.

In a normal freshening doe, calcium is drawn off the bone, where it is stored, as milk production begins in earnest. With the milk fever doe, the glands get lazy. They do not draw the calcium from the bone fast enough to replace the blood calcium, which is going into milk production; thus, the doe "collapses" with milk fever.

Prevention includes not fully milking out the udder upon freshening. Simply relieving the pressure on the udder several times a day for the first two days sometimes helps. A well-balanced diet is also necessary.

The only practical treatment for milk fever is an injectable calcium preparation, preferably given intravenously. It can be given intraperitoneally (into the abdominal cavity), but here it is absorbed slower and does not give as quick results. If you can reach your veterinarian, you should ask his advice in choosing the right treatment procedure. Ideally, you should have him come out to examine the doe. (Ketosis can be a complication of milk fever and needs to be treated, as well, often with a calcium-dextrose solution.)

If you live in the "boonies" and must treat your own does, it's smart to get a calcium preparation from your veterinarian to keep on hand. It nearly always comes in "cow-sized" bottles (500 cc), but use the dosage for sheep. Fifty to 100 cc of the calcium preparation is about right in most cases, depending on the size of the doe and the brand of calcium you are using; check the label.

When preparing to give an intravenous injection, be sure the needle (a 16-gauge, 2½-inch needle works fine) is well threaded into the vein and not just stuck precariously in the edge. Some calcium preparations are very irritating to the subcutaneous tissue, and if enough calcium leaks, it can cause a chunk of neck to slough off. It's also important to give the intravenous injection slowly because it can kill the animal if you give it too fast. It should go drip, drip, drip—not glug, glug, glug! (For more information on giving this kind of injection, see "Intravenous Injection" on page 371.)

Have an assistant hold the doe still because she may thrash after the dose begins to take effect. Once the doe has been treated, give her a little while to get oriented before you try to get her to her feet. If you slide a towel under her belly, one person on each side can lift and steady her, if necessary. There is no great rush in making her stand, however, so let her rest and munch on some grain and hay. She will also usually appreciate a drink. Most does get up unaided in a short time following treatment.

A doe can relapse with milk fever, so watch her closely for a day or so after she has had it. Also, watch her the next time she freshens because many does will have milk fever two or three years in a row—usually their peak production years. Her doelings will also be prone to this problem as they are more apt to be high producers than doelings out of just so-so producers. The more production we breed into our goats, the more troubles we run into. It is unnatural for a goat to produce more than 2 quarts a day, but we have bred them to produce more than 1 gallon. You just have to take the bad with the good!

Pneumonia

Pneumonia or a pneumonia complex is, in my opinion, one of the greatest causes of death and financial loss in goats. Not only can they die from the pneumonia, but if they survive, they are often useless as far as milk or meat production goes. If too much lung surface has been damaged by the pneumonia, the animal can only stand and pant for breath. This causes weight loss and a severe drop in milk production.

Pneumonia can be caused by several bacteria as well as viruses. It is not only found in a damp, cold, and drafty barn, although such a situation certainly is far from healthy. Pneumonia causes trouble everywhere, from spotless dairy barns to one-goat farms. As with many health problems, stress often brings it on.

One common cause of stress is a barn that's too warm, especially in the winter. Many goats are kept in a small building or an unused garage, which is well insulated and cozy. No drafts, no cold—but also no fresh air. Moisture from the goats' breathing, bodies, and urine can lead to dampness, chill, and stress if a barn is too airtight. Heating makes the condition worse as that will increase the humidity and the condensation. Goats can take a lot of cold, as long as it is *dry* cold, with plenty of shelter from wind and drafts and lots of dry bedding. Ventilation in a closed-in barn is a must!

Showing, breeding, and bringing home new animals are also common causes of stress. When animals exchange "germs" while under stress, pneumonia is a common result. And the more hosts a disease passes through, the "hotter" it gets, overcoming even resistant animals.

Miscellaneous stresses include changing owners, changing feed, and being chased by dogs or coyotes. Even weather extremes, such as sudden, severe cold snaps, rain with bad wind, hot, muggy summer days, or hot days followed by icy nights, can stress your goats and make them susceptible to pneumonia.

Pneumonia starts very quietly. The goat may just seem a little "off." It may lie down a little more than usual, refuse part of its grain, grunt, or not be quite as active as usual. *Please,* take its temperature right away; tomorrow it may be dead. Goats die more quickly than cattle from pneumonia, so you must act immediately to save them and their usefulness.

Most goats with pneumonia will run a high temperature—the average for pneumonia is 104° to 106°F (40° to 41.1°C). If one goat has a high temperature, check the others. I've seen goats with pneumonia and a 107°F (41.7°C) temperature *look* okay and be eating fine. Bear in mind, a goat's normal temperature can vary according to the individual. A goat that usually has a 102°F (38.9°C) temperature would be sick with a 103°F (39.4°C) temperature, which could be "normal" for another goat. Record your healthy goats' temperatures *before* they come down with something, so you'll have something to check against!

Goats can cough with pneumonia; but goats cough other times, too, so coughing isn't necessarily a symptom. Puffing for breath is, however. Don't ignore this. Isolate the sick goat, and then call your veterinarian right away. Pneumonia can quickly destroy the productivity of a goat and kill the animal fast, so don't fool around with home cures.

A broad-spectrum antibiotic, such as tetracycline or a sulfa combination, works in most cases. Tylosin, given for three to four days, can also give very good results. Some goats must be steamed (allowed to breathe the vapor from a bucket of boiling-hot water); others may need injectable expectorants, cortisone, or electrolytes. Let your vet make the choice of treatment based on his examination of the animal and its lungs.

Once a goat has had pneumonia, it may be more apt to get it again another year; so keep an eye on it, especially in times of stress.

Retained Placenta

The placenta, or afterbirth, is a milky membrane that envelops the fetus in the uterus. Most does expel the placenta with or just following the birth of each kid. But once in a while, a doe will not expel the afterbirth. It's generally easy to spot this problem as the placenta will be at least partially hanging out of the vulva. But sometimes there will be no sign of it; and unless you were there and noted the absence of it at birth, the doe could become toxic and die. These "hidden" retained placentas are the ones that cause the most trouble; the hanging ones keep the cervix open to pass drainage and pieces of afterbirth, which helps prevent toxemia.

If a doe hasn't passed the placenta in 12 hours after kidding, call your veterinarian. The placenta can stay in longer; but after 12 to 24 hours, some does close up too tightly to allow a hand in through the cervix to manually remove the placenta.

Don't be alarmed if your veterinarian decides to leave the placenta hanging. He will give the doe a shot (usually hormones to aid the natural release and expulsion of the placenta) and place boluses in the uterus to dissolve particles and protect against infection. If the placenta is not hanging out, the veterinarian will often pull the bulk of it through the cervix so that its weight, along with the hormones, will help release it. However, many veterinarians do not "clean" the doe (manually release the placenta from the uterus), because allowing the placenta to come away naturally helps ensure successful future breeding and the ability to carry the kids full term.

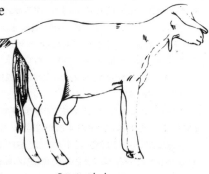

Retained placenta

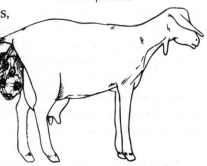

Eversion of the uterus

Never yank at the placenta or pull hard on it. Caruncles, the spongy-textured "buttons" or knobs on the uterus to which the placenta fastens, can be ripped off this way, causing fatal hemorrhage or sterility of the doe. If there is no vet-

Retained placenta and eversion of the uterus. *A retained placenta is thin and stringy. If the doe hasn't passed the placenta within 12 hours, call your veterinarian. An everted uterus looks like a red, fleshy bag with noticeable caruncles (buttons). This is definitely an emergency; call your veterinarian at once.*

erinarian available and you can't drive the doe to a veterinary clinic, you can attempt to draw as much placenta as possible through the cervix to keep it open; then place two sulfa-urea boluses in the uterus to help dissolve the pieces and prevent infection. To try to clean the doe without experience is like driving a car without experience—very difficult to do correctly and safely.

Ringworm

Ringworm is so named because it shows up as a circular crusty spot, a "ring," often on the face or neck. However, ringworm is not a worm, nor is it caused by a worm; it is caused by a fungus. It most often shows up in the winter months on goats kept inside. It is contagious, so you should isolate affected goats from other animals until it is cleared up. It is ugly but very seldom causes much of a problem, and it will disappear when the goats are turned outside in the spring. But the horrible-looking, grayish, crusty, bald patches can be a problem if you are trying to sell kids, breeding stock, or milk or if you have a buck standing at public service.

Iodine or a fungicide available through your veterinarian is often quite successful in treating ringworm. Many of the fungicides are in an oil base, which keeps the scab and crust softened so they are easier to remove. You'll want to remove the crust before each treatment in order to get down to the fungus, not just treat the surface. Soak the area with warm, soapy water, and then scrub it with a small brush to loosen the crust. Work from the outside of the affected area toward the center so you do not spread the fungus while treating it. When working around the eyes, always put a ring of bland ointment (such as petroleum jelly) around the eye before applying the medicine to prevent injury or burning.

Tetanus

Tetanus, or lockjaw, is fairly common in goats. This is not to say that goats are dying in droves from it, but it *is* a problem, one that is much easier to prevent than to cure.

Tetanus is caused by *Clostridium tetani,* which lives in the soil in many areas. It grows only in the absence of oxygen, and a deep wound or a puncture is an ideal incubator for the organism. The first symptoms you may notice are poor coordination, stiffness in the rear limbs, and refusal—inability, actually—to eat and drink. (Careful here, as these can also be symptoms of rabies.) The third eyelid becomes prominent, giving the eye a peculiar look. Bloat is another common symptom.

Call your veterinarian immediately if you suspect tetanus. By the time you notice the symptoms, the chances of recovery are poor, although massive doses of tetanus antitoxin and penicillin sometimes work. But many people cannot or will not put much money into an animal that is a poor risk.

Eighty percent or more of goats showing signs of tetanus die, even with treatment. But a yearly inexpensive booster of tetanus toxoid will protect against it. To prevent puncture wounds, keep all nails and wire away from the goat pasture. If you do spot any deep wounds or punctures, wash them out thoroughly. Flush the wound well, all the way to the bottom, with a syringe full of warm, soapy water and then again with an antiseptic like Betadine. Even though a wounded goat has had a toxoid booster, it is still a good idea to give it an injection of antitoxin, just to be safe.

Tetanus in goats is most common following dehorning or castration with an elastrator (the rubber band method). So if you use this method, be sure to have all goats protected by a tetanus booster a few weeks prior to doing the work or to give each an injection of tetanus antitoxin at the same time you dehorn or castrate.

Ticks

Ticks are larger than lice and more closely resemble a roundish watermelon seed. The body is hard, and colors range from gray through brown splotched to nearly black. The longer a tick is on a goat, the larger its body gets as it becomes engorged with blood. The body color becomes lighter as the tick swells. Unless they carry a disease or they are numerous on a goat, ticks usually don't cause a lot of trouble. They are quite easy to see, and it's fairly simple to remove them. In areas of the country where Lyme disease is a problem, keeping your goats free of ticks is particularly important because infected ticks may spread Lyme disease to humans.

If these pests are common in your area, keep in mind that they like to hide in long hair. Goats kept clipped are less bothered than nonclipped goats. There are also dairy wipe-on liquids or sprays that help to repel ticks. If ticks become a real problem, you can bathe your goats—they hate to be dipped—with a rotenone solution or similar preparation. Whatever you use, be sure it is safe for dairy animals; some insecticides leave a harmful residue in the milk. Personally, I do not like using any insecticide that is systemic or toxic except as a last resort for serious problems, which tick infestations seldom are.

If you do spot ticks on your goats, you can pull them off by hand or use tweezers (especially if you live where Lyme disease is a problem). Pull slowly. If you yank them, the head may break off. The head is not buried in the skin, but it stays attached to the skin and can cause irritation and infection.

Udder Edema

This condition, also known as caked bag, usually occurs just before freshening and just after, when there is a sudden increase in the circulation to the udder in preparation for milk production. The swelling shuts off vessels to a certain extent; thus, blood is being taken into the udder faster than it is being taken out of it. Fluid seeps out of the blood vessels into the surrounding tissue. This is a caked bag. It feels doughy to the touch, and fingerprints remain visible after you handle the udder. The udder may be painful to the doe.

Grain increases milk production or milk input to the bag, causing the udder to distend. So cutting the grain ration slightly a week or so before freshening may help prevent udder edema.

Some caked bags will just clear up naturally without treatment as the sudden increase in circulation slows down a few days after freshening. If the udder seems very badly caked, though, it needs treatment; it can be a stress and may end in acute mastitis, gangrene mastitis, or decreased production. Hot compresses, hot udder ointment, and massage all help reduce the swelling by increasing circulation. Diuretics such as Lasix (available from your veterinarian) have worked very well for dairy goats. These are available in both injectable and oral forms. Diuretics cause more frequent urination, drawing more fluid from the body (the udder). It usually takes only a couple of days of treatment before the udder is normal and stays normal without further therapy. If you are not sure whether the condition is bad enough to require treatment or which treatment you should use, consult with your veterinarian.

Do not confuse udder edema with the hard udder that's often found with does showing signs of mastitis caused by CAE. This udder seems "solid" and meaty—not doughy to the touch—and will not clear up with treatment. The doe with CAE-caused mastitis will seldom produce much milk, but the udder will usually remain hard. (For more information on this problem, see "Caprine Arthritis and Encephalitis" on page 122.)

Udder Injuries

Being low to the ground and carrying a large udder, the doe is a prime target for snags, tears, and cuts on the bag and teats. Goats and barbed wire are a bad mixture, as does (and bucks!) have little regard for it as a fence and will crawl or jump through. It's very easy for the does to snag their bags on the way through. Bloody scratches or worse usually result.

Because the udder is the place of milk production, it is richly supplied with blood and the skin is relatively tender. This is why many udder wounds bleed profusely. If you are not used to seeing blood, it can be quite a shock—but don't panic. Get a clean cloth: a dish towel, diaper, or anything clean and absorbent. Wipe the excess blood away, and then press the cloth on the wound. Most wounds will stop or nearly stop bleeding in 5 to 10 minutes. Don't move the cloth around even if it seems that the blood has stopped. When you disturb the clot that forms between the cut and cloth, the bleeding may start again. If the wound was not serious and the bleeding not profuse, carefully remove the cloth after all bleeding has stopped. If the bleeding was heavy, leave the cloth on the clotted cut for 12 hours or so; then soak it away.

When the cut is on the bag and is not deep, involving just skin, simple first aid measures are usually adequate. Rinse the injury well with warm, soapy water to flush out any dirt. Dry the area, and then apply an antiseptic, such as sulfa powder or iodine. Don't use ointments, because they attract and hold manure, dust, and dirt.

While many wounds fill in very nicely by themselves, you should have your veterinarian check most udder wounds. Cuts on the teats or udder that leak milk need prompt veterinary attention since they often will not heal by themselves (the milk interferes with healing). The skin may heal, but often a small hole remains, leaking milk continually.

If the cut is deep, gapes open, or leaks milk, it is usually best to have your veterinarian suture it closed. It is also many times advisable to sew up teat cuts because they heal quicker and smoother when sutured. Otherwise, they will be irritated by daily milking and handling, both of which can open the wound just as it begins to heal. Please, believe your veterinarian about whether or not to sew up an ugly rip. He wants the wound to heal as much as you do, and he will make the decision based on his experience of what will give the best results in the long run.

If you plan to call your veterinarian, don't put anything on a cut, except maybe soap and water, unless it is bleeding very badly and you have some astringent powder, the kind used when dehorning. Use the powder to stop the bleeding, if necessary. It is hard to examine or suture a wound if it is caked with gobs of powder or gooey salve.

When you suspect an injury needs sewing up, call your veterinarian right away. The longer an injury is left untreated, the harder it can be to repair successfully. Several hours after the wound has occurred, swelling begins to take place; then the edges begin to dry and finally start to heal. Any dirt in the wound is now part of the animal and may cause infection if sutured in. (By this point, it is nearly impossible to clean out the dirt.) To have an older injury heal well, your veterinarian may have to trim the edges of the wound or make them raw so they heal together.

White Muscle Disease

White muscle disease is quite common in some areas, especially where the soil is deficient in selenium. It usually affects kids, although fetal deaths during the later weeks of pregnancy can also occur. Symptoms include a stiff gait (often with an arched back), diarrhea, starvation (due to inability to nurse), an inability to rise, and finally death.

Treatment is often successful when you catch the condition in its early stages. Injections of selenium-vitamin E usually bring quite prompt relief.

But, as in most deficiencies, prevention is much better than treatment. Give all does in a selenium-deficient area a routine injection of selenium a month before they are due to kid; then follow with an injection for each kid at three months, four months, and five months of age. Supplementing the feed with selenium can be useful in some herds. Consult with your veterinarian to see if the area you live in is selenium deficient and if white muscle disease is a problem.

Worms

Given half a chance, goats are fairly worm-free. This is not to say that goats don't have worms but that due to their natural eating habits, goats come in less contact with worm eggs and larvae than do other animals. Goats don't eat as close to the ground (thereby picking up possible worm-infested grass) but prefer to nibble and browse when possible. Goats are also very fussy eaters. They will not eat feed with manure in it or drink manure-contaminated water unless very hungry or thirsty. Unfortunately, goats are seldom raised the way they would prefer to live, with plenty of space to roam and browse. And limited pasture and close housing can lead to worm problems.

There is a big controversy among goat owners over the best approach to worming. Some worm regularly with a broad-spectrum wormer, which kills most of the worms a goat has. Others wait until there is trouble from worms before treating their goats. Personally, I would recommend a routine six-month fecal exam by your veterinarian. He can examine the manure under a microscope to determine the presence of worm eggs and minute larvae. (Worms are seldom visible to the naked eye.)

Never just assume a sick goat is wormy and proceed to worm the hapless animal. All wormers are toxic to some extent—or they wouldn't kill the worms—and this added toxicity can harm a sick goat. Also, there are many worms that can infect goats, and you will want to be sure you choose a wormer that kills the worms your goat has. It is a waste of time and money to use a wormer that is not going to help, and it can be an unnecessary risk.

It will help your herd greatly if you aggressively work toward eliminating worm problems while kids are less than a year old. Provided that the adults in the herd are relatively untroubled by worms, taking fecal samples of the kids, then treating them as needed, can help keep a herd nearly parasite-free.

Some goats' internal parasites develop resistance to certain wormers, as can be the case when a herd is routinely wormed with the same wormer. And this is all too possible since there aren't many wormers "cleared" for use in goats. This is one reason to get after those kid parasites, as many wormers cannot be used on dairy animals of lactating age. (While several wormers, such as thibenzole, *are* approved for use in goats, others that have been used "experimentally" with good results, such as ivermectin, have *not* been cleared for use in dairy goats, owing to the expense of testing.)

To control most worms, it is necessary to use a wormer and then repeat treatment in two weeks. The larvae migrate through the bloodstream. While most wormers attack the worms in the stomach and intestines, they don't always kill those in the blood or destroy the eggs. These eggs hatch; and if the goat is not wormed again in two weeks, they can completely reinfest the animal even though it was just recently wormed. Ask your veterinarian, and read the label of your wormer very thoroughly for detailed treatment instructions.

Preventive measures can help greatly in reducing parasites in your goats. Rotating pastures will naturally keep down the amount of parasite eggs available where the goats graze. For even better results, plow and reseed your pastures regularly, move the animals to a new pasture before they graze the grass closely, and keep weeds clipped while a pasture is recovering from grazing.

Sanitation measures are also important. Give the animals adequate space to prevent crowding. Don't allow older kids to run with adults. Keep indoor pens dry and bedded with fresh bedding. Use keyhole mangers to keep animals from running in and out of the mangers. Salt blocks and water tanks need a keyhole access, too, for sanitation. Scrape away and remove barnyard manure often. Sprinkling borax every week or so in pens and barnyards can sometimes help because it kills worm larvae. And never allow goats access to manure piles; they love to climb and lie on them!

SHEEP

GENERAL CARE AND MANAGEMENT

$\mathcal{J}$t is far less costly to prevent problems than to treat them. And the most important aspect of preventing sheep diseases and problems is good general care and management.

Housing

Although sheep do not need elaborate housing, their shelter must be dry and draft-free. In the winter you need to be able to keep it above freezing during lambing. Sheep also need shade from the sun during the summer as they are prone to overheating.

A tight-woven wire fence is a must, not only to keep your sheep in but also to keep dogs out and to discourage coyotes. Dogs and coyotes are the worst predators of sheep. Wolves, bears, and an occasional bobcat or cougar will attack sheep, but nationwide, dogs are their biggest enemies. These dogs are often pets that chase sheep for "recreation"—the excitement of the chase—not for food.

A sheep or flock of sheep panics and runs easily, and a running sheep invites attack. Some sheep owners keep a goat or two—preferably bucks or wethers that are used to dogs, and with good sets of horns—with their pastured sheep. It is not so much the protection the goats offer but the fact that they don't panic and run. The sheep tend to gather around the goats, and standing sheep aren't so inviting. Donkeys and llama geldings are also used to protect sheep flocks. It helps greatly if you raise these protectors with the flock so they bond with the sheep. This increases their protective instincts and lessens the chance they will fight with the sheep.

Feeding

As sheep are often found in arid wastelands, many people get the mistaken idea that they can be raised cheaply on poor pasture. This idea has caused much disappointment and many first-time sheep raisers to go broke. To raise sheep, you will need just as good pasture and hay as cattle require. True, nomadic peoples raise sheep successfully, but they move the herds daily, giving them hundreds and hundreds of acres of fresh, albeit scant, pasture weekly. (This also helps keep down disease and parasite problems.) But most folks raise sheep on a much more limited pasture area, so that pasture must be good. Sheep also need grain at times—such as when the pasture is not lush, before and after breeding or lambing, and when the animals need to gain weight—or there's a great chance of losses due to ketosis or poor nutrition.

Also, keep a close watch on your sheeps' condition. Sheep can fool you, especially when carrying a good coat of wool; so part the wool and feel the skin. Sheep certainly should not be as fat as beef cattle,

PARTS OF A SHEEP

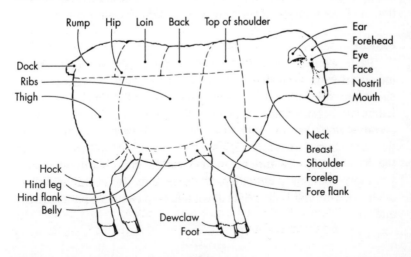

First Aid Kit for Sheep

Here are some basic ingredients that belong in a first aid kit for sheep. If you keep a herd of sheep, you should have all of the items below on hand. If you have only one or two sheep, you should at least keep the items marked with an asterisk. Of course, there is much more you can keep in your kit, but this is a good start. Ask your veterinarian for his advice for your situation. He might also be able to supply items that you can't find at your local farm supply store or in a farm veterinary supply catalog.

Balling gun (calf-sized)*
Blood stopper*
Dose syringe
Emasculatome or
    emasculator
Feeding tube*
Foot trimmers
Forceps/needle holder
Lamb nipples*
Mouth speculum
Rectal veterinary
    thermometer*
Scarlet oil*
Sheep clippers
Stomach tube
Three 18-gauge, 1½-inch
    needles*
12-cc syringe*
Veterinarian's phone
    number*

but they should not feel bony and thin, either. Check the body condition of all your sheep regularly, especially older ewes and rams.

Pasture

Pasture rotation is a vital part of raising healthy sheep. It is more important with them than with any other grazing animals because sheep are susceptible to internal parasites and their close grazing habits can be hard on pasture crops. When land is overgrazed, it soon becomes worthless and supports only noxious weeds. An ideal situation is to have at least four separate fenced pastures so you can rotate the flock to a new pasture before they eat the grass short. Soon after you move your sheep out of a pasture, run a mower over it as well as a harrow. This will keep weeds down and help eliminate parasite eggs and larvae.

Grain

Sheep do not like dry, ground feed like that fed to cattle. They much prefer either a coarser ground feed moistened with molasses or pelleted feed. Generally, sheep on good lush pasture do not require grain. If such pasture is not available, feed your animals good-quality legume hay (as much as they'll eat) along with 1½ to 2 pounds of good-grade mixed grain daily. In many areas sheep raisers feed their animals root crops, such as turnips, rutabagas, and carrots, with good results. (These vegetables should be chopped to improve palatability and to prevent choking.) Sheep can also do well on corn silage and on other feeds that are locally available. Your county Cooperative Extension Agent (usually located in your county seat) can help you make a good, economical choice. (He or she will also have many free booklets on different aspects of sheep raising.) Bear in mind that you must make any feed changes gradually, or digestive upsets and stress will result.

Water

Clean water is a must at all times. And although a creek is pretty and a handy water source, know where it comes from. If there are animals fairly close upstream, that stream can bring disease to your animals. It pays to check and think about this. If your neighbor upstream has had leptospirosis, for example, you might well choose to vaccinate your flock if they have access to the shared creek.

Creep-Feeding Lambs

Lambs will begin to munch on hay, grass, and grain shortly after they are born. At first, they will eat very little because they are still depending on the ewe for nourishment. But soon they will develop a taste for dry feed and be willing to nibble on grain off and on all day. To provide an eating arrangement that allows this yet does not let the ewes overload, it is best to provide a creep feeder. This is simply a pen in one corner, with openings that are big enough to allow the lambs to enter and eat but too small to admit the ewes. It has to be high enough that the more athletic ewes don't jump into the creep.

Clean up any leftover grain daily (feed it to the ewes) to prevent any moldy or sour feed from collecting in the corners of the feed troughs. It is also a good idea to cover the creep feeder if it is outside,

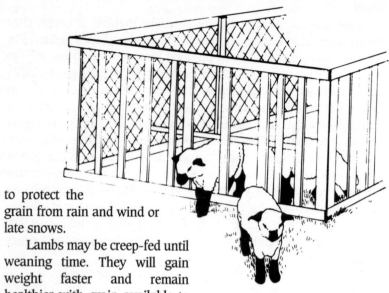

to protect the grain from rain and wind or late snows.

Lambs may be creep-fed until weaning time. They will gain weight faster and remain healthier with grain available to them free-choice, as opposed to simply feeding them as a group twice a day. However, you should still protect them against entero-toxemia to prevent overeating disease since some lambs tend to "hog" feed. (For more information on this disease, see "Enterotoxemia" on page 166.)

Creep feeder. *A creep feeder is a pen with openings that are big enough to allow the lambs to enter and eat but too small to admit the ewes. This permits the lambs to nibble on grain without competition from the ewes.*

Restraint

When you need to restrain sheep, either for examination or for treatment, the safest method is to calmly drive the whole flock or part of it into a small holding pen. It is very hard to cut out only one animal from the flock unless you are lucky enough to own a good sheepdog. Keep in mind that an excited sheep or flock is hard to drive; plus, running or exciting sheep, especially on a warm day, can kill them. Do not yell or run; just quietly move them to the pen.

If you use a dog to help with the flock, be sure it is trained and under your control. Some dogs can get a bit aggressive and "hard" on sheep while working them, and they should be supervised and en-

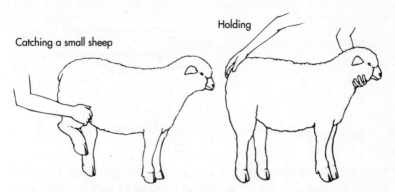

Catching a small sheep

Holding

Catching and holding sheep. *With a swift, sure movement, grasp the hind leg or the wool under the chin. To hold the animal, grasp a fold of flesh under the lower jaw. Placing your other hand over the dock can help to settle or move the animal.*

couraged to go lighter.

When the flock is penned, you may have to divide the pen if the flock is large. When you are ready to catch the sheep you need to work on or examine, walk toward it calmly. Don't look directly at it or try to "sneak" up on it—that only alarms the animal. Meander over in the animal's direction; then, when you are close enough, quickly reach out, grab the wool under the chin, and tip the head upward. This will keep a mature sheep off balance and make it easy to hold. (Lambs and smaller sheep are easier to catch by a hind leg.)

For longer restraint, such as needed for shearing, you can plunk the sheep down on its rear, with its back up against your legs. It's very handy to have an assistant's help here.

To drench a sheep (give it liquid medicine), catch it, retain the chin-hold with one hand, and swing a leg over the back, straddling the animal,

Restraining by sitting. *If you need to restrain a sheep for a period of time, sit it down with its back against your legs (or those of your assistant). Place one hand under the chin to tip the head up slightly; steady the shoulder with your other hand.*

Dose syringe

Balling gun

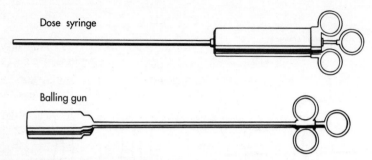

Tools for giving medication. *Use a dose syringe to give liquid medication. Restrain the animal, slip the syringe into the mouth, tip the head up slightly, and give the dose. To give a bolus, dip it in corn oil, place it in a balling gun, and slip the gun into the mouth of the restrained sheep. When the end of the gun is over the hump at the back of the tongue, eject the bolus.*

facing forward. Slip the dose syringe or bottle into the corner of the mouth and over the tongue, and give the liquid slowly. Don't tip the sheep's head way up, or there will be increased danger of it inhaling some of the fluid. And never squirt or pour the liquid in fast. The animal will struggle and choke, and if the liquid gets into the lungs, you will have a dead sheep.

To give a bolus (pronounced bowl-us), which is a large, oval-shaped pill, dip it in corn oil just prior to dosing. Place it in a balling gun, and then restrain the sheep as described above. Slip the balling gun into the mouth and over the hump at the back of the tongue, and then quickly eject the bolus. Hold the head up, with the mouth closed, and massage the throat downward until the animal swallows.

Giving an intramuscular injection to a sheep can be a challenge if you have never done it before. How do you find the sheep under all that wool? Hold the sheep in a corner and against a wall, with your knee in its flank; then divide the wool on the upper thigh until the skin is visible. Feel for the round, bulging muscle on the back of the thigh, and then slip the needle into the muscle. Draw back slightly to check for blood, which will tell you if you've hit a vein by mistake (remove the needle in that case), and inject the drug. Do *not* jab so deeply that you hit bone. The needle needs only to go well into the muscle. (For more details on giving this type of injection, see "Intramuscular Injection" on page 370.)

Breeding

The normal breeding season for sheep is in the fall and early winter (August to December). The ewe comes into heat every 21 to 26 days, and she usually remains in heat for 1 to 3 days. The gestation period is five months. Breed your ewes so they drop their lambs during the best months for your particular conditions. If your barn stays above freezing all winter or if your pens have supplemental heat and you are available to give extra care in cold snaps, you can breed your ewes in August to lamb in January. But if your barn is cold or you will not be able to give extra care at that time, it's better to breed in November or December so the ewes lamb in April or May.

A ram must be present to indicate heat in ewes because few ewes show signs of heat that are obvious to owners. It's best to keep him separate from the ewes, though, unless you want very early lambs, as some ewes come into heat earlier in the year than "normal." You absolutely must keep him separated from the others if older ewe lambs are with the flock, as these youngsters are too small and immature to be bred and will usually have trouble lambing.

There is some disagreement as to the best age to breed ewe lambs. Some owners breed 7- to 8-month-old ewe lambs in good flesh to increase the number of lambs each animal can produce during a lifetime. Others prefer the traditional first lambing of ewes at two years of age as the ewe is more mature and better framed and she has an easier time lambing. I like to see the ewe first bred when she reaches her adult frame and weight—whether at 8 months, if she matures early, or at 18 months, if she matures later.

Ewes should be "flushed" at breeding time. This means turning them out onto extragood pasture and giving nutritional supplements (such as grain or pellets) as needed so the animals are gaining weight when they are due to be bred. This does not mean having them fat at breeding but gaining, which increases ovulation.

One mature ram can serve 40 to 50 ewes in a breeding season if he is in good condition—neither thin nor overly fat. If you practice heat synchronization, the method of using hormones (often vaginal pessaries or implants) to artificially regulate heat cycles, it is best to have 2 rams for this number of ewes as they are all in heat at a relatively close time. A young ram can handle half as many ewes successfully.

During the winter feed the ewes good alfalfa or legume hay free-choice (as much as they'll eat) along with 1 to 1½ pounds of good mixed grain per animal daily. Raise or lower this amount as needed while you monitor the condition of the ewes. A month before lambing, you may have to increase the grain so the ewe is gaining weight slightly as lambing approaches. Many ewes are lost to ketosis or pregnancy disease due to feeding insufficient grain or poor-quality hay, which causes carbohydrate deficiency, especially in ewes carrying twins or triplets. Place the ewes' hay, grain, water, and salt in different areas so the ewes are forced to exercise mildly.

A ewe will usually show udder development about one to two weeks before lambing. Clip away the wool around her udder to make it easier for the new lambs to find the teats. This is called crutching, and it saves many slower or weaker lambs in a flock.

Lambing pens are an important part of successful lambing. Many lambs that are lost or rejected could have been saved by using pens. Lambing pens are small enclosures—about 5 × 6 feet—usually built by

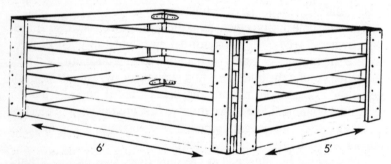

6' 5'

Lambing pen. A lambing pen will keep the ewe from being disturbed during delivery and will prevent the lambs from straying. Make these temporary pens by tying together a few gates.

fastening several gates together. Prepare them before your first ewe is due to lamb. Their purpose is to keep the ewe from being bothered by other ewes and to keep the lambs near the mother. When a ewe is nearly ready to lamb, put her in a pen. During cold snaps, when you may not be there during the birth, you can hang heat lamps *securely* over the pen. But, ideally, someone should be there to watch for lambing problems and to make sure that she cleans the lambs and allows them to nurse.

Normal Lambing

In the week before lambing, the ewe will build up a nice full udder. It should be pink and firm but not rock hard or bluish. (If the udder *is* very hard or discolored, have your veterinarian check the ewe at once for mastitis.) The ewe will move slower and may lie down more than usual. Her vulva will elongate and begin to relax. Approaching lambing, she may refuse feed and paw the ground; she may seek out a quiet corner, walking with her head down. But don't count on such warning signs: She may just lie down and pop out twins!

Once she throws out strings of mucus that are pink or tinged with blood, you will know she isn't fooling around. She will grunt and begin to strain hard. In 15 minutes or so, a dark bulge will appear in the vulva. This is the water bag. Closely following it will appear two feet, toes pointed down. When the legs are out nearly to the knees, the nose will appear. The ewe will usually work hard a few minutes and then force out the head and shoulders. She may rest a minute and then continue labor until the rest of the lamb is expelled. Remember, lambs are born with a long tail, which is later docked.

Most ewes of good size have twins, so the second lamb will probably soon follow. The ewe will then clean both lambs until they are white and dry. Some lambs are nearly black at birth, but they whiten as they get older. Within an hour they will be on their feet nursing, with their tails wagging.

Rear presentations (back feet and rump first) are quite common, as well. If the lamb is coming backward, the ewe will deliver it easily in most cases. But as soon as it is born, you must clean the nose and throat of mucus and afterbirth. The lamb begins to breathe as soon as the umbilical cord breaks, which sometimes happens when the backward lamb is only partway out. For this reason, it is best to assist the ewe to quickly deliver her lamb. Do *not* yank it out, but gently pull down as she pushes. If the lamb sounds bubbly as it breathes or is not breathing, you must pick it up by the hind feet and drain the mucus and fluid out of the throat and lungs, and the new lamb will usually start breathing normally. If the lamb doesn't breathe well, rub it vigorously with a warm towel while holding the hind legs higher than the head, and keep wiping the fluid out of the nose and mouth.

Abnormal Lambing

When the ewe labors more than a half hour and does not produce a lamb, you should examine her manually to check the position of the lamb. Scrub your hands first, and use some liquid dish soap as a lubricant.

Often a leg gets deflected on the brim of the ewe's pelvis. If the head and only one leg are in the birth canal, you will have to bring up the missing leg. Be careful to get the leg belonging to that lamb, not its twin! It is often necessary to force the lamb back so you have room to bring the leg into the birth canal. Be careful not to lose the head back into the uterus in the process and to protect the uterus from the lamb's foot by slipping your hand over it while prying it into place.

If the front legs appear but no head, you can be almost assured that the head has been turned back inside the uterus. Here you must push the legs back to gain room while trying to reach the head with your other hand. Often you can cup the head in your hand and pry it around. If this doesn't work, try getting a finger and thumb in the lower jaw, like a fishhook, and draw the head around with that hold. Once the head is in position, draw head and legs out gently. Again, be sure the head belongs to the right twin. Two lambs cannot be born at the same time!

When a lamb is just too big to fit through the birth canal or if it has a retained head or leg that you cannot reach in a few minutes, it's best to call your veterinarian. He may be able to deliver the lamb normally or else perform a cesarean section. Don't work on the ewe until she is exhausted. Exhaustion can throw a ewe into shock, and sheep die easily from shock. Whether you plan to take your ewe to the veterinarian or have the veterinarian come to your place, give them both a better chance by doing so early in the difficult labor.

(For other problems related to pregnancy and lambing, see "Eversion of the Uterus" on page 166, "Ketosis" on page 169, "Retained Placenta" on page 173, and "White Muscle Disease" on page 175.)

Caring for Lambs

Twins or triplets are sometimes a problem because a few ewes tend to ignore one of the lambs. It can be necessary to keep shoving the ignored one to her nose or even to take the other lamb away temporarily until she begins cleaning up and mothering the ignored one. Some weak lambs must be tube-fed. (See "Caring for Kids" on page 103 for details.) Extra heat, like a heat lamp or heating pad, also helps perk up these lambs. You can often stop this special care after three or four feedings, when the lamb is stronger.

Orphan and Rejected Lambs

It is fairly common for a ewe to reject her lamb. Often it is a young ewe with her first birth. She will completely and firmly refuse to have anything to do with it, kicking and butting it away when it tries to nurse. Sometimes these ewes can be fooled by smearing Vicks VapoRub on the lamb's body and the ewe's nose. She then cannot smell the lamb and may nurse it. (This also works when you are trying to foster an abandoned lamb on another ewe with plenty of milk and only one lamb or on one whose lamb has died.)

Slipping a piece of twine around the ewe's hind legs in a figure eight and forcing her to let the lamb nurse will often eventually work. Do not tie the twine, but hold it in your hand to prevent injury to the legs.

When a ewe completely rejects a lamb or a lamb is left an orphan and you do not have another ewe for a foster mother, you will have to bottle-feed the lamb. Place it in a warm, draft-free pen or a cardboard box in the kitchen. (My grandmother raised many a lamb behind her wood kitchen range!)

It is necessary for this lamb to receive colostrum for at least three feedings. If you can force the ewe to let it nurse this first milk or milk it from her, fine. Otherwise, try to find a neighbor with a goat that has just freshened, and use that colostrum. Lacking that, there are dry colostrum products on the market. Ask your veterinarian, or look in your farm veterinary supply catalog. It is smart to have a product like this on hand before lambing time, just in case. Keeping a few containers of colostrum frozen in the freezer is a good idea, as well. When ewe's milk is not available for feeding after the colostrum stage, goat milk is an ideal substitute. Lacking that, cow milk or a good-quality dry lamb milk replacer will work.

For the first week after birth, feed the lamb at least every four hours around the clock. It will take from 1 to 2 ounces soon after birth. Through the first week, gradually increase the feedings. By the end of the week, you can feed twice a day, giving a 16-ounce bottle at each meal. The lamb should be almost full but still be eager for more milk when the bottle is empty. If the lamb develops scours (diarrhea), cut the amount of milk per feeding in half, and dose with Kaopectate according to label directions. Encourage the lamb to nibble on non-medicated calf pellets and mixed sweet feed as well as grass or good-quality legume hay. When the lamb is eating a good amount of pasture or good-quality hay in addition to 1 pound of mixed sweet feed twice daily, you can wean it from the bottle. (For details on feeding lambs as they get older, see "Creep-Feeding Lambs" on page 153.)

Castration

Castrate all ram lambs that you are not keeping for breeding. The meat cuts will gain faster, and the meat will have better flavor. If you plan to castrate surgically, do it while the lambs are young, before fly season arrives. It is often easiest to castrate at the same time as docking to save labor.

Surgical Castration

Have an assistant hold the lamb on his or her lap, with the hind legs drawn up. Wash the scrotum with warm, soapy water, and then dry it. With a single-edged razor, scalpel, or sharp knife, make an incision across the bottom of the scrotum over each testicle. (For help in making a proper cut, see the illustration "Surgical Castration" on page 106.) It helps if you push the testicle toward the bottom so it bulges the scrotum somewhat. Pull out the testicle and tunic (the whitish membrane surrounding the testicle) until the cord breaks. There should be nothing left hanging through the incision. When the testicle is pulled out until the cord snaps, there is very little bleeding. If the cord is too tough to break, as in the case of older lambs, scrape it with a knife until it breaks. This also results in little bleeding as opposed to cutting it right off. If the lamb is large, it's best to cut the cord with an emasculator, which crushes the cord and blood vessels as it cuts, preventing bleeding. Whichever method you use, repeat the process with the second testicle.

It is very wise to give each lamb an injection of tetanus toxoid before or at the time of castration. It is inexpensive insurance against this deadly disease, which is often seen following these procedures.

Clamping, or "Pinching"

Using an emasculatome is a very good alternative to surgical castration. This instrument, often referred to as a Burdizzo (the originating company, and still the best), produces bloodless, quick castration. It simply crushes the blood vessels and the cords so the testicles wither away, with no chance of infection, bleeding, or prolonged pain. Take care to do each testicle individually, and do *not* include the separation between the testicles in the "pinch." (For detailed information on using an emasculatome, see "Clamping, or 'Pinching'"on page 37.)

Using the Elastrator or "Banding"

Banding involves using an inexpensive elastrator, which is used to slip a special, heavy rubber band over the scrotum and testicles. The band is slipped off the holding pegs of the instrument above the testicles, shutting off circulation to the area. After several weeks, the whole scrotum dies, dries up, and falls off. It is quite painless, inexpensive, and easy to learn.

The young lamb is easiest held by an assistant, cradled upside down on their lap. The elastrator is squeezed open and slipped over the testicles. The operator carefully inspects them to ensure that both testicles are outside the elastrator band, with the elastrator being held as close to the body as possible. The band is then rolled off the pegs and the elastrator removed. There is a slight wound around the band site as the scrotum dries, readying to fall away. Therefore, it is a good idea to give the lamb an injection of tetanus toxoid at banding time, just to be safe, as tetanus is always possible with any wound. Do NOT "help" the scrotum fall off by pulling on it or you may cause bleeding and pain.

Docking

All lambs (except long-tailed breeds, such as the Fat Tail) should be docked. Long tails harbor dampness and filth, which can attract flies and encourage maggots. Sheep carrying long tails are not showable, nor do they bring good prices when sold; in addition, the tails can cause breeding difficulties in ewes. It's easiest to dock lambs from one week to one month old. The younger the lamb is, the quicker the procedure is and the less bleeding that will occur. Done quickly and right, there is very little pain, shock, or bloodshed from docking, and it will prevent many problems later on.

While many old-time sheep raisers cut off the tail with an ax, chisel, or knife, the best way is to use an emasculator. This quickly cuts the tail off and also crushes the blood vessels, resulting in a bloodless dock. Try to position the emasculator between the bones in the tail so that they are not crushed. Take the tail off very short, leaving only an inch or so on the lamb—just enough to cover the rectum. Following docking, dip the stump in an antiseptic to prevent infection. An injection of tetanus toxoid before, or at the time of, docking is also recommended. The lamb may also be docked by using an elastrator, as described in castration ("banding"). Be sure to leave enough tail to cover the rectum and position the band between the bones of the tail for easier and better docking.

DISEASES AND OTHER PROBLEMS

Even with excellent care, your sheep flock may eventually have some disease or problem. With knowledge and experience, you'll be able to spot early symptoms of trouble and decide whether to treat the problem yourself or call your veterinarian. It's also important to know the normal temperature of your sheep so you can check for fever or other abnormalities. The normal body temperature of a sheep is 101° to 102°F (38.3° to 38.9°C).

Caseous Lymphadenitis

This is an infection of the lymph glands caused by *Corynebacterium pseudotuberculosis*. Occasionally, visible abscesses form in the lymph glands near the skin, but generally, there are internal abscesses in the intestines, liver, kidneys, or lungs. Caseous lymphadenitis has been called the wasting disease because most affected animals simply become emaciated or waste away. The best way to get an accurate diagnosis is to have your veterinarian culture the external abscesses (if there are any) or do an autopsy.

Sheep may become infected at shearing time if caseous lymphadenitis is common in the area and the shearer does not disinfect the equipment between flocks. A vaccination can help to protect your animals. Also, never buy animals from a flock showing any signs of caseous lymphadenitis.

There is no treatment; so if the disease occurs in your flock, be very aggressive in taking preventive measures to protect your other animals. Isolate obviously affected animals, culling them when possible, and raise lambs apart from older animals. If you notice abscesses, drain them and flush them out with Betadine. (See "Abscesses" on page 114 for treatment details.)

Coccidiosis

Coccidia are protozoa (one-celled parasites) that thrive in crowded conditions, damp bedding, and dirty barn lots. Often attacking lambs, they cause diarrhea, unthriftiness, and stunted growth, and they can

Suggested Vaccination Schedule for Sheep

Here are some guidelines to show which vaccinations you should consider and when to give them. Different problems are common in different areas, though, so check with your veterinarian to work out a specific schedule for your animals.

	DISEASE	WHEN TO VACCINATE
LAMBS	Enterotoxemia (*Clostridium perfringens* Types C and D)	10 to 12 weeks; booster 14 days later
	Tetanus (toxoid)	At or before docking
EWES	Caseous lymphadenitis	Yearly
	Enterotoxemia (*C. perfringens* Types C and D)	Yearly
	Tetanus (toxoid)	Yearly
RAMS	Caseous lymphadenitis	Yearly
	Enterotoxemia (*C. perfringens* Types C and D)	Yearly
	Tetanus (toxoid)	Yearly

eventually kill an animal. Because many cases of coccidiosis go unrecognized, this disease causes many economic losses in the sheep industry.

If you notice any lambs that are not "doing well" (thriving and gaining weight), have your veterinarian examine their manure for coccidiosis. Treatment is often very successful if you catch the infestation early. Sulfas, such as sulfaquinoxaline, give good results. Amprolium has also proved effective.

Prevention is extremely important. Strict cleanliness is essential. Always feed your sheep from feeders, not on the ground in the barn or barn lot, and do not allow lambs to run in feed troughs or mangers. Also, keep the water fresh and free from fecal contamination. Keep all stress at a minimum, especially in lambs. And, where possible, keep all sheep on a clean, dry pasture, not in a feedlot or in the barn lot.

Enterotoxemia

Enterotoxemia, also known as overeating disease, is caused by *Clostridium perfringens* Type D, which is related to the organism that causes tetanus. It is most common in show or feedlot lambs being grained heavily for fast weight gain. It often strikes the biggest lambs first and is occasionally seen in adults. Affected animals show signs such as circling, pushing their heads against a wall, convulsions, and unsteadiness. They often die suddenly. As with tetanus, there is no successful treatment for enterotoxemia. But you can protect your animals with routine vaccinations, especially for lambs from weaning to eight months of age and ewes four to six weeks before lambing.

Related to the organism causing enterotoxemia are *C. chauvoei*, which causes blackleg in sheep, and *C. novyi*, which causes bighead, a swelling of the head, usually in rams. (For more information on blackleg, see "Blackleg" on page 44.) Bighead gets started when rams play hard and fight, causing bruising and injury—perfect conditions for *Clostridium* organisms to multiply in. Neither of these diseases is very common in sheep, but they *are* found in certain locales, and the spores live a long time in the soil. Ask your veterinarian if these diseases are a problem in your area. He may recommend using a combination vaccination for enterotoxemia that contains protection for blackleg and bighead, as well.

Eversion of the Uterus

An eversion occurs when the uterus is turned inside out as it is pushed out of the body by contractions during or soon after lambing. The visible uterus is a heavy, oval-shaped, reddish mass. It is studded with knobs that look like fleshy sponges. (These knobs, technically known as caruncles, serve to hold the placenta to the wall of the uterus during pregnancy.) The uterus must be replaced very soon, or the shock will kill the ewe. This situation is definitely an emergency.

When you discover a ewe with an everted uterus, slowly move her into a small pen where she will be alone. Many ewes are lost when other sheep walk over their ejected uteri. An everted uterus is fragile, and if it is torn or punctured, the ewe will very likely die. After you get her penned, call your veterinarian immediately. Keep the uterus clean and covered with a warm, moist towel while you wait. Gather several clean towels, a bale of hay or straw to rest the uterus on during replacement, and a pail of hot water.

When your veterinarian arrives, he may use a hormone injection to help shrink the uterus to near normal size. This makes it a bit easier to replace the uterus, as it is fragile, heavy, and awkward. This injection will also help after the uterus is in place, preventing the ewe from feeling something she must push on. Lacing the lips of the vulva can help keep the uterus in place, but the ewe can still push it back out if she strains too hard. It helps greatly to elevate her hindquarters by standing her on a piece of plywood that's propped up in back with hay or a few bricks. This takes pressure off her uterus and makes it easier for her to keep it in. Watch her for several hours. If you see her straining, call your veterinarian right away. He may need to give her a spinal block to stop the straining.

After a ewe experiences an everted uterus, do not plan on keeping her or her lambs for breeding. This can be an inherited weakness and will often be repeated yearly until death results.

Flies

Sheep are more often bothered with maggots than are other farm animals. This is because the dense wool covering their bodies makes a good hiding place, especially if the sheep has had diarrhea or a cut, which provides moisture and attracts the flies. Flies lay their eggs in the cuts or damp, foul wool that's been soiled by diarrhea or blood. Fly eggs are seen as tiny yellowish white specks. There can be hundreds in a small area. Soon—sometimes in just a day—these eggs hatch into small maggots. These maggots not only clean up any foul matter, but they go on, eating the living, healthy flesh.

This problem is the main reason why lambs' tails are docked. The tails are heavy and hang below the rectum, gathering any moist fecal material and holding the moisture. Of course, not all undocked sheep get maggots; but once you've seen an otherwise healthy sheep with its whole hind end seething with maggots, you'll be a believer in docking. (For details on this procedure, see "Docking" on page 163.)

If a sheep shows dark wool around the hindquarters, catch it and find out why. If the fleece is soiled badly with filth, wash it thoroughly and keep the sheep in until it is fully dried, or at least shear off the soiled portion of the fleece, exposing the skin to fresh air. It's better to lose part of the fleece than the whole sheep! If diarrhea is the problem, treat it, as well. Treat any cuts at once with a fly repellent-antiseptic, such as scarlet oil.

Foot Rot

Two types of foot rot are common in sheep. Benign, or common, foot rot, often found when sheep are pastured in damp or rough areas, causes small chapped areas in the space between the toes. Virulent foot rot is more dangerous and is very contagious. It seems to start out like common foot rot, but if two particular bacteria are present, it becomes very "hot" and does more damage to affected animals. It also spreads quickly and is much harder to treat effectively.

Symptoms of both types of foot rot are alike in the beginning stages. Affected sheep will become lame on one or more feet. They may not want to move about or even rise. There is often a foul odor in the feet and dead tissue between the toes. In advanced cases the horn of the toes may separate from the foot.

When you notice these symptoms, move the sheep to cleaner, drier, less rough pasture. Remove the dead material by scraping with a pocketknife, trim the foot, and treat the feet with a 5 percent formalin solution. If only a few sheep are affected, bring them in, soak their feet in warm water containing dish detergent, rinse, and then treat with a drying antiseptic-astringent.

If the condition is simple foot rot, it should improve in three to four days. If it doesn't, call your veterinarian to make sure you are not dealing with virulent foot rot. If that *is* the problem, he will suggest treatment and preventive measures. These often include isolating all affected animals, treatment with injectable antibiotics, and soaking in foot baths with antibiotic solutions.

Needless to say, prevention is the key to both types of foot rot. Pasturing your flock in damp or rough areas is asking for trouble. When you bring new animals into your flock, isolate them for at least a month; then examine their feet to make sure no problems are present before you let them run with the other animals. In areas where foot rot is common, you may vaccinate routinely; ask your veterinarian for his opinion.

Ketosis

Ketosis is a condition that arises when ewes don't receive adequate carbohydrates in the latter stages of pregnancy. Groups of ewes receiving only mixed grass hay and little or no grain can experience 75 percent ketosis, while increasing the grain and providing legume hay can reduce the incidence to less than 5 percent.

Ewes should not be overweight at breeding, but gaining. To keep your ewes gaining, gradually increase their grain as needed as the pregnancy goes on. Regular feeding is critical. Missing feedings due to moving, having poor help, or penning without feed overnight often throws ewes into ketosis.

The first symptoms are facial twitching, acting "dopey," circling, loss of balance, pushing up against a wall, or any other sort of unusual behavior during the last few weeks of pregnancy. Later, the animal goes down and cannot rise; she lapses into a coma and dies. Once an animal goes down, treatment is seldom successful.

Ketosis treatment is usually effective when you catch the problem before symptoms are evident. To check for possible ketosis, slowly drive the flock daily for a short distance, and watch carefully for any ewes that are acting abnormally. Cut any "slow" ewes from the flock, and pen them where you can give them special attention. Providing extra grain mixed with molasses, and even special treats—such as chopped carrots, turnips, stale bread, or greens, fed several times daily—can often relieve the symptoms.

If this special care does not relieve a ewe, it is best to call your veterinarian. Treatment with oral propylene glycol and fluid therapy often works wonders. When the ewe does not respond and is at the end of her pregnancy, a cesarean or induced labor will often save her life.

To help prevent ketosis, check your ewe flock for weight as they approach the eight-week period before lambing. Feel their backs and sides, under the fleece. Some ewes appear fat with a heavy fleece and a load of lambs but are, in reality, quite thin. They need adequate grain before lambing to prevent ketosis. Remember, cold weather makes the ewes eat more, and they may need the extra grain to keep warm; there may not be enough carbohydrates left over to nourish the ewe and her lambs. However, do not make the mistake of giving ewes access to free-choice grain with the idea that more is better. This practice often causes laminitis, or founder.

Leptospirosis

Leptospirosis is a contagious bacterial disease in sheep as well as in many other animals, including humans. It usually spreads through contact with streams, ponds, or surface water contaminated with the feces or urine of affected animals.

Symptoms include fever, weakness, anemia, and abortion. The urine may contain blood, turning it a red or wine color. If you suspect leptospirosis in your flock, call your veterinarian at once. With prompt testing and treatment, you can usually stop this disease. Treatment commonly includes antibiotics, blood transfusions for anemic animals, and good nursing. It's highly recommended that you isolate affected animals to protect the rest of your herd. You'll also want to vaccinate the animals that are not showing signs of the disease.

Prevention includes routine vaccinations as well as fencing to keep animals away from contaminated ponds and streams. Keep sheep feed free of rodent contamination. Buy replacement animals from flocks that are vaccinated yearly and that have had no cases of leptospirosis.

Lice

Lice are small, grayish, soft-bodied parasites that attack sheep, most often during the winter. Infested animals will rub and scratch, often damaging the fleece. Lice can become so numerous that they can actually bleed a sheep to death, even before you really notice there is a problem. Less dramatically, lice cause anemia, unthriftiness, loss of fleece, and wasted feed as the sheep must eat for itself and the lice.

It is generally best to routinely powder or dip your flock *before* you notice lice trouble. Many sheep raisers dip their flocks following shearing to head off problems with lice that may occur later in the year, when the fleece is heavier. A rotenone or pyrethrin powder is safe and effective. It is best to powder once a week for three weeks in the early winter and then again in January or February before lambing.

If you notice lice becoming a problem in your flock, you may choose to use a more strenuous control, such as a pour-on or an injectable product. Ask your veterinarian for his recommendations for a control program. Follow his directions, and read all labels carefully.

Mange

The most common type of mange in sheep is chorioptic mange. It is caused by tiny mites that burrow into the skin, usually on the hind legs or near the feet. Another possible problem is itch mite infestation, which causes the affected sheep to bite and rub (and thereby damage) their fleece. Sheep scabies, formerly a very damaging type of mange, has not been reported in the United States since 1970, but it is still found in many other countries.

Treatment consists of dipping in a 1 percent lime-sulfur solution or injecting ivermectin. If you suspect mange, contact your veterinarian at once for diagnosis and correct treatment. Mange can be a real headache to deal with, but you can eradicate it with aggressive treatment.

Pneumonia

Pneumonia claims many sheep yearly and causes economic loss in those that survive. After a bout of pneumonia, large amounts of scar tissue can form in the lungs, and the animal must fight for oxygen. It loses weight and can seldom stand a

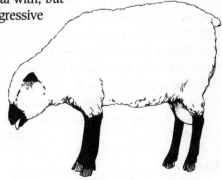

Sheep with pneumonia. *A sheep with pneumonia will show signs of dejection and puffing for breath. If the animal is running a fever, you'll need to start treatment immediately.*

pregnancy or the added strain of raising lambs. Even less severely affected animals are still stressed and are more prone to internal parasites, metabolic diseases (such as ketosis), and other bacterial infections.

Several bacteria and viruses can cause pneumonia in sheep. The most frequent kind is bacterial pneumonia, brought on by a period of stress.This stress can be anything from changes in the weather to being chased by dogs.

A sick sheep will stand, usually puffing a bit. It may stop eating or just act a little slow. Take the animal's temperature right away. A sheep with pneumonia generally runs a temperature of 103° to 107°F (39.4° to 41.7°C). If the sick sheep was with the flock, take the temperatures of several others. Often other sheep will not exactly look sick, but they can be on their way, with temperatures of 103° to 104.5°F (39.4° to 40.3°C) or so. It is critical to start treating all sick sheep immediately. Sheep have the least stamina—some call it "will to live"—of any animal on the farm. Once down and sick, many seem to refuse to live.

Isolate all sick sheep to reduce the chances of pneumonia spreading in your flock. Others may be coming down with it, which means they are incubating the disease without showing symptoms yet. So watch the rest of the flock even after you've removed all the sick ones.

When this disease strikes, call your veterinarian for advice, as there are many factors to consider when treating pneumonia. Antibiotic therapy, for instance, will not check a viral pneumonia. An injectable expectorant may help in some cases to break up the consolidation in the lungs. Cortisone sometimes helps, but in other cases it may cause harm. Often, steaming (allowing the animal to breathe the vapor from a bucket of boiling water) or light exercise and sunshine will help. Your veterinarian will know if a bacterial pneumonia is "going around" and what antibiotic has been effective in treatment.

Anything you can feed to keep a sick sheep eating will help. Try offering very small amounts of chopped carrots, chopped apples, soda crackers, stale bread, lettuce, rolled oats with molasses, or other goodies.

Prevention is very important. When you bring home animals, isolate them for at least two weeks. This includes any sheep that have been to shows, fairs, or away for breeding, as well as newly acquired animals. Provide your animals with dry, well-ventilated quarters that are free of drafts. Preventing stress at all times will also help prevent pneumonia. Keep feed changes gradual. Don't let the flock out on days that there is icy wind or freezing rain, and make sure you provide adequate shade in the summer. Keep stray dogs from harassing your sheep, and always handle the animals calmly and gently.

Retained Placenta

After each lamb is born, the placenta, or afterbirth, should follow. Occasionally one of the placentas does not come away from the uterus. This condition is usually quite obvious, with the placenta hanging a foot or more out of the vulva. Once in a while, a part rips off, and the rest remains in the uterus, hidden from sight. This is the most significant reason for observing the afterbirths at lambing time.

It is important to differentiate between a retained placenta and an eversion of the uterus. The placenta is a clear or nearly silver membrane, long and stringy; an everted uterus is a heavy, reddish mass. A retained placenta is something you'll want to keep an eye on; an eversion of the uterus is a definite emergency. (For more information on the latter, see "Eversion of the Uterus" on page 166.)

If a ewe retains her placenta for more than 12 hours, call your veterinarian. The placenta must come away from the uterus to prevent infection. (If the uterus holds pieces of the placenta and the cervix closes tightly, the discharge is trapped and quickly becomes infected.) When the placenta does not come away by itself, your veterinarian can either remove it manually or give an injection of hormones to encourage it to come away, while also placing boluses in the uterus to help dissolve bits and pieces and prevent infection.

Scours

Scours (diarrhea) is most common in lambs that are one to three weeks old. Several bacteria can cause scours, as can viruses or just plain overeating. Milk is irritating to the intestines, and if a lamb eats too much at once, the irritation may bring on scours. This most often happens when lambs are bottle-fed with dry milk replacer. Normally, a lamb nursing on the mother takes only a few sucks at a time, all day long. But on the bottle, it gets more milk, fed only two or three times a day, which causes overloading. (If you must bottle-feed and ewe's milk is not available, be sure to use the best substitute for ewe's milk obtainable: goat milk, cow milk, or very good milk replacer. For more details on proper feeding, see "Caring for Lambs" on page 161.)

Always keep watch for any lambs with wet or sticky tails or backsides. If you spot the scouring early, reducing the milk intake and providing a few doses of Kaopectate will usually remedy the problem. (Be sure to give water in place of the milk, or the lamb may dehydrate.) A small- to medium-sized lamb can take 2 to 4 tablespoons of Kaopectate every 4 hours. If the stool is not firmer after 12 hours of treatment, consult your veterinarian. Sometimes you'll need to give antibiotics, as well, and you may have to replace the milk with oral electrolytes until the scours has cleared up. A lamb cannot have severe diarrhea for much longer than two days without being in serious trouble.

Diarrhea in older lambs and adults can come from overeating grain or lush pasture, eating slightly toxic plants, or overeating salt-mineral mixes. But it can also be a symptom of coccidiosis, worms, enterotoxemia, and other problems. A general rule to follow is to bring the affected sheep into a dry lot, clean off the wool to prevent fly problems, and treat the animal for a day with a simple astringent antidiarrheal, such as copper sulfate, iron sulfate, or catechu (kaopectate). This will remedy simple diarrhea. If the diarrhea persists, take a stool sample (a tablespoonful or so) to your veterinarian. He can examine it for internal parasites and advise the correct treatment.

Soremouth

Soremouth is a very contagious disease. It is caused by a virus that is transmissible to humans. It can be brought to a farm by sheepshearers or new sheep. There are plenty of signs when a flock is infected. The lips swell and scab. The scabs may extend into the mouth, and there may be scabs on the feet, between the toes, and on the nose.

Once it has broken out, no treatment is effective. Feeding moist, easily mouthed foods and even drenching with gruel may be necessary to keep the animals' strength up until the virus runs its course. If the lesions are severe and numerous, antibiotics can help prevent secondary infections. When handling a sheep with soremouth, take routine sanitary precautions, such as wearing gloves when working with the animal and washing your hands afterward.

Fortunately, vaccination will prevent soremouth in areas where it is common. Vaccinate all new sheep, and isolate them for two to three weeks before turning them out with the flock. It is a good idea to isolate any sheep that have been away for showing or breeding, even if they've been vaccinated, as they could carry the virus in on their bodies.

Tetanus

Tetanus, or lockjaw, is caused by *Clostridium tetani.* This organism lives in the soil in many areas, gaining entrance to the body through punctures or other deep wounds that are not exposed to the air. It is quite common in sheep following docking and castration, especially after using an elastrator (the rubber band method). For information about symptoms, treatment, and prevention, see "Tetanus" on page 144.

Ticks

Ticks can be a problem in many geographical areas. Usually they cause trouble only as a parasite, sucking the animals' blood; but in some localities they can spread disease. And as deer ticks can transmit Lyme disease to people, it's even more important to control ticks on your sheep.

Ask your veterinarian about the ticks in your part of the country. In areas with severe tick infestations, you may need to dip your sheep several times a year. Where ticks are a minor problem, a single dip after shearing may be enough. More recent control methods involve the use of systemic pour-on insecticides and vaccination. Your veterinarian can recommend the best approach for your situation.

White Muscle Disease

White muscle disease is not a true "disease" but instead is caused by a selenium deficiency, often due to a lack of selenium in the soil. It is most common in lambs, sometimes occurring soon after birth. Symptoms include stiffness (usually starting first with the hind legs), an arched back, an inability to nurse, an inability to rise, diarrhea, and sudden death.

Treatment is often successful if you catch the problem in the early stages. While it is a good idea to have your veterinarian out to correctly diagnose and suggest treatment for any suspected problem, the symptoms of white muscle disease are frequently very clear. Injections of selenium and vitamin E can bring about a quick recovery, and they won't hurt anything if your diagnosis was incorrect.

To prevent white muscle disease, give ewes an injection of selenium a week or so before lambing to protect newborn lambs. Then give lambs an injection of selenium at about three weeks of age; repeat the injections at monthly intervals until the lambs are weaned and eating from a salt-and-mineral lick. Sometimes it also helps to provide selenium and vitamin E in a mineral mixture. Ask your veterinarian about the incidence of white muscle disease in your area, and see what supplements he recommends, if any. (Some areas have an overabundance of selenium, and providing a supplement can cause toxic reactions.)

Worms

Here we approach the biggest problem in sheep. Many different kinds of parasites affect sheep, and some are hard to get rid of completely. Some of the most common internal parasites include bankrupt worm, brown stomach worm, common liver fluke, common stomach worm, common tapeworm, hair lungworm, nodular worm, thread lungworm, and thread-necked worm. For information on coccidia, another common parasite, see "Coccidiosis" on page 164.

A sheep gets parasites, or is reinfested with them, by grazing on and swallowing grass on which there are eggs or cysts, small larvae, or snails (which carry some parasites). This is why pasture rotation is so important for sheep. They tend to graze closely, thus picking up more parasites. If the pasture is good, the grass is long, and the sheep don't feed on it for long periods, there's much less of a chance of contamination. After moving your sheep off a pasture, mow and harrow it to break up the manure. This will expose the manure to the sun and naturally help kill parasite eggs.

Even if you worm your sheep routinely, they can still be less than worm-free under normal farm or range conditions, and thus reinfestation is always possible. No wormer gets all internal parasites; in fact, some folks inadvertently kill a lot of sheep when they mistakenly assume that since they worm every two months, their trouble can't be internal parasites.

Worms and other internal parasites make trouble by causing anemia and unthriftiness, destroying organs, making the animal prone to disease, and sometimes causing death. Lambs are infected by worms through the bloodstream and may die soon after birth.

Worm Control

There is no one worm medicine that is effective against all parasites. Therefore, it is best to take a fecal sample to your veterinarian and ask his opinion if you suspect worms or other internal parasites. This way, you know what worms your sheep have before treating them, so you can use the most effective wormer available for that particular worm and the most effective worming schedule to rid your flock of it. This will save your sheep and save you much money and time in the long run.

Putting a phenothiazine-trace mineral-salt mix (10 pounds phenothiazine to 100 pounds of salt) in the pasture after lambing will greatly help to reduce worm problems, but bear in mind that it does not kill all worms. You should still have your veterinarian check your sheep and worm them with a broad-spectrum wormer, as needed, in the early summer and late fall. If a real worm problem is evident, using ivermectin will often bring about relief. Remember that many worms have developed resistance to certain routinely used wormers, so it is wise to rotate wormers, as needed. Follow your veterinarian's recommendations, as he is familiar with the types of sheep parasites commonly found in your area.

Liver Fluke

This parasite is a deadly one, infesting the liver. Sheep can pick up flukes from infected deer and snails. Much liver fluke damage is seen in sheep grazing on marshy or swampy ground. The liver fluke destroys the liver of the affected animal, often before you see any symptom of trouble.

Treatment is now quite successful, with several new drugs available. Contact your veterinarian if you suspect liver fluke. Often diagnosis is successful only on autopsy, although sometimes the eggs are visible in the manure.

Prevention consists of keeping animals off swampy pasture and away from deer—if deer are known hosts in your area. It may be necessary to routinely use a drug proven to kill flukes in sheep; follow your veterinarian's recommendations.

Horses

General Care and Management

$\mathcal{K}$nowledgeable care and management are very important in keeping your horses bright, healthy, and performing well. With good husbandry practices, there is seldom much need for veterinary expenses other than for minor, routine work.

Housing

Healthy horses are sturdy animals, and more are over-housed—kept in all winter and even during the summer—than underhoused. Horses need shelter from cold, driving rain, and heavy snow. But they also need exercise and sunshine.

Box Stalls

A box stall is the best kind of stall for a horse. It should be 12 feet square or larger. This will allow the animal to move around freely and lie flat if it wants to. Bedding can be straw, wood shavings, old (but not moldy) hay, or moss. (Dried moss, available in some areas, is great for bedding and makes the manure dandy compost for your garden!) Bank the bedding deeper toward the sides as horses can get cast, or stuck, if they roll into a low spot by the stall wall. The bedding should be 4 inches deep over a gravel or clay floor, 6 inches deep over wood, and 8 inches deep over cement.

The very best arrangement is a box stall with a door outside to the pasture. Even in the winter, horses will run, play, and wander about, enjoying the nippy weather. If free outdoor access is not possible, a box stall in a barn is fine, provided the horse can be turned out every morning that the weather is fit.

Tie, or Standing, Stalls

If you can't provide box stalls, you can keep your horses in tie, or standing, stalls. These stalls are 5 feet wide × 8 to 10 feet long, with a place to tie the horse to a manger that's supplied with hay and a box for grain. Tie stalls demand more work on your part than box stalls. You'll need to exercise the horse daily, regardless of the weather. You *must* also clean and bed tie stalls daily. (With a box stall, you can cheat if you're in a hurry one day: Just remove the wettest bedding, throw in a little more dry bedding, and then clean the stall thoroughly the next day.) Another disadvantage of tie stalls is that horses can more easily become cast when they lie down since the sides are closer.

PARTS OF A HORSE

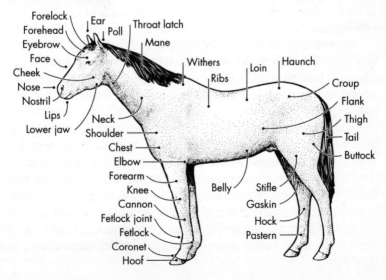

If you must rely on tie stalls, construct the sides and manger with 2 × 6 lumber—preferably hardwood. Make the sides solid, or at least with spaces less than 2 inches wide, and build them high enough to reach higher than the horse's side, nearly to the back. The section where you tie the horse should be hardwood, or at least reinforced, and *very* solidly built. It is also a good idea to make a higher divider toward the front of adjoining tie stalls. This higher section can be solid or built of bars to allow free air movement and the horses to see each other. Make the divider higher than the horse can reach when tied. This prevents fighting between adjoining tied horses, especially at feeding time. It also keeps one horse from stealing another's hay.

To tie a horse securely, use a ¾-inch nylon rope that's 2 to 3 feet long with a heavy bull snap. Using a longer rope is asking for trouble as the horse will usually get a front leg over the rope and struggle violently. Leave the rope tied in the stall at all times, and use a separate lead shank to lead the horse outside and bring it in.

It is a good idea to place a heel chain across the back of the tie stall. Use a piece of hay rope with a very heavy snap, or a heavy chain and snap, strung across the open end of the stall, just below the buttocks of the horse. This will prevent the horse from backing into the aisle or keep another loose horse from crowding in with it, causing injury.

Fencing

Most horses are fairly easy to fence in. There is no 100 percent safe fence for horses, but any tight, strong, well-built fence is usually quite adequate and safe for the average horse. The more tightly horses are confined, the stronger and safer the fence needs to be. A pole, pipe, or board fence is excellent for a paddock, a corral, or an exercise ring, but it is often expensive to use around the whole pasture. A stone fence or wall is ideal, but it requires experience, hard work, and, of course, lots of stones. The most practical fence is woven wire. It is safe, fairly easy to put up, economical, and long-lasting. Woven wire fence needs good solid corners and line posts, and you may have to top it with a board or strand of barbed or electric wire to keep the horses from leaning over it. You'll also need to tighten the fence yearly to prevent sags in which horses can catch their feet.

Tight barbed wire is cheaper than woven wire and just as safe, in most instances, when used in a pasture. It has gotten a bad name because many horses have been badly injured by it. But I've had large pastures fenced with barbed wire for years and have never had a cut animal. Four strands of tight barbed wire are a minimum for safety, and five are better. This keeps the horses from reaching through the fence, preventing cuts. Do not use cheaper light-gauge barbed wire to save money. Insist on "Made in the U.S.A." wire because foreign wire often sags after a period of time and loose barbed wire is a menace. Many horses are injured badly by getting tangled up in barbed wire that is half-buried in the grass. They panic and pull, tearing gashes all over their bodies. Also, do not use barbed wire in a stallion's paddock or in a colt pasture. Colts and fillies are nervous, playful, and nosy. They may hit the fence in their play or while frightened and become injured.

Electric fencing also works well for horses. Like anything else, the more money you spend, the better a fence you can build. There are excellent, albeit more expensive, electric fences with coated wire and fiberglass posts that look solid, last, and are safe as well. More often an electric fence is built for economy, using lightweight posts and few wires. Use this type of fence only as something temporary until you can build a better fence. A single strand, hung just above the knee level of the horse, will often work, but three strands are better. With this type of electric fence, you can count on loose horses from time to time because of shorts in the fence, breaks (sometimes caused by wild animals, such as deer), or an excited horse just forgetting the fence and running through it. Keep this in mind if your farm is on a well-traveled road. Not only can a horse be killed on the road, but the people owning the car can sue you.

Temporary electric fences can also cause fires. Once, one of my horses or a wild animal broke down a section of electric fence in my back pasture, half a mile from the house. It was during the summer, and the grass was dry. When I checked the horses the next day, there was a black, fire-burned area 50 feet long, with the fence still sparking. I shudder to think of what might have happened had there been any wind. An electric wire strung on top of a barbed wire, wood, or woven wire fence is safer all around. The fire hazard is much less, and if a short does occur, the other fence will hold the animals in.

First Aid Kit for Horses

Here are some suggestions for a basic equine first aid kit. The ones marked with an asterisk belong in every barn with a horse. The other items are not critical, but it's helpful to have them on hand in case you need them. Ask your veterinarian for his recommendations for your particular area and situation.

Balling gun
Bot block/knife*
Breeding hobbles
Clippers
Dental float
Fly repellent*
Forceps/needle
   holder
4-inch gauze*
Hoof dressing*
Hoof packing
Hoof pick*
Leg wraps

Liniment
Rectal veterinary
   thermometer*
Roll of cotton
Scarlet oil*
Sheath cleaner
Sturdy halter*
Three 18-gauge, 1/2-inch
   needles*
Tie rope and bull snap*
12-cc syringe*
Twitch*
Veterinarian's phone
   number*

Feeding

Feed your horses according to the amount of stress they are subjected to. This stress can range from standing in a sunny pasture (zero stress) to racing or showing regularly, which involves considerable stress from hard work, transportation, change in water, excitement, and other factors.

Pasture

A horse that is idle, or very near so, does very well on just pasture during the spring, summer, and fall—provided that the pasture is adequate. In some areas 2 acres of land is adequate; in other areas 100 acres may not be enough to provide sufficient grazing. The horse should never eat its pasture right to the ground, leaving only large, unpalatable weeds. If your grazing area is limited, divide it into two pastures, and rotate your horse between them. After you take the horse off one pasture, mow the area to remove any weeds or coarse grass, and harrow it to scatter the manure. This will prevent weeds from taking over the pasture grass, and it also helps kill any parasite eggs in the manure by exposing them to sunlight and air.

Hay and Grain

In some locales horses can survive on pasture all year. But as most grass is low in nutrients in the winter, it is often necessary to supplement with grain or good-quality hay. When heavy frost, ice, or snow covers the winter grass, provide good-quality, clean, mixed hay. Feed the hay free-choice (as much hay as the horse will eat) or just twice daily if the animal tends to gain too much weight on free-choice.

I generally don't recommend pelleted complete feed, even though it is nutritionally sound, because a horse will eat its pellets quickly and then become bored. A horse is naturally adapted to continual grazing, and that lack of activity leads to many bad habits. Boredom causes cribbing, pawing, stall walking, weaving, and other bad behaviors that are often nearly impossible to cure once they start.

The growing colt or filly, the mare heavy in foal, and the stallion at service should receive grain daily, even if on good pasture. Generally speaking, a horse doing light work daily can use about 6 pounds of mixed grain per day. This amount is also good for growing colts, mares in foal, and stallions at medium service. A horse worked fairly hard every day, such as in pleasure training or showing, a mare heavy in foal, and a stallion at heavy service can use 10 pounds daily. A horse at hard work, such as racing, rodeo, ranch work, hunting, or contesting, can use up to 16 pounds or more daily, depending on the horse's conformation and disposition. A close-coupled horse of stocky build will need less feed to stay in good shape than a tall, long-backed horse. And a "hot" horse that worries and gets worked up easily will use more grain than a calm horse.

While most horses needing grain do well on a basic corn-oats mixture, old, sick, or thin horses benefit from a more palatable and more fattening ration, such as steamed, rolled, or crimped grains with molasses added. You can provide additional fat by adding corn oil to the grain. (Add it slowly at first as it can cause diarrhea. If you notice this problem, cut back a bit on the oil.) You can also feed pelleted hay to provide nutrition with less chewing effort. Start pellets slowly, too, to avoid colic and other digestive upsets. Old horses or horses with mouth injuries do well on ground hay or pellets that are soaked in hot water until they become soft.

Salt and Water

A salt block containing trace minerals should be available at all times, as should fresh, clean water. Although many horses survive on eating just snow during the winter, they will stay in better shape and have fewer digestive upsets if they have access to water. Some horses do not eat enough snow to furnish their bodies with adequate water, and they become dehydrated. A big pailful of snow melts down to very little water, and a horse uses a lot of calories to melt that snow. Eating snow or ice can also cause severe colic in horses.

Do not allow a hot, sweating horse to drink until you've walked it gently or let it graze awhile to cool down. A hot horse that gulps water will often get colic or founder, possibly even dying as a result. For that reason, it is best to keep the last part of your ride slow and gentle so the horse will cool off before returning to the barn.

Exercise

A horse needs daily exercise. This could be walking about in the pasture, playing in a paddock for a few hours, or actively working. If you plan to work your horse hard, you need to build it up gradually. A great many horses are ruined daily from too much strain and exertion when out of condition. True, a horse can run for a couple of miles; but when a horse is soft (not conditioned by daily training), it's dangerous to jump on its back and tear off at a gallop. It's a sure way to kill or seriously disable your horse. Heaves, founder, lameness, and broken bones in the feet are only a few of the ills brought on by violent weekend exercise. Let the movie cowboys tear around: They aren't riding your horse! (Those movie horses really weren't running for miles—only a few feet per "shoot"—or those horses sure wouldn't have lasted long!)

Even the stallion and brood mare, heavy in foal, need daily exercise. If you can't turn them out every day, work them (if they are broken to ride or drive), or exercise them on a long line. You can also lead the mare alongside another quiet horse.

A horse in good shape will feel hard. The ribs should be just barely visible as the horse moves, and the backbone and hips should be well covered and rounded. The horse should not be fully rounded with soft fat, like a beef steer. Excess fat leads to health problems in horses, just as it does in humans. A horse in top condition for working or breeding is seldom plump, any more than a top human athlete would be. Fat mares have breeding and foaling trouble, and fat stallions are often unwilling to breed or are less fertile than lean, well-conditioned stallions.

Restraint

Because of the horse's well-developed nervous system and power, you need a little more knowledge to properly restrain one than you do for most other livestock. If not properly restrained, an agitated horse can break loose and injure people or itself.

When moving a horse from place to place, *always* use a lead shank, even with a gentle horse. If the horse shies while you are just holding the halter, you can dislocate your fingers or a shoulder. No horse lives that can't be scared by something, and the lead shank provides some "give."

Tying Safely

Tying a horse safely is an art in itself. Many gentle, well-trained horses can be tied with a light rope and halter. But if you have a fractious horse or if you need to keep the horse relatively still, you'll have to take stronger measures. First, use a sturdy halter. Few halters made today will hold a horse set on breaking loose. One exception is a triple-thickness, flat nylon halter with good-quality rings; this generally will hold. Lacking this, you can make do with an ordinary halter if you use it with a neck rope. This is a strong rope with a loop that has a heavy ring tied

Tying a horse safely. A neck rope, used in conjunction with a halter, will hold just about any horse. Tie the rope to a post, run the snap through the halter and around the neck, and then fasten the snap to the ring.

in it about 2 feet up from the heavy bull snap. Tie the rope to a post, run the snap through the halter and around the neck, and then fasten the snap to the ring. This way, the horse can pull back without breaking the halter or choking.

The tie rope should be long enough to allow the horse to touch its knees with its muzzle, but no longer. Longer ropes invite injuries as somehow the horse gets a foot over the rope and then panics, thrashing around. Fasten the rope to something solid at eye height when the horse is standing relaxed. Tying higher or much lower may result in neck injuries if the animal should pull back hard. Always tie a horse so you can release it right away if need be. Keep in mind that a tight rope in trouble makes a regular knot harder to release. A jerk knot or safety knot works best because you won't need slack to release the horse quickly in an emergency situation.

Cross Ties

Cross ties are highly overrated in restraining horses for treatment. Cross ties—one rope extending from each side of an aisle and clipped to the side rings of the halter—are great for grooming, saddling, or harnessing because they prevent the horse from wandering back and forth. But they are dangerous when worming or giving injections or other treatment to uncooperative horses. In the first place, the ropes or chains are usually too light to hold a fractious horse. In the second place, the horse can back against the ties or leap forward, hitting people or striking out with its front feet.

Twitch

The twitch is a device that is slipped over the fleshy part of the horse's nose and tightened. It does not hurt the horse but confuses it, so the animal keeps its mind on the twitch, not the treatment. There are two kinds of twitches. One is a hardwood handle about 18 inches long, with a chain loop on one end. This loop is slipped over the horse's upper lip and twisted until quite tight. While you treat the horse, you'll need an assistant to hold the twitch tight. If you need to distract the horse further, shake the twitch lightly. Slightly less effective is the one-person twitch, which is more like a clamp made of lightweight aluminum. Put it over the horse's nose and upper lip, clamp it tightly, wind the attached nylon string tightly around the handles, and clip the string to the halter. This type of twitch allows you to treat the horse without an assistant.

When using the chain twitch, be sure you have a dependable helper who will hang on to the handle, regardless of any movement the horse may make. I've been hit in the head too many times because someone became frightened and let go, allowing the twitch to become a flying missile.

Rope in the Mouth

Here you simply take a lariat and place the noose behind the ears and through the mouth. Wind the rope tightly—don't overdo it—until the whole rope, or a greater part of it, is in the mouth, cramming it open. This acts like a twitch, but in most instances you can restrain and treat the horse by yourself. There is no pain with this method, only confusion.

Chain over the Nose

A chain shank—a lead shank with a section of chain before the snap—can be useful to control a pushy or difficult horse. Used correctly, it will keep all but the rankest horse under control, with its front feet on the ground. Yank the chain gently or quite hard, depending on the horse, to bring sharp pressure on the bridge of the nose. Just pulling on the lead shank is of no use and may cut the skin. *Never tie a horse with a chain over its nose.* Many horses are severely injured by this; and when in severe pain, the horse will strike and yank back, breaking free. Some handlers run the chain under the chin instead, but I don't like this method as it will often cause or encourage the horse to rear.

Hobbles

There are three uses of hobbles: to keep a horse from moving off while grazing, to prevent kicking or striking during restraint, and to attach ropes for "throwing" the horse.

Simple hobbles prevent the horse from wandering while grazing or, in some cases, from moving around while you are working on it. They fit around the front pasterns. Most are made of heavy leather or nylon arranged in a figure eight or are two separate hobbles connected by a strong, short piece of chain. If your horse has never been hobbled before, get someone with experience to work with it the first time;

some horses become panic-stricken when they are pulled up short by the hobbles, and they thrash around.

Other kinds of hobbles, including front leg hobbles, breeding hobbles, and Scotch hobbles, are designed specifically for restraining a horse for treatment to prevent kicking or striking. If you need additional restraint, you can use a twitch in conjunction with any of these.

A front leg hobble is simply a rope or strap placed around the doubled-up front leg, just above the knee. This makes minor operations, like cleaning a cut or clipping a flap of loose skin from a wound, easier.

Breeding hobbles can be purchased or made from a ¾-inch nylon rope. The ropes, or hobbles, keep a horse from kicking back; but remember that the horse can still cow-kick (kick forward with the hind feet). Breeding hobbles are used for rectal or vaginal examinations, artificial insemination, surgery on the tail, and service by the stallion.

A Scotch hobble is designed to keep one hind leg up so the horse is relatively immobile. This makes it easier and, in many cases, safer

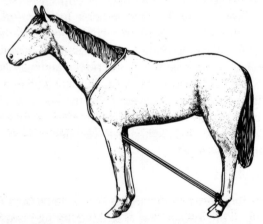

Breeding hobbles. *Commercial or homemade breeding hobbles will prevent a mare from kicking back during breeding, artificial insemination, and rectal or vaginal examinations.*

to work on the horse. Using a soft, strong rope, begin rubbing the hindquarters; then slowly but firmly work on down the leg. (Do not touch the horse's lower hind leg unexpectedly, as it is a good way to get kicked.) Fasten the rope around the pastern, and then slowly draw the leg up and forward, tying it with a jerk knot to a separate neck rope.

A throwing rig is a combination of ropes and hobbles used to "throw" a horse to the ground. Any horse can be put down safely using this rig, but it should be done by someone experienced, or else the horse may be injured or unnecessarily frightened. Veterinarians often use a throwing rig for castration or more major surgical procedures, often in conjunction with a tranquilizer or an anesthetic. Place the hobbles on either the front or the back legs; then run a rope from one hobble, through a belly band, down to the other hobble, back through the band, and on to the person doing the restraining. A horse thrown correctly will not fight much but will sort of "tip over." A panicked horse, however, can bruise itself badly. Once the horse is down, you must tie its legs correctly—in a completely flexed position—or it can strain or break a leg.

Restraining Foals

To restrain a small foal, put one arm under its neck and another behind the buttocks, as if you planned to pick it up—sort of a "whole foal hug." With a larger foal, elevate the nose with one hand, and use your other hand to push against the neck or shoulder to keep the foal off balance when it tries to move. Crowding a foal into a corner works well; but you must really crowd it, or you may get a kick or two from those fast little feet.

Always keep an eye on the mare when working on a new foal. Even the gentlest mare may become a little overprotective when her offspring appears threatened.

Breeding

Of course, you mule owners must pass this section, as 99 percent of mules are sterile, being a hybrid cross between a jack and a mare.

The Heat Cycle

Mares come into heat every 21 to 27 days. They remain in heat for 2 to 10 days, although they show the strongest signs for 2 to 3 days. A mare in heat will urinate frequently and will tease other horses, and her temperament may change. A well-trained, easygoing mare may get nervous or temperamental, for instance. A gelding may mount or show interest in a mare in heat. When taken to a stallion, the mare will squat and urinate when teased. (Teasing involves leading a stallion on one side of a fence or gate while the mare is on the other; he is not permitted to mount her.)

Mares begin to come into heat early in the spring or about 9 days after foaling. Many mares will continue heat cycles all year if not bred; others experience heat only in the spring and summer. A mare will foal 11 months after conception, so keep the month of foaling in mind when planning a breeding. If your barn is cold, for instance, you won't want the mare to foal in January or February.

Keeping Stallions

Keeping a stallion is a pain! Don't do it unless you are a horseperson with experience and patience—and a *very* good stallion. A stallion is first a breeding animal. It is his instinct and purpose in life, and he can never be completely dependable because of it. No matter how well trained he is, something can set him off unexpectedly. Most stallions regard a strange gelding as a stallion and will attack one at every chance. Owning a stallion means going to bed wondering if an irate phone call will awaken you with the news that your stallion broke out and is in with the neighbor's mares or fighting with the gelding. It means having superstrong fences, being careful of who rides to your place on a horse, and watching any kids that are around. And it means the stallion will never be all yours: He belongs to his instincts. A good stallion will make a better gelding, without all the worries.

Instead of keeping a stallion in your barn, take your mare to someone else's stallion that is standing at stud. Believe me, paying a stud fee beats the worry of owning a stallion. Plus, you will not have to incur the expense of feeding that stallion, vaccinating him, worming him, and having his feet worked on all year—all of which usually cost more than most stud fees! In addition, you have your choice of stallions each year.

Make arrangements ahead of time to breed your mare since many owners book their stallions' breeding schedules in advance. You will have to ship your mare to the stallion because very few stud owners will risk exposing their stallions to disease, stress, and injury by hauling them to mares. Also, find out what the stallion owner expects. Many want the mares to have negative Coggins tests for swamp fever. The stallion owner may also require a veterinarian to examine your mare for vaginal or uterine infections before you bring her to the stallion, as one mare can bring trouble to a breeding farm.

Normal Foaling

Eleven months from the time of a successful breeding, your mare will be ready to foal. Of course, you can test her much earlier than that to be sure she is in foal. Missed heat periods are a strong indicator. Blood tests also show very early, and there are now "home pregnancy tests" that are quite dependable. Or have your veterinarian do a rectal examination of the mare.

As the mare approaches her foaling date, her udder will become quite full, and a drop or two of colostrum may ooze out and harden. This is called waxing. Just a day or two before foaling, the ligaments will slacken above the mare's tail, and her belly will drop, looking almost pointed at the bottom.

Most mares foal at night or early in the morning, so don't count on seeing the foal born unless you sleep with your mare! If the mare is due in the late spring or early summer, the best place for her to foal is in the pasture or grassy paddock. These are clean and free of obstructions and booby traps for the brand-new foal. In bad weather house the mare in a large, well-bedded box stall. Bank bedding against the wall so it's a foot or so deeper around the sides than in the center, like a shallow bird nest. This will keep the mare from lying with her rump to the wall when beginning to foal, blocking the birth. Remove all feed boxes and pails soon after they are used; it's not unusual for a foal to die from suffocation after being dumped into them. Likewise, do not keep a water tank in the stall or even a large water tub. I've heard of more than one foal that drowned in one at birth.

Just prior to foaling, the mare may go to an isolated corner of the pasture or act restless in the box stall. She may paw or pace in the stall. She will often begin to sweat, and she may act a bit colicky. Most mares will lie down to foal, and most foal quickly, only 15 to 20 minutes elapsing between the onset of labor and the time the foal is dropped. The water bag and two front feet are closely followed by the nose. Don't worry that the feet look "abnormal" (soft and flaky); this is normal and protects the mare's uterus and vagina. The hooves will harden in a day.

Front Presentation

The front presentation foal will be born in three stages: the front feet and head, the shoulders and brisket, and last the hips and hind legs. The mare generally rests in between stages for a moment. Most often the placenta (afterbirth) will pass with the foal. This is the whitish membrane covering the fetus in the uterus. The membrane usually breaks as the foal is expelled into the world. If it does not break, the mare generally takes care of this after the birth. If she doesn't, you should quickly rupture the membrane at the foal's head so that it doesn't suffocate.

Clean the foal, paying special attention to clearing any mucus from the nose and mouth. The umbilical cord usually breaks at birth, leaving a foot or so of cord hanging. Dunk this cord thoroughly in iodine. If too much cord is left hanging, you may tie it off with a nylon line and trim the cord shorter; then treat it with iodine. This helps prevent not only navel infection but joint ill and scours (diarrhea), as well. Giving the newborn foal an injection of tetanus antitoxin is also a good idea as some foals have picked up tetanus at birth, usually through the umbilical stump.

After the foal is perky, leave it to the mother's care. Too much interference can make a mare nervous.

Be sure to carefully examine the placenta at this time, checking to see that it is all there and that there are no missing pieces. Mares are very prone to toxic reactions when pieces of the placenta are left in the uterus. If you are unsure, save the placenta, and call your veterinarian.

Rear Presentation

With a normal rear presentation, the hind feet show first. You can tell the difference as the toes will point up instead of down, showing the frogs and soles of the hooves. The backward foal is usually born quite rapidly and with little trouble. The one problem is possible suffocation or inhalation of fluids. A foal begins to breathe as the umbilical cord breaks. This is fine in a front presentation, but in the rear presentation, the foal's head is often still in the birth canal after the cord breaks.

During a rear presentation birth, help the mare as soon as the hind legs are through the vagina: Firm traction downward as she pushes will hasten the birth. As soon as the foal is dropped, clean out the mouth and nostrils with a dry towel. If the foal is breathing irregularly or not at all, smack its chest on the side, hard, with the flat of your hand. It is sometimes necessary to hold the foal up by the hind legs to drain the lungs. For a normal-sized adult, the easiest way is to grasp the hind feet while you are squatting, back to the foal, and then stand up. This will hang the foal from your shoulders, allowing the lungs to drain. A helper, if present, can clean out the fluid as it drains. When the foal begins to struggle, let it down.

Abnormal Foaling

While 90 percent of mares foal without human help or with minimal assistance, it's wise to know just when there is a problem and what to do about it. Prompt help from you, or from your veterinarian in difficult cases, can save the life of both the mare and the foal.

Front Presentation—Leg Back

When the mare strains, producing the head and only one foot, suspect that one knee has caught on the brim of the pelvis and has been deflected back into the uterus. Scrub and lubricate your hand and arm with liquid dish soap; then examine the mare to check the position of the foal. Locate the deflected leg and foot, and cover the hoof with your hand to protect the uterus. Push back on the foal's chest to gain some room, and pull the leg up, keeping your hand over the hoof. Straighten the foal into the normal birth position. As the mare strains, pull down gently on the foal to help her.

Front Presentation—Head Back

When you see two feet but no head, suspect that the head has been deflected back. This is the most difficult position commonly found in foaling difficulties. A foal's neck is very long, as are its limbs, and the head can get a long way from the pelvic opening, making it difficult to reach.

I'll suggest how home delivery can be helped, but you really should have a veterinarian with obstetrical equipment for this. Scrub and lubricate your hand and arm with liquid dish soap; then examine the mare to check the foal's position. Follow the neck from the foal's chest to its head. Slip an obstetrical chain (or a rope, if you lack a chain) in the shape of a noose through the foal's mouth and behind the ears. With this grip try to work the head around, the way the neck naturally flexes. You may have to push the legs back some to gain enough room to bring the foal's head into the normal birth position.

Do *not* try to pull a head-back foal with a fence stretcher, tractor, or other forcible means. You will kill the foal and injure or kill the mare. And do *not* work longer than 15 minutes without results before calling the veterinarian. If you wait, the mare will probably become exhausted and go into shock.

Rear Presentation—One or Both Legs Retained

When the mare strains, producing only one hind foot or nothing but the water bag, suspect an abnormal rear presentation. Scrub and lubricate your hand and arm with liquid dish soap; then examine the mare to check the foal's position. If both hind legs are retained, push the buttocks back with one hand while pulling up one leg at a time. Guard each hoof with your hand to protect the uterus. Once both legs are in the birth canal, firm traction will aid the mare in delivery, for she may be tired. Treat the foal for mucus retention, as in a normal rear delivery.

Calling the Veterinarian

Delivering a foal by cesarean section is an awfully risky operation at best, so it is important to obtain skillful help if your mare is having foaling trouble. Never attempt force, because a foal jammed into the birth canal can seldom be delivered alive, even by a veterinarian. Some laypersons are great in aiding a hard foaling. Such people are generally grooms who have spent their lives with horses and have gained experience helping mares foal. But do not entrust your mare to a "helpful" neighbor unless you know he or she has had a lot of experience.

Mares are nervous and easily thrown into shock, which can be fatal. They are very prone to peritonitis, caused by uterine tears or shreds of afterbirth left in the uterus. If the mare cannot deliver her foal in 15 minutes or if she is not making progress, examine her to check the position of the foal. If you do not feel competent to correct the problem, call your veterinarian immediately. At any rate, do not work on the mare for more than 15 minutes without seeing results.

(For other problems related to foaling, see "Edema" on page 209 and "Retained Placenta" on page 219.)

Caring for Foals

In most cases the mare will care for her foal just fine with no help from you. Once in a while, a mare dies or is killed soon after foaling, or she just refuses to accept her foal. Left on your hands, a foal is one of the hardest animal babies to raise. A foal is large and strong but at the same time very delicate.

If a mare rejects her foal, you can sometimes persuade her to let it nurse, using tranquilizers, a twitch, Scotch hobbles, and plenty of determination and patience. Rubbing some of her milk on the foal's muzzle and rump sometimes also helps. A few maiden (first-foal) mares do not seem to know what the foal is, and their udders are swollen painfully, making any attempt to nurse uncomfortable to them. If this is the case, milking the udder partway out by hand—saving the colostrum for bottle feeding, if necessary—may bring about relief. When the new foal begins to nurse, the mare will often sigh as if she has figured it all out.

The best substitute for the foal's dam is another mare or a jenny burro. But unfortunately, even if a nurse mare is available, many violently refuse (even when restrained) to accept an orphan. Rubbing camphorated oil, peppermint, or some of the mare's milk on the foal's muzzle and rump can sometimes help. Twitching or hobbling the mare may also be helpful. If the mare seems to let the foal nurse, still keep an eye on the pair for a day or two. She may suddenly decide she's had enough of the newcomer and injure it.

Lacking a nurse mare, locate a milking doe goat, or two if one is not a good producer. Goat's milk is easier for the foal to digest than cow's milk because the fat particles are smaller. When the foal has been without milk for several hours, dilute the goat's milk with an equal amount of warm water. When possible, allow the foal to nurse directly from the goat. Most does allow this, and they make very good dam substitutes. If that isn't an option, feed the foal with a lamb nipple on a soda bottle; pail feeding causes digestive upsets that can be fatal. You may have to tube-feed a very weak foal until it seems perkier and has the desire to nurse. (For details, see "Caring for Kids" on page 103.) If you are unable to find a doe goat to provide milk, there are several powdered milk replacers on the market for foals that are quite good. Choose the best you can find.

The foal must be fed every two hours. Gradually increase the milk at each feeding, giving just enough so that the foal is still hungry but almost satisfied. It's important to get the foal onto solid feed as soon as possible. At the end of each feeding, slip a few pellets of Calf Manna (*not* medicated calf pellets) into its mouth. At first the foal will mostly spit them out. But soon the foal chews some of them and then learns to relish them, as well as nibble on grass, bits of good, clean hay, and sweet feed. As soon as the foal eats a pound of pellets a day, you can drop the every-two-hours night feedings, feeding milk only once a night. Feed the pellets free-choice (as much as the foal will eat) until the foal cleans them up rapidly. Then begin mixing a little horse feed—high-protein mixed grains, such as rolled oats, cracked corn, bran, and alfalfa pellets, plus vitamins and minerals—with the Calf Manna pellets. You should also give the foal a calcium-vitamin D supplement daily to prevent rickets.

Get a bale or two of the best hay you can find, and let the foal nibble on that. I'd stay away from straight alfalfa as it can cause loose bowels and scouring in some orphan foals. If there is grass up, let the foal graze at will. Sunshine will really put pep into the baby, so be sure it gets lots of it. But, of course, be sure it does have access to shade and fresh, clean water.

If the foal should begin scouring (experiencing diarrhea), cut out the milk, and feed an oral electrolyte solution in its place. Kaopectate, an ounce or two every four hours, will also help. Foals often scour briefly a week after birth. At one time this scouring in foals was thought to be caused by the changes in the mare's milk when she experienced the foal heat (the heat period about a week after foaling), but orphan foals undergo it, also. If the foal scours badly, consult your veterinarian; intravenous or intraperitoneal injections of electrolytes will often help.

Castration

Unless you are an accomplished horseperson, it is wisest to have any stud colts gelded, no matter how tempting it is to leave them stallions. There is too much trouble involved in keeping a stallion around. Although a colt can be castrated when quite young, most people prefer to have a little more masculinity in their geldings. A colt gelded young may not develop the full neck and masculine build that a colt gelded as a two year old will have. And it is often easier for the veterinarian to castrate the two year old because some colts' testicles are not large or do not descend into the scrotum until they are near that age. But if the colt is acting up and is hard to handle as a yearling because he's beginning to feel his hormones, it is far better to have him altered earlier than to have someone hurt by his exuberance. (Remember, however, that any colt can act full of life at that age, and gelding him will not take the spunk out of him if he is just naturally high-spirited.)

The horse is one farm animal that I recommend having your veterinarian castrate. In the first place, you have a large animal with very quick reflexes. He is also hard to restrain sufficiently to do a decent job without an anesthetic. In the struggle to get him restrained and operated on, you or the horse can easily be injured.

Call your veterinarian a few days in advance of the time you would like him gelded. Also, have a strong, experienced helper on hand the day you plan to have the horse castrated. This person may not be needed, but sometimes it is necessary to have someone hold a rope or sit on the colt's head for added restraint, even with an anesthetic. Some horses under an anesthetic move as if asleep and jerk their legs. For this reason, most veterinarians use a throwing rig to secure the horse safely on the ground and restrain its legs.

Nearly all veterinarians use surgical castration. When the operation is finished and the horse has recovered, do not put him in a stall for the rest of the day—turn him out in a paddock or small pasture instead. Standing in one place after castration only encourages swelling and stocking up (edema) of the hind legs. Most new geldings will graze as soon as they are up from the operation and will act fine and full of energy in a day. They should not run or tear around for a couple of days to avoid hemorrhage. Do not turn the new gelding in with mares for a month or so as it is possible that the horse will breed a mare. Also, he will not be completely healed and may become injured by kicks.

Caring for Hooves

The saying "No foot—no horse" is all too true. Good hoof care is a vital part of keeping your horse healthy and useful. But keep in mind that good care does not necessarily mean shoeing. If you don't ride your horse on rocky, gravelly, or hard surfaces or if you don't race, show, or work it daily, it may not need shoes.

Many pleasure horses need only to have their feet cleaned and checked regularly, plus a periodic trim, to keep them in top shape. If you keep your horse in a stall, clean its feet daily. Without daily cleaning, stabled horses' hooves can pack with manure and wet, foul bedding, providing ideal conditions for thrush (a problem similar to foot rot). Pastured horses with feet that are trimmed regularly usually do not need daily cleaning as they "self-clean" their feet while moving about—provided that they do not stand in a wet barnyard for extended periods. You should still check the feet daily, though, as a stone, thorn, or puncture wound can cause trouble if left untreated. Even a puncture that does not cause lameness can kill the horse through tetanus.

Hooves normally grow out and require regular trimming unless the horse is pastured on gravel. And even then, it is wise to have the hooves checked for uneven wear, which can cause stress to joints. It is not too hard to learn to trim your own horses' feet, but at the price most farriers charge, it is best to have a professional job done. The farrier will not only cut off the extra growth but also trim to correct any faults in gait and help you head off any future troubles with the feet that you might overlook.

Some horses, like people, have brittle nails (hooves) and have a tendency to develop cracks, splits, and chips. You can usually minimize these problems by painting the hoof and frog (the spongy triangle-shaped pad on the underside of the hoof, which absorbs shock while the animal is moving) with a good hoof conditioner. Be careful you don't buy a hoof black or hoof shine by mistake; these make the hoof "pretty" but will not help condition it. If the brittleness is due to a dry pasture, it helps to let the water tank run over onto a clay base, which the horse will stand in several times a day when drinking. This automatically moistens the feet.

When any cracks occur, call your blacksmith at once since hoof cracks can usually be quickly repaired if treated as soon as they are noticed. There are several quite good hoof patch materials that will repair even a large chip or crack. If you leave a crack untreated, it can get much worse, even causing your horse to go lame.

Trailering

Some of the most common injuries to horses occur while the horse is being hauled. And 99 percent of them could be prevented. Following a few basic safety steps may help to save your horse's life.

First, always inspect the trailer floor before loading the horse. Poke a jackknife here and there, near the front, rear, and sides. If any spots in the floor seem punky (soft), replace the floor. Many horses poke a leg through the floor, resulting in severe and horrible injuries. Prevent rotting floors by removing mats and all manure after every trip, hosing the floor well, and allowing it to dry before putting the mats back in. Treat the floor with a preservative at least yearly.

Teach your horse to load and haul by taking short, pleasant trips before going on its first long trip. Always close the escape door while you are loading and afterward. Many panicked horses try to leap out of this small opening, resulting in bad injuries.

When hauling one horse in a two-horse trailer, load it on the left side. This is the high side of most roads, which often are crowned a bit for drainage. This will prevent a lot of rollover accidents where the swerving trailer becomes top-heavy and rolls over.

Tie the horse short in a one- or two-horse trailer. I leave a strong tie rope, with a heavy bull snap, permanently tied in the manger. This way, you can quickly fasten the head securely while someone else fastens the butt chains, preventing the horse from becoming frightened and backing out. A bit of feed helps keep the animal occupied at this time.

Encourage a reluctant loader to enter with a butt rope. Fasten the rope to the gate post of the trailer, pass the rope beneath the horse's buttocks, and bring it around to the other gate post or the center post. Keep steady pressure on the free end to tighten the rope and encourage the horse to walk forward. Never use a whip on it, lose your temper, or yell at it: Someone—often the horse—will get hurt.

When hauling a horse that is "spooky" or has never been hauled, a stock trailer is a better option than a two-horse trailer. A stock trailer gives the horse more room, and it does not have to be tied. It loads much easier and will not fight the restraint of being tied while frightened. A much-hauled buddy can be loaded in the rear part of the trailer, separated from your horse by the center gate. This has a calming effect and makes a much pleasanter trip for all concerned.

Provide sand for bedding on a long haul. Straw gets slippery, and horses can fall on sudden turns, swerves, and stops. Sand also provides cushioning if you don't cover the floor with trailer mats. Wrapping the legs or using shipping boots, primarily on the hind legs, may prevent injuries, especially when you are backing the horse out of a two-horse trailer. Be careful not to wrap the legs too tightly, though.

Never tie your horse to the outside of a trailer on anything but the solid frame, near eye level. Watch for things it might get a foot through, such as the brace bars to the back end of the trailer, which form triangles that can easily injure a pawing forefoot. Also, don't tie the horse where it can reach the license plate. This cuts a lot of horses in a show season. A hay net can be used for feeding outside the trailer. Never tie the horse long "so it can eat"; it'll end up tangled and injured. And don't tie the horse to a trailer that is not hooked to your truck. A spooked horse can drag a trailer a long distance.

On long trips remember to provide water at least twice a day— more often in hot weather. Dehydration is hard on a horse.

DISEASES AND OTHER PROBLEMS

While horses are generally quite hardy and disease-free, it's smart to be aware of diseases and health problems that *might* happen. This will help you prevent many problems and choose the best course of action for those that do occur. It's also important to know the normal temperature of your horse so you can check for fever or other abnormalities. The normal body temperature of a horse is 99° to 101°F (37.2° to 38.3°C).

Breaks

Today, many horses can and do recover well from broken legs, if given the chance. A horse can break a leg from an accident, such as running into a hole, an open culvert, or a tangle of brush, or just while running in a paddock. Many stallions have been crippled while attempting to serve a mare that was unrestrained by breeding hobbles. One kick is all it takes to snap a bone. It is well worth the trouble to slip a set of hobbles on even the quietest mare before bringing the stallion out.

Broken bones may be very obvious. In a compound fracture, for example, the sharp end of a bone sticks out of a wound in the skin. But often fractures are harder to detect, as when the bone is severely

Suggested Vaccination Schedule for Horses

Below is a suggested schedule for vaccinating your horse against common diseases. But keep in mind that different diseases are common in different locations, so you should ask your veterinarian for his recommendations for your situation. If you are a one-horse owner and your horse never is in contact with other horses, your vaccination program will be different from that used by a multiple-horse owner who travels to shows, races, or breeding farms.

	DISEASE	WHEN TO VACCINATE
FOALS	Equine encephalomyelitis (Eastern and Western)	3 months
	Influenza	3 to 4 months
	Rhinopneumonitis (EHV-4)	2 to 4 months
	Tetanus (antitoxin)	Soon after birth
	Tetanus (toxoid)	3 months
MARES	Equine encephalomyelitis (Eastern and Western)	Yearly, before mosquito season
	Rhinopneumonitis (EHV-1)	2d, 5th, 7th, and 9th months of pregnancy
	Strangles	Yearly, before possible exposure (i.e., shows or breeding)
	Tetanus (toxoid)	Yearly, 6 weeks before foaling
STALLIONS/ GELDINGS	Equine encephalomyelitis (Eastern and Western)	Yearly, before mosquito season
	Rhinopneumonitis (EHV-4)	Yearly
	Tetanus (toxoid)	Yearly

cracked but not apart. If a horse suddenly becomes severely lame, suspect a broken limb, and have your veterinarian take an X ray immediately. A horse with a badly broken limb will hobble about, and the leg will often dangle badly or flop around when the horse moves.

Try to keep such a horse quiet. A broken leg will often panic a horse, which in turn can cause the animal to do irreparable damage to itself. If you must move the horse, do so very slowly and carefully. But in most cases, it is best to leave the horse where you find it until the veterinarian arrives.

Broken legs can often be repaired by use of plaster casts, intramedullary pins, and plates and screws. New technology allows many horses with broken limbs to be saved. Your veterinarian will often stabilize the break and help you make arrangements to send the injured horse to a specialist or large university with an excellent equine orthopedic surgeon.

Fractures in Feet

The small foot under that 1,000-pound horse is not just one bone but several small ones. Under trauma, such as stepping on a rock while running or shock from jumping, one or more of these small bones can crack or break apart. A very common, and often overlooked, stress is lunging (working the horse on a lunge line) a young horse for long periods of time. This causes the bones in the foot of the horse to work at a continual angle. Sometimes a bone will twist and snap, causing severe lameness.

With the exception of the navicular bone, many of these fractures will heal well with treatment and rest. Navicular fractures will seldom heal, although much can be done to relieve the condition and allow the horse to be used without pain. If you suspect a foot fracture, call your veterinarian.

Amputation

Some breaks are so severe that the horse must either be destroyed or have the leg amputated above the break. There is much new work being done on artificial limbs for horses, and you should consider this option before putting down a much-loved companion or valuable breeding animal. Although you won't be able to ride the horse, a prosthesis will allow the animal to be bred and enjoy a very normal life. It does entail expense and a good amount of care, but many people think it provides an excellent alternative to having a horse destroyed because of a broken bone. Ask your veterinarian for referral to a specialist.

Casting

Any horse, regardless of care, can become cast (stuck while lying down). A horse normally gets up by first sitting on its haunches and then throwing its neck forward to balance when the rear end lurches up. If there is no place to throw its neck forward, the horse sometimes is unable to rise, no matter how strong it is.

Some situations are particularly conducive to casting. In a tie stall, for instance, a clumsy horse or an older horse with a touch of arthritis may have a difficult time rising after lying down. Other horses tend to lie down in a corner of a box stall or paddock and get stuck that way. Horses sometimes become cast when they lie down to roll on ice or in deep snow or mud. I've seen a lot of horses cast in fences, too. A horse often eats over a fence, getting its feet tangled. When it tries to back away, it trips, falls, and is unable to rise.

A horse can also become cast when tied on too long a rope. If the rope gets tangled around its legs, the horse can panic and fall. Tie your horse with just enough rope to let it touch its knees with its muzzle. If you tie it even a little longer, a hind foot can get over the rope and throw the horse when it becomes unbalanced. If this happens in a tie stall, the horse is in trouble, especially if it happens in the middle of the night.

The worst thing about a cast horse is the panic. A horse will bang itself around, throwing its head out again and again as it tries to get up, pounding its head against the walls and ground. The longer the animal is down, the more battered it will become. Concussions, eye injuries, and other trauma often result. *Never* go into the stall or in close quarters with a cast horse; you could get pinned under a panic-stricken, thrashing animal. Instead, climb in through the manger, or hang over a partition—but keep yourself protected. It doesn't matter how much the horse likes you or how gentle it is. It is frightened, and it may kill you.

It is critical to get a cast horse up soon after you find it as horses are animals that cannot lie down for long periods of time without dying. Get a lead rope on the halter, and then release the tie rope if the horse is tied. Encourage it to get up, helping to steady it with the lead or boosting its hindquarters by the tail.

If the horse is really stuck, you may have to pull it back out of the stall to enable it to rise. A come-along or fence stretcher will slowly pull the horse backward. A horse that weighs under 800 pounds can be pulled out by knotting the tail—but don't twist the bone—and hooking onto that. On a larger horse, you may have to slip a rope across the chest, like a breast collar, and scoot it back with this.

Once the horse is free of the stall, let it rest awhile. Keep it rolled

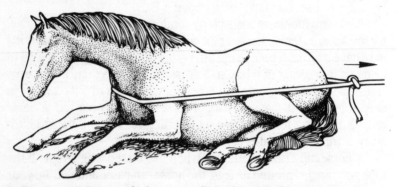

Pulling a cast horse. *If a horse is really stuck in its stall, you may need to slide it back to give it room to get up. Working carefully, slip a rope across the horse's chest, and pull back, using a come-along or tractor, if necessary.*

up on its brisket, not out flat on its side; prop it up, if need be, using a bale of hay. A horse left on its side for any time gives up and will die. Offer the animal a drink; then feed it some hay and grain. When it is rested, urge it to stand. A horse that is a bit weak benefits from a boost via the tail. If it is unable to rise, call your veterinarian instead of continually trying to get the horse up. You will only tire and possibly injure it. The veterinarian will be able to administer injections—possibly cortisone or dextrose to give added strength—and can provide much experience in helping the cast horse up. Once it is up, let it stand a few minutes while you massage its legs to increase feeling and circulation. When the horse quits shaking and seems stronger, lead it slowly around until it seems normal. Keep a careful eye on the horse, though, as it is weak and usually tired and could get cast again.

Colic

To put it simply, colic is a bellyache. It is common in horses and is quite painful, but in most cases it is easy to treat when caught early and seldom fatal. A number of things can cause colic, including overeating, drinking large quantities of water after eating grain, eating sand along with feed or grass, internal parasites, constipation, eating iced or frosted pasture, and drinking water while overheated. An affected horse will pace about uncomfortably, seldom eat or drink, paw, sweat, and squat, as if undecided about whether to lie down or not. It may kick or look at its belly, breathe hard, and often roll. Rolling can cause a torsion (twisting) of the bowel, which is often fatal. Thrashing can cause rupture of the bowel or stomach as well as external injuries, especially to the head. When the colic is caused by an impaction that is not relieved, the horse may become toxic and die.

If you find a colicky horse down in a tie stall, never walk in alongside it as you could be severely injured, no matter how calm the horse normally is. Pain can make the most gentle horse crazy. Instead, crawl in through the manger or from over the stall partition. Release the horse, and fasten a long lead shank to the halter. Then encourage the horse to get up. Back it out of the stall, but be careful not to get pinned against the wall. Once you get it out of the stall, begin walking it while someone else calls the veterinarian.

Walking will usually keep the horse on its feet and out of severe pain until the veterinarian arrives. While you are waiting, try to determine the cause of the colic, and tell the veterinarian your ideas when he arrives. Correct diagnosis is an important part of successful treatment. If it is a simple digestive upset due to the horse eating a new food, the treatment will be aimed at easing the cramps until the feed passes. If an impaction is suspected, such as from eating sand, oral or injectable laxatives will relieve the blockage and the pain.

It is a very good idea to have a bottle of colic remedy in your tack room first aid kit, just for an emergency when a veterinarian is not available. You can ask your veterinarian if an injectable pain reliever for colic might also be advisable. If a commercial product is not available, you can make your own by combining 1 pint of oil (corn, mineral, or vegetable) with 2 tablespoons of cayenne pepper, 2 tablespoons of ginger, and 2 tablespoons of baking soda. Mix the ingredients well, place the mixture in a sturdy, long-necked bottle, and give it as a drench. Horses hate this drench (wouldn't you?), and it is not the easiest to administer. But this old-time remedy does work well in most cases.

Have your veterinarian out as soon as he can come because colic can sometimes be the symptom of a serious problem, such as a torsion of the bowel, severe internal parasite load, or a sand impaction that will recur unless prevented. If colic is just let go or mistreated, you'll often have yourself a dead horse.

After the horse is treated, either watch it closely or walk it gently until all pains have passed. If the horse is sweaty and hot, be sure to throw a sheet or blanket over it—it is easy for a hot horse to get chilled.

Many colics can be prevented. Do not make sudden feed changes, such as trying new grain mixes or changing from a dry to lush pasture. Do not let your horse graze on icy pasture when it is hungry or on sandy pasture that has very short grass. It is better to feed hay than contend with sand colic. Sometimes a horse can get sand colic after drinking from a stream with a heavy sand or sediment content. Check your horse's water supply often to make sure it is clean. Never water a hot horse or water immediately after feeding grain. Do not work a horse heavily after a full feeding. And keep the feed bin locked. Many colics result from a horse escaping its stall and gobbling grain.

Cuts

Glass, tin, and barbed wire account for many cuts on horses. Right behind these, I would list running into wooden fences or partitions, which splinter and gash the horse. Kicks, bites, and rips on nails also cause many injuries to horses. To be as safe as possible, all fences should be strong and tight. Never park machinery in a field containing horses, especially near a fence or in a corner where a horse could get cut up running through at close quarters. Keep pastures free of loose boards, junk, and brush piles, and repair any ragged culverts. Fill any holes with rocks, and then pack them with soil. If you shelter your horse in a metal shed, plank up the inside at least 4 feet high as many horses are cut badly after kicking through a metal wall. And never turn a horse out wearing its halter because many horses get tangled up by the halter, severely cutting or otherwise injuring themselves.

If a cut does occur, catch the horse, wash off the blood, and really check the injury. If the blood is running or dripping, pack the wound with a dry, sterile cloth. Leave it in place for 5 to 10 minutes, and the bleeding will usually stop. When a wound spurts blood, an artery may be cut, so you'll need to apply more pressure. Press a cloth hard onto the wound by hand, or, if you can, tie it in place with a few wraps of gauze. A wound like this needs prompt treatment by your veterinarian, or the horse could lose enough blood to be in serious trouble.

Once you've controlled the bleeding, you must decide whether the injury will heal better left open or sutured. If you are not experienced, ask the opinion of your veterinarian. Many wounds do heal best when left alone, other than for cleaning and application of an antiseptic. Then there can be better drainage, less swelling, and often less scarring. Some wounds must have a flap of skin clipped off to make healing smoother and more complete. Small, three-cornered tears or ragged cuts, for instance, often benefit from being trimmed.

Whether or not you plan to suture the wound, always trim the hair away. Hair is irritating, collects dirt and bacteria, and will very much retard healing, if not cause infections. Even with a show horse, it is best to clip that hair away. The hair in a clipped area will grow in a lot quicker than that in a bald area around a wound where serum and pus have been seeping.

Keeping a wound cleaned out daily with plain warm, soapy water will greatly speed healing. This is much better than smearing salve on top of salve every day. Fresh air, no bandage, and daily cleaning, plus systemic or topical antibiotic solution or powder, are the best treatments.

Cuts on Feet and Legs

If your horse is wounded on a foot or lower leg, have your veterinarian check it out. These wounds are especially prone to development of "proud flesh," or exuberant granulation, producing tissue that resembles a tumor. From an inch-long cut, a mass of proud flesh the size of a basketball can form. This oozes serum, is easily injured, bleeds easily, and will continue to enlarge. It very seldom just "goes away." When surgically removed, it often grows right back. It is best to do everything possible to prevent this problem from starting in the first place.

With your veterinarian's advice, however, you can treat proud flesh successfully. I have had very good luck using Kopertox, soaking the area well with warm water between treatments, and carefully keeping the area clean. In very bad cases, you may need to clean the area and then wrap it lightly with 4-inch gauze soaked well in Kopertox. Leave the gauze in place for two days; then carefully peel it off, removing a thin layer of dead proud flesh. Repeat this treatment until the proud flesh is gone. It takes weeks, during which time you must keep the horse clean and dry.

It is advisable to give any wounded horse an injection of tetanus antitoxin, just to be safe from this deadly disease.

Dental Problems

A horse chews and grinds its food in such a way that it wears down the edges of its molars, making sharp edges at times. These points often cut the cheek or tongue, causing poor eating that can result in weight loss, indigestion, and wasted grain. When a horse takes a mouthful of grass (or, more noticeably, grain) and chews with an exaggerated motion, dropping gobs of half-chewed food, suspect that it has sharp teeth.

It is wise to have your veterinarian inspect the teeth and float them, if necessary. Floating is filing the teeth down smooth with a special file about 4 inches long on the end of a long handle. While many horse owners can learn to routinely float the teeth, it is best to have your veterinarian inspect the teeth of any horse that is having dental trouble, as it may be more than just sharp teeth. Horses, especially older ones, are prone to abscessed teeth, which need pulling. Other problems commonly mistaken for sharp teeth include ulcers in the mouth, foreign objects wedged between the teeth, and foxtails and burrs in the gums and tongue.

Many veterinarians use a mouth speculum to hold the mouth open while floating the teeth. Others have an assistant hold the tongue out of the mouth and to one side, with the other hand holding the side of the halter. Some horses must be twitched to keep their attention on their noses instead of on what's going on inside their mouths, as floating does make a grating sound.

You should inspect the inside of your horses' mouths twice yearly for sharp edges and points. Use a flashlight so that you can see well. If you're unsure of what you are looking at, ask your veterinarian to explain the next time he is out to your place for another call.

Edema

Edema in horses is also commonly called stocking up. It commonly happens in the legs. You can differentiate edema from swelling by the doughy feeling of the flesh. If you squeeze your fingers around or into the area with edema, dents will remain where your fingers pressed.

Basically, most edema, or stocking up, is due to something shutting off part of the circulation in an area. Sprains, injuries, hard or jarring work, bee stings, and leg wraps or boots applied too tightly can all bring on edema. Mares often stock up just before or just after foaling because the increased size of the udder shuts off circulation to some extent, causing fluid to seep out of the blood vessels and into the surrounding tissue. The penis of a gelding or stallion will sometimes swell with edema due to an accumulation of body secretions and dirt in the sheath. You can prevent this by cleaning the sheath periodically.

Diuretics, such as Lasix or Naquasone, work very well to remedy edema by stimulating the kidneys. This causes more frequent urination, which draws fluid—the edema—from the body.

Equine Encephalomyelitis

Equine encephalomyelitis is commonly known as sleeping sickness. There are three kinds that you should know about: Eastern equine encephalomyelitis (EEE), Western equine encephalomyelitis (WEE), and Venezuelan equine encephalomyelitis (VEE).

Eastern Equine Encephalomyelitis

EEE is a virus-produced disease, most often spread by mosquitoes. Although named Eastern, it has been found in Mexico and Central and South America as well as in western locations in the United States. It spreads from mosquitoes to birds, back to mosquitoes, and then to horses and sometimes humans. Common symptoms include depression, incoordination, drooping lip, high fever, pushing against a wall or fence, and being down, unable to rise. The disease is short, lasting only two to four days before the horse dies. The few horses that do live are often "dummies," having suffered brain damage from the disease.

If you suspect this disease, isolate the horse, and call your veterinarian at once. Any horses living in, or passing through, an area where EEE has been reported should be vaccinated. It is a good idea to vaccinate *all* horses yearly with an EEE-WEE vaccine. With horses on the move across country and across continents today, encephalomyelitis could break out nearly anywhere, sometimes with little warning.

Western Equine Encephalomyelitis

WEE is quite similar to EEE, but it is found chiefly in the West and Midwest of the United States. The symptoms are also similar, but the disease is not quite as fatal, with perhaps half of the afflicted horses surviving. WEE is more often seen in humans than EEE.

Caused by a virus, WEE cannot be treated with antibiotics. However, good nursing will save many horses that might die otherwise. Keeping the horse standing up by means of a chute, slings, or padded stocks helps. Heavy bedding, aspirin to lower the fever (a high fever can cause brain damage), and intravenous electrolytes are often helpful. Feeding good hay and a good grain mix, by hand if need be, sometimes helps keep the horse's strength up until the disease has run its course.

Vaccination is the only preventive, other than complete isolation in a "bug-free" barn. I strongly recommend an EEE-WEE vaccination yearly for *all* horses.

Venezuelan Equine Encephalomyelitis

VEE is a fairly new disease in northern areas. Most of us never heard of it until the outbreak in Mexico and along the U.S. border states in the 1970s. The symptoms are similar to those of EEE and WEE. Although never a problem far north of the Mexican border, it is a disease to keep in mind when hauling a horse to or from this area. While VEE is thought to be pretty much under control in Mexico, another recent outbreak alerted us to the possibility of future problems.

A vaccine is available and recommended if you keep or haul horses in the southwestern U.S. border states. Otherwise, the EEE-WEE vaccine is recommended for protection against sleeping sickness.

Flies

Several kinds of flies bother horses. In addition to annoying horses, biting insects can spread diseases, such as swamp fever, equine encephalomyelitis, and Rocky Mountain spotted fever.

You can prevent a lot of the stable fly problem by keeping the manure away from the stable. (Spread it on your fields, and work it in with a harrow.) Fly parasites, which are tiny flies that parasitize the eggs of stable flies but do not annoy people or horses, also work quite well. In conjunction with these treatments, use fly traps in or around the barn and barnyard. Draining low spots near the barn and pasture or filling them in will help keep down mosquitoes as well as flies.

Sometimes flies become a problem despite preventive measures. In this case you'll need to use a wipe-on or spray fly repellent. Apply it in the morning and then again in late afternoon. Some horses will require an additional wipe or spray in the middle of the day.

If your horses are shy of the sprayer, you can spray some of the repellent on a cloth to use on the ears and face. Spraying away from the body (that is, not touching the horse with the spray at first) will waste a little spray, but it will get the horse used to the sprayer's noise and the sight of the mist coming at it. Do not use force, as that will only make the horse fear the spraying.

Fly bonnets and fly chasers, which are attached to the halter, are two alternatives to spraying for face flies. The only problem here is that you must leave the halter on in the pasture—a very real danger.

For information on controlling bot flies, see "Worms and Internal Parasites" on page 225.

Influenza

With more horses moving from state to state and country to country, equine influenza is becoming more common. Caused by a virus, equine influenza is very contagious and moves quickly through susceptible horses. Although affected horses are quite sick in many cases, showing symptoms such as a high fever, coughing, nasal discharge, lack of appetite, and weakness, few animals die.

Isolate any horse affected with influenza. There is no cure, but good nursing can help aid recovery. Give aspirin to reduce the fever, antibiotics to treat any secondary infection, extra good feed, and rest.

Regular vaccinations can prevent equine influenza. After the initial injection, give another two months later and a booster six months after that; then vaccinate yearly. Keeping any new, unvaccinated horses isolated for one month will also help.

Lameness

There are hundreds of causes of lameness in horses, and there have been entire books written on just this subject. (I recommend *Lameness in Horses* by O. R. Adams, D.V.M., M.S., and *The Lame Horse* by James R. Rooney.) Here I will just touch on the subject, covering the most common causes of lameness.

If your horse suddenly acts lame, examine its foot. Use a hoof pick to clean manure and dirt from the hoof. Work from heel to toe along the frog to avoid injury to the heel. Check for stones, sticks wedged in between the frog and the sole, slivers, glass, thorns, nails, cuts, and punctures, which often show as black spots. Also, check for swellings, considering snakebite by a venomous snake in the lower leg. If the horse wears shoes, check them to see if they are loose or need to be reset. Shoes must be replaced or reset every 8 to 12 weeks. If the hoof grows too long, the shoes do no good and can cause lameness by forcing an unnatural angle to the pastern. If the horse became lame soon after shoeing, have the farrier check for a possible nail puncture.

After making an initial examination, call your veterinarian unless you have discovered an obvious nonthreatening cause, like a stone wedged in the frog. Some forms of lameness are only temporary, such as when the horse has been kicked in a muscle of the upper leg. Others are temporary with simple treatment but may become permanent unsoundness if left untreated. Following is an overview of some of the more common causes of lameness in horses, with their symptoms and treatments.

Azoturia

This condition, also known as Monday morning sickness, can appear when you allow a regularly worked horse to rest for a day or two (such as over a weekend) while keeping it on its regular grain ration. When you work the horse again, it becomes lame, trembles, sweats profusely, and loses its coordination. Its urine may become dark, from a dark orange to almost black. Most moderate cases recover with the help of complete rest, oral electrolytes, sodium bicarbonate, and injectable thiamine. To prevent azoturia, cut back on the horse's grain ration when resting it from normal work for a day or two.

Bowed Tendon

In this case a tendon, often in a front leg below the knee, appears to bow outward. Soreness and severe lameness result. It is caused by severe strain or overwork. To help relieve the soreness, stand the horse in cold water (a creek is ideal) for at least an hour daily. Ice packs and complete stall rest help. Your veterinarian may recommend an external blister (an ointment or salve rubbed into the skin to produce heat in the area) or firing (applying a firing pin or electrical hot point to the skin over the affected area) to increase circulation and aid healing. Anti-inflammatories help to reduce pain and swelling. Do not work the horse for at least six months.

Capped Elbow or Hock

With a capped elbow or hock, the lameness is accompanied by a large swelling, which may feel full of fluid, on either the point of the elbow or the hock. It is caused by bruising, possibly due to insufficient bedding or to striking with toe or heel, as seen in trotters or gaited horses. Treatment includes ice packs, cortisone, mild exercise (such as hand walking), and total rest from work. You may also need to give antibiotics if injuries accompany the bruise.

Founder

A horse suffering from founder, or laminitis, is severely lame and reluctant to move. It will stand with its feet in front of its body to take weight off the toes and may have an above-normal temperature. One common cause, especially with ponies, is overeating lush pasture. Other causes include overeating grain and drinking water when over-heated. In mares a retained placenta can lead to laminitis. Treatments include injectable antihistamines, rest in a well-bedded stall, standing in cold water, and ice packs. When a foundered horse begins to move around again, provide mild daily exercise, and have it shod by a far-rier who does corrective shoeing.

Bowed tendon

Small wind puffs

Splint

Ringbone

Several common leg injuries.
Horses are prone to a variety of leg injuries. Treatments vary depending on the particular injury and the cause, although most require at least some rest from work.

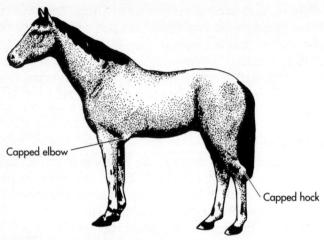

Capped elbow

Capped hock

Capped hock and elbow. *A capped hock manifests as lameness and a large swelling on the point of the hock. A similar swelling on the point of the elbow is called a capped elbow. Both problems are caused by bruising.*

Navicular Disease

A horse with navicular disease does not "move out" freely but takes shorter strides and may stumble. It stands unnaturally and may "point" with the bad foot. Left untreated, the hooves may become narrow and long. Navicular disease is caused by trauma to the feet. This can include stepping on a rock while running or jumping, hard work on unyielding surfaces, faulty conformation, lunging too long on hard surfaces, and other shocks, any of which can crack small bones in the foot. Surgery, corrective shoeing, and cortisone injections can help prolong the usefulness of the horse, but nothing cures this condition.

Ringbone

Ringbone appears as lameness with swelling or ridges in the pastern area. At first the horse may be less lame after you work it for a while. Eventually, though, the joint movement is often impaired as calcium deposits form. Possible causes include hard work, stress, kicks or blows, arthritis, and infection following an injury. Pull the horse's shoes, and allow complete pasture rest along with cortisone and anti-inflammatory drugs. When the inflammation subsides, you can return the horse to light work; but you must have it shod by a competent farrier who does corrective shoeing. Some horses are never sound again, depending upon the position and size of the calcification.

Sand, or Quarter, Crack

Many horses have dry, cracked hooves without lameness; but when the toes grow too long, the weight of the horse can force the crack to widen. This in itself can be painful, but it also lets stones and grit work into the sensitive inner layers of the hoof. You'll usually notice these cracks on the front of the hoof, from the toe nearly up to the coronet. Infection and severe lameness may result. Have your farrier trim the feet and work on the crack. Often a groove is burned or cut across the top of the crack to stop the ascension, allowing the crack to eventually grow out. (Remember, the new horn grows down from the coronet to the toe, so it can take from 9 to 14 months to completely replace the old horn.) Your farrier may also use light shoes to distribute the weight more evenly and keep the crack from widening, along with hoof patch preparations to prevent complications. If your pasture tends to be dry, let the water tank overflow, creating a moist spot in which the horse must stand daily. It also helps to paint the hooves with good hoof dressing.

Splints

In this case lameness is accompanied by small inflamed spots that later harden owing to calcium deposits. Splints are caused by hard work on hard or rough surfaces, blows, or injuries. Treatment includes pasture rest and liniment, possibly along with surgery or firing.

Stifling

A stifled horse appears to have its hind leg "stuck" straight, usually backward, when you lead it from a stall or work it. You may also see stifling, or luxation of the patella, on a young horse playing in a field. It's caused by a conformation weakness—a stifle that's too straight—and is often hereditary. To replace the dislocation and keep the joint from slipping apart, draw the leg forward by running a rope from it through a neck loop. Rest the horse from work. Blistering is often used, as well. Treatment does not always work, however, and a horse that has been stifled is not a safe horse for hard work, such as racing, jumping, or contesting. The condition may occur again and be disastrous for both horse and rider as there is no warning. Do not use the horse for breeding, because the condition may be passed on.

Thrush

With thrush, lameness is accompanied by foul foot odor. It is caused by unclean or damp bedding, especially when you fail to clean the hooves out regularly. Pare down any necrotic tissue, often around the frog, clean the feet well, and apply astringent thrush remedy daily. Provide clean, dry bedding, and keep the stall clean to prevent future problems.

The stifled horse. This condition is caused by a weakness in conformation. Drawing the leg forward with a rope can replace the dislocation, although the condition may occur again without warning.

Wind Puffs

Wind puffs appear as puffy swellings on the lower leg, along with lameness. They are caused by strain. Rest the horse completely until the swellings subside. Astringents may help, as can standing the horse in cold running water. In severe cases you may have to use liniment or a blister.

Lice

Lice are gray, soft-bodied parasites that are smaller than a grain of rice. They are usually a problem during the winter months when there is little sunlight and the horse has longer hair. You'll most often see lice on the neck and chest of a horse and sometimes near the tail. In addition to causing intense itching and unsightly, bald, moth-eaten-looking patches, lice can actually bleed a horse to death if they are numerous enough.

Check your horses thoroughly for these parasites every week from fall to spring. Part the hair on the neck, and take a good look at the skin. Pick off any suspicious specks, and place them on a piece of white paper for more thorough inspection.

If you find lice on your horse, purchase a good louse powder. (One that's safe for dairy cows is safe for horses—and you. I'd advise one containing rotenone or pyrethrins.) Dust the horse thoroughly from head to tail. Repeat weekly for three weeks so you get all the lice that hatch out after the first application. You should also dust any other horses in close contact with the infested horse even if you don't see lice on them.

Mange

Mange is caused by tiny mites that burrow into the skin. These mites cause extreme itching, which makes the horse rub itself until bloody, crusty scabs form. These scabs are in turn rubbed raw, and the infestation spreads. Secondary infections, often bacterial or fungal, can follow. If enough of the skin becomes nonfunctional, the horse will become emaciated and die. Mange spreads quickly and will travel from one horse to another easily.

Fortunately, mange is not a common problem. But if you do suspect it, isolate the horse, and call your veterinarian. Most cases of "mange" turn out to be other things, such as summer sores or allergies to parasites or to fly spray. Your veterinarian can take a skin scraping that, when examined under a microscope, will reveal the true problem.

If you catch mange early, it is usually easy to treat, but you must treat it thoroughly and religiously. Clipping the entire area before treatment is a great help. Products containing rotenone and lime-sulfur often work well, provided you scrub them into the skin and leave them on for an adequate time. Your veterinarian will prescribe a miticide that he feels will do the job. Always follow the directions, no matter what product you use. Also, be sure to thoroughly clean and treat clipper blades after clipping the horse, or you may spread the infestation to other horses.

Puncture Wounds

Puncture wounds occur often in horses, most times in the foot because of its structure. Puncture wounds are more dangerous to a horse than to other animals because of their susceptibility to tetanus.

When a horse begins to limp, be sure to thoroughly examine the foot from heel to toe for a puncture. This may look like only a tiny black hole. But on closer examination, you may notice soreness on squeezing, pus, or slight bleeding. I once took a 4-inch piece of smooth wire out of the frog of a Belgian gelding. He had been limping for a week, and the owner could find nothing wrong with his foot. There was only a minute black spot on the side of his frog. On probing the spot, I found the wire and pulled it out. I crossed my fingers as the horse received his tetanus antitoxin. After all, the wire had been rusty, covered with manure, and in the foot for a week! Luckily, the horse recovered fully. (He did receive antibiotics for a week following the extraction of the wire.)

Use a syringe to *thoroughly* flush out any puncture wound, first with warm, soapy water and then with Betadine or another antiseptic. Remember, the antiseptic must reach to the bottom of the wound, not just remain on the top. Also, call your veterinarian to check the wound and to start a week of antibiotic injections to prevent infection.

Every horse should have a yearly tetanus booster plus an injection of tetanus antitoxin when you know it has been injured. (For more information on this disease, see "Tetanus" on page 224.)

Retained Placenta

Most mares expel the placenta (afterbirth) at the time of foaling or very soon afterward. You or your veterinarian should examine it at once to make sure that it is intact, with no missing pieces. (If part of the placenta stays in the uterus, the mare can become toxic and die in a very short time.)

When a mare does not expel her placenta after 10 hours, call your veterinarian. The placenta should not be in the uterus more than 12 hours after foaling; otherwise, the mare may become toxic and develop founder or septicemia (blood poisoning), possibly resulting in permanent disability or death. Horses are *not* like cows or other animals in this respect—a retained placenta in a horse is an *emergency*.

It may be necessary to remove a retained placenta manually. Have your veterinarian do this, if at all possible, because leaving in even one small piece can mean disaster. If you absolutely can't get a veterinarian, you may have to tackle the job yourself. Scrub and lubricate your hand and arm with liquid dish soap; then insert it into the mare. Carefully work your hand between the placenta and the wall of the uterus. *Never* yank or pull on the afterbirth to remove it; peel the placenta away very carefully, leaving it in one piece. Work slowly and carefully, keeping tension on the placenta with your other hand. Placing uterine boluses in the uterus, after you remove the placenta, helps prevent infection. But let me say again: Removing a mare's retained placenta is not a "do-it-yourself" job. Get a veterinarian if at all possible!

Rhinopneumonitis

Rhino is the commonly used name for a complicated viral disease correctly known as equine viral rhinopneumonitis, equine abortion virus, or equine herpesvirus 1 (EHV-1). There are two strains of EHV-1, formerly classified as two separate viruses (EHV-1 and EHV-4). Both of these cause respiratory problems, nasal discharge, fever, coughing, and lack of appetite. Mares with EHV will abort, often in their seventh to tenth month of gestation. Mares that do not abort can produce foals with the virus, which quickly causes a severe respiratory infection, often killing the foals quickly. In severe outbreaks horses may become uncoordinated and partially or totally paralyzed in the hindquarters. Mares may or may not have genital lesions.

EHV-1 is very contagious, and it is increasing in incidence as horses are traveling more and more to shows, sales, breeding farms, races, and other equine events around the country and the world. If you suspect your horse has this problem, call your veterinarian to get a correct diagnosis. There is no treatment other than good nursing, antibiotics to help treat or prevent secondary infections, and aspirin to lower the fever.

All horses should be vaccinated yearly for EHV. However, this will not provide total protection, as a hot virus (one that has passed through several animals, gaining strength) can overcome even a vaccinated horse. Therefore, you should take good preventive measures at all times. Isolate all horses (and donkeys and mules) coming to your place for one month. This includes horses returning from equine events. House pregnant mares separately from horses that travel routinely, such as race horses and show horses. EHV is a serious problem in horses, and you should treat it with respect and caution. Once it's on your premises, it is very hard to get rid of.

Saddle Sores

Sores on the back are often caused by cheaply made saddles that are nailed together underneath. Other possible causes include debris under the saddle pad, wrinkles in the pad, and a pad that is crusted with sweat and dirt.

Pressure sores on the withers (at the base of the neck) are often caused by a saddle that sits too low on the withers. A saddletree built for a round-backed horse like a Quarter Horse will not fit a high-withered horse like a Saddlebred, no matter how many thick saddle pads you use.

If you don't often work your horse with a saddle on its back, it may get a sore near the elbow, where the girth passes around the barrel. The rubbing of the girth on the tender skin in the area causes a condition that is very similar to a blister on a human's heel from a pair of new shoes. To prevent this from happening, use the saddle for only short periods of time daily until the horse's skin toughens up. You can often "hurry" this time up a bit by soaking the spot with damp tea bags after every ride. While riding, check the area for any puffiness or soreness, as these are the first signs of a sore. If you see these signs, stop riding because further work will cause the sore to erupt.

To prevent saddle sores, always check a new saddle, no matter what it cost or how "pretty" it is, to be sure there are no nail heads underneath. Always use a clean pad and a clean girth, or cinch. Also, keep in mind that synthetic girths may cause sores in some horses due to the material's inability to breathe.

If you don't have time to brush the whole horse thoroughly before riding, at least brush the horse's back and sides as well as under the girth area. When placing the saddle on the back, always lay the saddle and pad a bit forward and then slide them back into place. This eliminates rough hair bunching up and causing sores. After you draw the girth tight, make sure there is no fold of skin bunched under it. If necessary, stretch the front legs out one at a time, as if shaking hands with the horse. This will pull the folds smooth.

The saddle should always be snug on the back. A saddle sliding back and forth will cause sores, just as too large a shoe will cause blisters on your foot. When riding in mountainous country, use a breast collar along with a britching if your saddle slips too far forward when riding down steep slopes.

If your horse does develop a saddle sore, the quickest cure is rest from the saddle. When you must work the horse, ride it bareback if possible. If you have to use the saddle, you could cut out part of a felt saddle pad around the sore spot and then use another pad over that one. But this is not advisable, because the pads do slip with use and the sore may become worse. As with many other conditions, prevention is much better than any treatment.

Scratches

Scratches, also called grease heel, occurs most often in the summer months. Suspect scratches if you see sores or roughness appear on the back of the horse's pastern. This condition is often confused with rope burns or cuts from fencing. But scratches often starts as dermatitis due to skin irritation caused by stubble, dry hard weeds, lime, gravel, or damp bedding. When the dermatitis becomes infected with a fungus or bacteria, the area becomes swollen, hot, and tender, and lameness often results. The area becomes crusted with dried serum, and the hair sticks stiffly outward.

Wash the affected area daily with warm, soapy water to loosen the crust. Clip the hair in the area short to keep it from irritating the skin. Using an astringent and antibiotic ointment alternately—three days with one and then three days with the other—usually clears up most cases quickly. If the condition does not improve after four days of home treatment or if it gets worse during that time, call your veterinarian; the horse may need systemic treatment with an antibiotic and cortisone.

Sprains

Due to their natural activity plus the work people give them, horses are quite prone to sprains. Often its speed and strength, not to mention its weight, work against a horse, and it becomes unbalanced. To regain balance, the horse overexerts and sprains a leg or shoulder. Like humans, the horse with a sprain will suddenly pull up lame. Soon you may be able to feel heat in the area of the sprain. Pressure on the spot will often cause the horse to flinch or pull its leg away.

With a fresh sprain, apply cold in the form of cold water or ice packs. Standing the horse in a cold stream or running a hose on the leg continuously for half an hour will help. To apply ice to a lower leg sprain, make an ice bag from a pant leg cut from an old pair of jeans by sewing the cuff end together. Slip the bag over the horse's hoof and up the leg, and then fill it with crushed ice. Alcohol, cooling liniment, and cortisone injections are also used to treat new sprains.

Once swelling has developed, apply heat instead of cold. Heat will increase circulation in the area and reduce swelling. Hot packs, heating liniment, and hot udder ointment work well. Apply these treatments at least twice a day. Massage will also bring relief. Rest the horse completely until it is sound again; then resume work very slowly.

Strangles

Strangles, or distemper, is also called shipping fever in horses because it often occurs after horses have been shipped or moved, such as to shows, tracks, sale barns, or trail rides. It is very contagious. The contagion spreads through contaminated water tanks, hay racks, and small pastures. An affected horse will often have a heavy mucous secretion from the nose, a cough, and a fever. You may also notice enlargement or abscess of the lymph glands under and between the jaws. This is where the disease gets the name strangles.

Completely isolate any horse you suspect may have strangles so it has no contact of any kind with other horses. This includes keeping it away from any water tank, pail, or pond accessible to healthy horses. Keep the sick horse in warm, draft-free surroundings, give it adequate feed and water, and watch it carefully for symptoms of distress or weakness.

Once the animal shows signs of sickness, there is not much you can do to stop the disease, but you should still call your veterinarian. Antibiotics, while not really a "cure" in this case, will help keep down secondary infections, such as pneumonia, in the already-stressed animal. Strangles in horses is about as severe as mumps in people. Although there have been fatalities, they are rare, and the disease is more one of misery than danger.

Prevention is very important. It's smart to vaccinate horses that will be traveling, but do this well in advance of traveling as it can produce an abscess at the injection site. (Vaccination will not always prevent strangles, but it will result in a milder case.) Isolate all new horses, including those that have traveled, for one month. When you are at equine events, do not let your horse drink from a community watering tank, and do not loan water or feed pails, bridles, or hay nets to others unless you thoroughly wash and disinfect them afterward. Remember that a horse can spread strangles before really appearing sick.

Swamp Fever

Swamp fever, also known as equine infectious anemia (EIA), is caused by a virus. It is spread by biting insects or by accidentally injecting minute amounts of virulent blood (as when using an old, nonsterile syringe and needle). The most common outbreaks occur at racetracks, show stables, and breeding farms. This is the reason why many states require traveling horses to have their blood tested with the Coggins test and many breeding farms and trainers require blood tests before accepting horses.

There are several forms of the disease: acute, subacute, and inactive. Acute EIA develops suddenly, producing high fever, weakness, incoordination, and quick death. Subacute EIA is less severe and appears in a series of "attacks"—the horse may just seem to be a "poor doer." Inactive EIA is perhaps the most dangerous phase, as the horse usually is sick only once and then appears well for the rest of its life while remaining a carrier to other horses in the area.

There is no treatment or vaccination for EIA, and it can spread very fast through a barnful of horses. Any new horses, even those visiting for a week or so, should have had a recent negative Coggins test before they are brought to the farm. Destroy infected horses, or isolate them completely and permanently in an insect-proof stable and take aggressive measures to reduce biting insects in the area. This protects neighboring equines from infection from the isolated animals.

Tetanus

Tetanus is a too-common problem in horses as they are highly susceptible to the organism that causes it and they often sustain injuries that encourage its growth. The tetanus organism is anaerobic, meaning that it grows in the absence of oxygen; so a deep wound or a puncture wound provides the ideal incubator. The first signs of tetanus are usually stiffness in the limbs and refusal to eat. The nictitating membrane, or third eyelid, is often prominent.

Treatment is nearly useless unless started very early in the course of the disease, usually before obvious signs are seen. Systemic treatment with antitoxin and antibiotics in massive doses sometimes works. But the real "cure" is prevention. Every horse should receive an annual tetanus toxoid booster—which prevents most tetanus in hidden injuries—plus an injection of tetanus antitoxin in the event of a known injury or puncture wound. And always keep nails, wire, pitchforks, and machinery away from horses. One tiny poke from a small nail can be the start of a terrible death for a horse. (For more information on this problem, see "Puncture Wounds" on page 218.)

Warts

Warts are sometimes a problem on horses, and as they are caused by a virus, they are often quite contagious. You'll most often see them on the muzzle and face. Although warts are seldom very injurious, they can be a problem affecting the usefulness of the animal. Warts rubbed by the bridle or bit can irritate the horse to the point of making it uncomfortable and hard to control. Warts, of course, also spoil the looks of a show horse. And it is at shows and fairs that many outbreaks occur. Never borrow tack or pails for water and feed. And never stable your horse next to or across from one with warts.

The only treatment that seems to work well on most horses is the use of wart vaccine. Often, one injection will effect a cure, but sometimes a repeat injection is necessary two weeks later. Ask your veterinarian for his recommendations.

West Nile Virus

West Nile Virus first occurred in the United States in 1999. It is spread by mosquitoes and carried by birds. West Nile Virus causes swelling of the brain in horses (and occasionally people bitten by affected mosquitoes), which shows as dullness, incoordination, facial paralysis (drooping eye lids, lip), sleepiness, and death. There is no cure, other than supportive treatment.

West Nile Virus can be prevented by keeping insects from horses by use of sprays, stabling during heavy mosquito periods, and vaccination. The one problem with vaccination is that it is not 100 percent sure to prevent the disease and that once vaccinated, the horse's blood will test positive for West Nile Virus when tested in the future. Therefore, a vaccinated horse exhibiting symptoms similar to West Nile Virus can not be tested with accuracy. However, in ares with West Nile Virus present, vaccination is definitely your best option. Consult your veterinarian about the prevalence of this disease in your area.

Worms

A horse can be quite severely infested with worms and show few or no symptoms visible to the naked eye. A wormy horse may look slick and shiny and be full of spirit, or it can look dopey and rough. The only sure way to know your horse is not wormy is to have your veterinarian check a sample of its manure. Many people develop a false sense of security by worming routinely, several times a year, without having a fecal sample tested. However, some worms develop resistance to many commonly used wormers after a period of time, making those wormers nearly useless. And some wormers get only a few kinds of worms, leaving others to cause harm. If a horse is not doing well, don't just assume it must be wormy and proceed to dose it. Worm medicine is toxic and can kill a sick horse. And, please, if your horse is wormy, use a wormer that will kill the worms it does have, not just something you got cheap at a local store!

Three basic types of wormers are commonly used: liquid given by stomach tube, products to be mixed with the feed, and—most frequently used—paste wormers. Some products will kill bots as well as most other common worms; others just hit bots or one or two worms. Unless you have had some experience in choosing wormers, it would be wise to consult your veterinarian for advice. He can help you set up a routine worming schedule to benefit your horses in addition to providing yearly fecal examinations.

Ascarids

These are the large worms sometimes seen in the manure. They resemble bean sprouts and are from 5 to 8 inches long. Ascarids, or roundworms, cause the most damage in young horses, mainly foals. An affected foal will not do well and may slowly go downhill, showing loss of appetite and activity, unthriftiness, and a potbelly.

Bots

These are fairly large, grublike worms (actually fly larvae of the bot fly) that attach themselves to the stomach lining. During summer and fall, the adult flies lay their eggs on the hairs of the legs and belly of the horse. Here they remain, tightly fastened, until they are ingested by the horse and end up in the stomach, where they attach themselves and cause their damage. They pit and scar the lining of the stomach, sometimes causing colic and perforation of the stomach, resulting in peritonitis, which is often fatal. If the horse is not wormed, the larvae are passed in the manure, settle into the ground, and later emerge as adult flies, ready to lay more eggs and continue the cycle.

To prevent a large amount of bots from entering the stomach, remove the bot eggs from the hair daily. Scraping the area with a hacksaw blade or bot block works well and does a fast job. Then after the first hard freeze of the fall, give your horse a wormer effective against bots. A fecal examination now is a good idea, not for the bots but for other parasites. (Since you will be worming anyway, you could rid your horse of any other parasites it has at the same time by using a combination wormer.)

Pinworms

Pinworms cause intense itching around the anus, leading the horse to rub its buttocks on a fence, tree, or anything else handy. The hair across the buttocks and on the tail soon becomes scanty and rough. There may be a yellowish crust around the anus. (Check thoroughly for lice around the dock as they can also produce these symptoms.) Pinworms seldom cause much actual damage, but their presence is annoying to both the horse and the owner. Occasionally the horse will develop a secondary infection, bacterial or fungal, when the area becomes raw and irritated.

Strongyles

This fairly large group of worms is divided into two groups: large and small strongyles. These worms are smaller than ascarids and bots and less often seen in the manure. They do, however, present a danger to your horse. They migrate through the bloodstream, causing scarring of the vessel walls, occasional colic, aneurysm, and thrombosis. Some horses get down and are unable to rise owing to migrations of strongyles blocking off the blood flow in the hind legs. These parasites also cause anemia and damage to the liver, lungs, and heart. It has been estimated that between 70 and 80 percent of all horses are infested to some degree with a type of strongyles.

Other Parasites

Horses can become infested with several other intestinal parasites, including tapeworm, *Habronema*, lungworm, and liver fluke. To be safe, have your veterinarian give your horse a yearly checkup. Most internal parasites can be diagnosed and treated successfully with a fecal exam and the correct wormer.

PIGS

General Care and Management

Pigs have a reputation for being dirty animals, but this is not true. In fact, given the chance, they are among the cleanest of all farm animals. It's just that they are often housed in pens where they are unable to remain clean. Pigs will naturally pick one area for their "toilet" and use that spot only. They will not manure in their food or lie in filth, if given anywhere else to lie.

Housing

Pigs are quite easy to house since all they require is a snug, draft-free, dry area. You can keep them in a stall in a barn, with access to an outside yard or pasture, or in an elaborate hog house complete with custom farrowing pens and slatted floors. As long as the pig is warm in the winter and cool in the summer, has dry bedding, and is given good food and plenty of fresh, clean water, it will do well.

Indoor Pens

Pigs are strong animals; so when building a hog pen or fence, be sure to make it strong. One-inch lumber or flimsy plywood will not hold a pig, nor will saggy woven wire or an old, rotten board fence. Build the inside pen of 2-inch lumber, and nail it together with 16-penny spikes. Nail the boards on the *inside* of the posts as pigs are strong enough to root the boards right off the nails. Stretch all woven wire fencing as tight as possible, with a strand of barbed wire at the top and bottom, also stretched tightly.

Farrowing Pens

A farrowing pen should be at least 8 feet square for average-sized sows and larger for very big sows. Sometimes it is better to have a longer, rectangular pen for more protection for the little pigs. There should be a railing around the inside walls of the pen, 10 inches high and 10 inches away from the walls, to offer protection to the new pigs. Otherwise, the mother could flop down in a position that would pin the pigs to the wall, crushing them. This railing must be strongly constructed of pipe or hardwood and bolts.

It is a good idea to block off one corner or end of the pen and hang a heat lamp into it. This offers a refuge for the little pigs to go to soon after birth to keep warm, dry off, and stay out of the sow's way while she has the other pigs. This nursery corner saves many young pigs from being flopped down on, chilled, or stepped on. Be very careful to protect the lamp from breakage as many fires are caused by fallen or damaged heat lamps.

Disinfect the farrowing pen thoroughly before moving the sow into it, and lay down a good deep layer of fresh bedding (such as 4 to 6 inches of sawdust or shavings).

PARTS OF A HOG

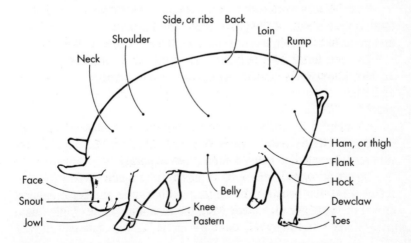

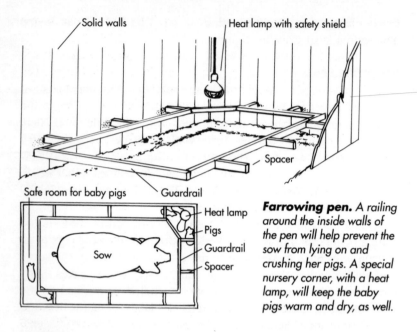

Solid walls

Heat lamp with safety shield

Spacer

Safe room for baby pigs

Guardrail

Heat lamp

Pigs

Guardrail

Sow

Spacer

Farrowing pen. *A railing around the inside walls of the pen will help prevent the sow from lying on and crushing her pigs. A special nursery corner, with a heat lamp, will keep the baby pigs warm and dry, as well.*

Outdoor Areas

Electric fences will contain many pigs, but make them of barbed wire. String the two strands about 18 inches apart, with the lowest strand about 12 inches off the ground. "Train" each pig to the fence by placing a pan of feed on the other side of the wire, leaving it for the pig to learn the shocking power of those little wires.

Board fences work well for hogs if you use solid boards and place them on the inside of the posts. Make the fence at least 3 feet high, and preferably higher, as some pigs vault a 3-foot fence like athletes.

The best fence for pigs is made of sturdy posts and hog panels—16-foot-long panels made of welded steel rods. They are very strong and easy to work with, last a very long time, and are truly "hog-proof."

It's helpful to have movable houses for your pigs so you can move your pigs from one pasture or yard to another. This lets the pasture recover and also helps control internal parasites.

Do not allow different sizes of pigs to run together. Many injuries result from this because the larger pigs boss the smaller ones and crowd the younger pigs away from the feed and shade. A pig has a powerful jaw and a good sharp set of teeth that can cause severe damage.

If the pig has a pasture area or roots up its yard badly, you will need to ring it. Ringing pigs is simple and similar to getting pierced ears yourself. Buy a box of rings and a ringer (both inexpensive) at a hardware or farm supply store. Restrain the pig; with a ring in the ringer, position the ringer above the nostril, on the edge of the rooter. (The rooter is the hard ridge of cartilage that the pig roots with.) Quickly close the ringer, and the ring sinks into place. The most effective method of ringing is to place one or two rings above each nostril. Be careful not to ring so deep that the bone is scraped, because this can cause infection. Ringing makes it uncomfortable for the pig to root. Although rooting is natural behavior, it will quickly ruin a good pasture and cause holes in the yard, which will quickly fill up with rainwater, making a real mess.

Feeding

It is true that you can feed pigs on garbage, but keep in mind that the quality of the food will be the quality of the meat and the little pigs they produce. This is not to say that you can't feed your potato peel-

First Aid Kit for Swine

Here's a basic list of items to keep on hand for caring for pigs. Anyone with a pig should at least have the items marked with an asterisk. If you breed pigs, it's smart to have all the items below on hand. There are many other things you could add to this kit; ask your veterinarian for his recommendations.

Betadine*

Forceps/needle holder

Heat lamp or pig heat mat

Hog ring pliers and rings

Pig obstetrical forceps

Pig tooth nippers

Rectal veterinary
    thermometer*

Scalpel and blades

Scarlet oil*

Three 18-gauge, 1½-inch
    needles*

12-cc syringe*

Veterinarian's phone
    number*

ings or stale bread and garden waste to your pigs, but a balanced diet is just as important in raising pigs as any other animal. Use table and garden scraps only as an addition to their regular feed.

You can successfully raise pigs on a wide variety of feeds and combinations of feeds, but the thing to remember is the value and use of each feed. Corn is useful for fattening hogs that are nearing the slaughter size of 250 pounds, but corn alone is not an adequate diet for growing pigs or breeding stock. They need protein for growth and reproduction, carbohydrates for warmth and weight gain, and vitamins and minerals to ensure good health. A good book to consult when looking for a balanced ration to fit your particular area is *Feeds and Feeding* by Frank B. Morrison. You can also pay a visit to your county Cooperative Extension Agent (usually located in your county seat). The agent can give you information on a good feeding program for your area and will have many free booklets on various aspects of pigs, as well.

Pigs benefit from access to good pasture, which they seldom get these days. But quality pasture makes for healthier pigs, carrying less body fat and more muscle; this is a good thing today, with folks becoming more and more health conscious. Plus, it is more economical: Your pigs will get a lot of feed on a good pasture, so you won't have to buy as much dry feed. Rape, alfalfa, clover, and rye are all good choices for pasture crops. Pigs will also eat good-quality legume hay fed free-choice (as much as they'll clean up). They also enjoy having skim milk or whey added to their dry food, and these materials are very beneficial.

Restraint

Pigs are often difficult to restrain effectively without the proper pig-handling equipment. If you keep many pigs, a good pig crate with a head gate is a necessity. If you raise only a few pigs, however, you can get by using ropes or gates for occasional restraint. A fairly large pig can be restrained by slipping a rope noose around the upper jaw, behind the tusks,

Restraint with a noose. *To restrain a fairly large pig, slip a rope noose around the snout, behind the tusks. Fasten the rope about 1 to 2 feet above the ground on a sturdy post.*

and then fastening it to a sturdy post about a foot or so from the ground. When tied, the pig will most often back up against the rope and be held for treatment. Crowding a pig into a corner using a strong, portable gate about the same length and height as the pig also works well for examination and treatment that is not extensive.

The easiest way to restrain little pigs is to hold them up by their hind legs, with their front feet just off the ground. For operations such as rupture repair and castration, have an assistant hold the pig upside down by the back legs and brace the animal between the knees or lay the pig on its back in a V-shaped trough.

Restraint with a rope. *A rope-throwing rig is handy when you need to restrain a large pig. Slowly pull on the free end of the rope to bring the pig down, and have an assistant hold onto the rope while you treat the animal.*

A very large boar may be restrained for castration by using a 55-gallon drum with one end cut out. Withhold feed for a day, giving only water. The next day, with two or three strong helpers present, carry the empty drum to the boar's yard. Place some feed in the closed end of the barrel. When the boar dives in after the feed, have your assistants tip the barrel up on end, leaving the boar ready for surgery. If necessary, you can restrain the boar further using a block and tackle and

Restraint with hobbles. *Another way to restrain a large pig is with hobbles. Restrain the front end of the animal with a noose, then attach the hobbles to the back legs, and pull to turn the pig on its side.*

ropes, although having one person hold each hind leg is usually enough restraint for castration.

A large hog can also be restrained with a rope-throwing rig or hobbles. Both of these methods provide secure restraint for longer times. If you need to get a hog into confined quarters for treatment or if you need to haul it to your veterinarian, you can often drive it into a trailer by slipping a bushel basket over its head and backing it up the ramp.

Breeding

Understanding the breeding cycles of your pigs is important if you want to make money. It will also help you save money by avoiding unnecessary veterinary calls.

Boars

When choosing a boar, either for service or to buy, keep in mind how you plan to use his offspring. You will want pigs with strong legs, meaty shoulders, and large hams. And you will want a long pig, with plenty of lean bacon and pork chops. A very fat boar will likely sire fat-prone pigs, which are not desirable for today's health-conscious consumers. If you're raising gilts (young female pigs), you'll want a boar that produces gilts with at least 12, and preferably 14, functioning teats. (These characteristics are passed from the boar as well as the sow or gilt.) The boar should also have a good disposition. It is no excuse to say the boar is mean "because he's a boar."

Never use a boar for breeding that has unevenly developed testicles or is ruptured (with testicles that appear extralarge and quite flabby). The tendency to rupture is an inherited factor and greatly reduces the sale value of the young pigs. Do not keep a boar from a litter that has had a ruptured pig in it or from future breedings of the same bloodlines.

A boar is generally ready for light service at about seven months of age, but this depends on the boar's development and previous care.

Gilts and Sows

A gilt is a young female pig that has not farrowed or has just farrowed her first litter. When she is ready to have her second litter, she is no longer a gilt but a sow.

There is controversy among pig raisers over whether it is more profitable to breed gilts, raise a litter, and then sell them and buy more gilts or to retain them and keep breeding them as sows. Gilts tend to have fewer and slightly smaller pigs, but they are safer mothers: A big, heavy sow has a tendency to lie on her pigs, crushing or smothering them. Also, a gilt is often cheaper to buy, and she increases in value as she farrows and gains weight. The older sow is usually a better milker, however, and she is more predictable as far as production goes. It is easier to make a close guess as to how many pigs she will have and the quality of them as they grow older.

Whether you choose a sow or a gilt, you may be able to raise two litters a year from her. In fact, with very good management, you can have them farrow every four to five months. This requires excellent care, good records, and good facilities.

Sows come into heat every three weeks and three to five days after their litter is weaned. Sows should be "flushed" two weeks before breeding. This means putting them on full feed and usually lush pasture so they are rapidly gaining weight when they are bred. This increases ovulation, which means the sow will bear more baby pigs.

A sow shows her heat by riding other sows, grunting, and urinating frequently. She may often show a red, swollen vulva. She will also stand quietly when you press a hand on her back, provided a boar is nearby. Take her to the boar as soon as you notice her heat so she'll be settled down by the time she's bred. After breeding, the sow needs a high-protein ration, at least a 13 percent supplement. Give her all the top-quality pasture or alfalfa hay she will eat, along with a trace mineral supplement. Plenty of fresh, clean water is a must as this will add to her condition and help make milk. Do *not* overfeed during the first 30 days of her pregnancy, however, because this is suspected to cause embryo death.

Farrowing

Three months, 3 weeks, and 3 days (114 days) after breeding, the sow will be ready to farrow. A week before she is due, clean her off thoroughly. Washing her udders well with warm, soapy water will help prevent parasite infestation of new pigs. Move her gently to a farrowing pen, as she will need time to settle down and become accustomed to her new surroundings to be ready to take care of her new pigs. Sows that eat, lie on, or disown their pigs are often sows that have been upset just prior to farrowing.

If at all possible, you should be present at farrowing time. Gather some supplies, including several clean, dry towels, a small wide-mouthed jar of iodine, a pair of side cutters (for trimming the teeth of the young pigs), a pair of scissors, and a spool of thread.

A sow will usually work for 15 to 30 minutes to produce the first pig in the litter. Most often the following pigs will come faster. If the sow works for longer than half an hour on a pig, failing to make any progress, she should be examined. A person with a small hand should scrub up well, lubricate the hand and arm with liquid dish soap, and check the progress of the pig. If it seems lodged, gentle but firm traction will often bring it out. If this does not work, call your veterinarian as too much work on a lodged pig can exhaust the sow and cause the death of one or more pigs. Sometimes a forceps delivery is necessary. There are special baby pig forceps that can be a great aid, in skillful hands. Many people who raise pigs in great numbers keep a pair in their first aid box. But if you are not experienced, call your veterinarian. In some cases all that is needed is an injection of posterior pituitary, which helps the sow deliver her pigs normally.

Some sows require a tranquilizer shortly after farrowing: They become agitated and thrash about, trying to escape their pigs or eat them. In such cases it's best to take the pigs away until the tranquilizer is working, to prevent further excitement and injury to the babies.

Caring for Baby Pigs

As the pigs are born, it is a good idea to clean each one, dip the navel in iodine, clip the sharp needle teeth to prevent injury to the sow's udder, and place the pig under the heat lamp until labor is finished. If the umbilical cord is long, tie it off an inch or so from the pig's belly with strong thread, and then cut off the rest, leaving a stump 2 inches long. Dip this stump in iodine.

To prevent anemia, which is quite common in baby pigs, give the young pigs an iron supplement orally, by injection, or by painting the preparation on the sow's udder. Allow baby pigs access to a heat lamp for two weeks. At two weeks of age, they will usually begin to eat enough grain or pelleted feed to give them a free-choice creep-fed ration. (See "Creep-Feeding Lambs" on page 153 for more information on setting up a creep-feeding system.) Adding skim milk to a little ground pig starter will encourage week-old pigs to start nibbling at feed. At first they will walk in it and play with it more than eat it, but soon they will be making short work of the mash and be ready to start pellets. From the pellets they easily graduate to a good mixed growing ration, and they are ready to wean when eight weeks old.

(For problems related to breeding and farrowing, see "Anemia" on page 241, "Failure to Let Down Milk" and "Hypocalcemia" on page 243, and "Mastitis" on page 245.)

Castration

All male pigs—except those you plan to save for breeding boars—should be castrated between the ages of one and five weeks. At this age there is very little, if any, setback and very little bleeding, shock, or pain. The meat of an adult boar is rank and just about inedible to most people. Therefore, for home use as well as for future sales, a barrow (castrated male pig) is much more valuable for meat than a boar. (Actually, you can have it both ways, if you desire: I have often kept a young boar to breed one or two sows and then, after they were safely pregnant, castrated him, raised him to butchering weight, and put the meat in the freezer.)

To castrate a small pig, first gather your supplies: a pail of warm, soapy water, a bottle of antiseptic, a wash cloth, and a towel. Also have a sharp instrument—a scalpel, single-edged razor blade, or sharp pocketknife—sterilized and ready. Have an assistant hold up the young pig by the hind legs, with the belly outward; you stand facing the pig.

Scrub the area with the soapy water, and dry it. With one hand push the testicles toward the belly and outward against the skin. Make an incision in the scrotum over a testicle, grasp the testicle, and pull it out as far as the cord will allow. In small pigs you can pull the cord until it snaps. With larger pigs cut the cord very close to the body so that when you release the tension, the stump pulls back into the incision. (If you cut the cord with a scraping motion instead of a clean cut, there will be less bleeding.) Be sure you also remove all of the tunic (the tough white membrane surrounding the testicle), and do not leave any of it sticking out through the incision. Otherwise, healing will be incomplete and lead to a condition called scirrhous cord. In this condition the scrotum fills with fibrous tissue, which must be dissected away from the skin and body tissue with the fin-

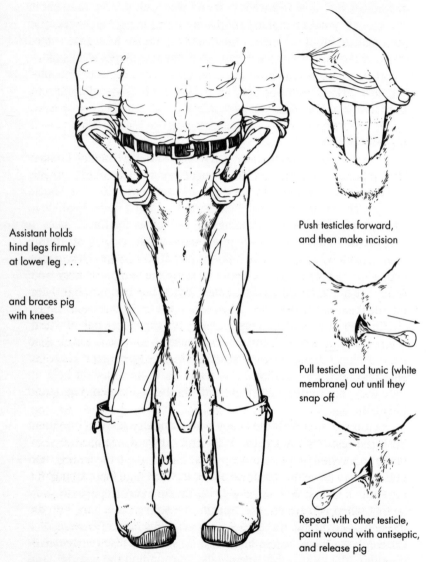

Assistant holds
hind legs firmly
at lower leg . . .

and braces pig
with knees

Push testicles forward,
and then make incision

Pull testicle and tunic (white
membrane) out until they
snap off

Repeat with other testicle,
paint wound with antiseptic,
and release pig

Castrating a pig. *It's best to castrate male pigs when they are one to five weeks old. While an assistant holds the pig, wash the scrotum with soapy water, and dry it. Push the testicles forward, make the incisions with a sharp, sterilized instrument, and pull out each testicle and tunic until the cord snaps. Treat the wound with antiseptic before releasing the animal.*

gers to prevent hemorrhage. It is a miserable, finger-cramping job that no veterinarian enjoys.

After castration be sure the incisions are large enough: across the entire bottom of the scrotum over each testicle and a bit up each side. If you make too small an incision, the skin will close up before healing is complete, and infection or tetanus may occur. Also, be sure to pour in some antiseptic after castration, such as Betadine. If you castrate during fly season, consider using a fly repellent to prevent maggots. Scarlet oil works well for this because it repels flies as well as prevents infection.

Large boars should be castrated by your veterinarian, as it takes more experience to handle a large animal and the use of an emasculator to prevent bleeding.

The Ruptured Pig

Once in a while, you may run across a ruptured pig at castrating time. With a ruptured pig, often one testicle will be larger and feel softer than the other. Sometimes both testicles will appear large and sloppy. The enlargement and softness are due to the fact that there are intestines in the scrotum along with the testicle. And sometimes you do not have warning of a rupture until you castrate the pig—and a few minutes later, you find the intestines sticking out or dragging behind the pig. It is a shocking surprise but seldom fatal if you discover it at once.

If this happens, the inguinal canal must be sewn closed after the intestines are cleaned and pushed back into the body. Some hog raisers simply castrate as usual and sew the scrotum shut to contain the intestines. This works in some cases but may still lower the market price if the rupture is large, making the pig look "entire." Or worse, it may allow the strangulation of the intestinal loop, killing the pig. For this reason, it is safest either to take a ruptured pig in to your veterinarian for castration and immediate repair or to sell the pig "as is" at an early market and take the lower price. If you raise many litters of pigs, ask your veterinarian to show you how to correctly repair a rupture.

The tendency to rupture is an inherited defect. It's best never to use a boar out of a litter that contained even one ruptured pig and never to choose a replacement gilt out of that litter. Once rupture is a part of your herd, it is hard to get rid of it, and it is much easier to routinely castrate baby pigs without the worry and headache of having to repair ruptures.

DISEASES AND OTHER PROBLEMS

Learning about the diseases and injuries that are likely to affect your pigs will help you avoid many common problems. In addition, you'll be more apt to notice and deal with problems that *do* occur before they become life-threatening. It's also important to know the normal temperature of your pig so you can check for fever or other abnormalities. The normal body temperature of a pig is 101° to 102.5°F (38.3° to 39.2°C).

Sample Vaccination Schedule for Swine

Generally, the more swine you have, the more stringent vaccination schedule you need due to the movement and introduction of new animals to the place. Here's a suggested vaccination schedule, but keep in mind that other diseases can also be a problem if you live in certain areas. For this reason, you should ask your veterinarian to recommend a vaccination program based on your situation and location.

	DISEASE	WHEN TO VACCINATE
GILTS BEFORE BREEDING	Leptospirosis Parvovirus Erysipelas	Twice before breeding
SOWS BEFORE BREEDING	Leptospirosis Parvovirus (at weening) Erysipelas	Twice before breeding
BOARS	Leptospirosis Parvovirus Erysipelas	Twice a year

	DISEASE	WHEN TO VACCINATE
GILTS	E. Coli Atophic rhinitis	Twice before farrowing
SOWS	E. Coli Atophic rhinitis	Before farrowing
BABY PIGS	Atophic rhinitis	Once or twice before weaning
FEEDER PIGS	Erysipelas (40-100#)	When purchased as feeder pigs

Anemia

No matter how much iron supplement you feed to a sow, milk is naturally low in iron, so young pigs are prone to anemia when they are mainly on a milk diet. Anemia is a costly condition, for once pigs become anemic, they don't gain as well as pigs that have been given iron injections or oral iron supplements. They are also stressed, making them prone to diseases and other problems, such as *Escherichia coli* infection, parasite infestation, and weakness.

Anemic pigs will at first look like the best pigs in the litter: very plump and round. But unfortunately, this is not fat or healthy tissue but edema due to poor circulation.

To prevent anemia, give new pigs oral iron, swab the sow's udder daily with an iron-and-honey or -molasses mixture, or give the babies iron injections. Once the pigs have access to pasture or green feed, the danger is greatly reduced.

Brucellosis

Brucellosis in pigs is caused by the organism *Brucella suis.* It not only affects pigs but also can infect cattle and humans. (This is not, however, the brucellosis commonly affecting cattle—that is *B. abortus,* causing so-called Bang's disease.) Pigs affected with brucellosis will abort, have weak pigs that often die, show lameness, or even have hindquarter paralysis. Some affected boars show swollen testicles.

There is no treatment for brucellosis other than slaughter. Test all new pigs when you bring them to your place, or make sure they come from a brucellosis-free herd. Do not just accept the owner's word for the health status of the herd: See the paperwork. Many brucellosis-infected herds do not show any obvious signs of the disease.

If you have a boar standing for service, make sure all sows or gilts brought in by others have tested free of brucellosis before breeding. And do not loan out your boar to another's herd unless that herd is brucellosis-free.

Coccidiosis

While not a severe problem in swine, coccidiosis can give trouble in certain locales. It is caused by protozoa (one-celled animals) that are parasites invading the intestine. Coccidia cause unthriftiness, diarrhea, and stunted growth. This condition is most common in damp, dirty pens or hog lots.

If you suspect coccidiosis or if your pigs are just not doing as well as they should, take a fecal sample from several animals to your veterinarian for examination under a microscope. He will check for coccidiosis as well as other internal parasites and suggest the proper treatment. In many cases you can greatly reduce the incidence of coccidiosis by moving your pigs to clean, dry pens, feeding a good, balanced diet, and treating the animals with intestinal sulfas or nitrofurazone.

Prevention of consists of extreme cleanliness coupled with routine fecal examinations. Never allow fecal contamination of feed or water containers. (Contamination is particularly a problem with trough-type feeders. It's best to use feeders of the self-feeding type, with a lid that automatically falls shut when the pigs are not eating. Similar styles of waterers are available.) If manure does get into the feeder or waterer, flush it out well with water. Keep pens dry and well bedded. Rotate pastures frequently, and do not allow the pigs to congregate in muddy, manure-covered yards.

Erysipelas

Erysipelas can be a serious problem in young pigs in many locales. With the acute form of the disease, death may be quick, from one to four days after the first signs appear. Infected pigs will have a high temperature, be in pain, squeal, and show diamond-shaped purple blotches on the sides, belly, and back. After the disease has run its course, sometimes these diamond-shaped lesions will slough off. Following an acute attack, some of the pigs that have survived will become carriers, being chronically infected with the organism, which lives in the joints or heart.

If identified early, erysipelas treatment is often successful, so call your veterinarian right away if you suspect this problem. Penicillin and serum are both used, either alone or in combination. But, as with many diseases, it is safer and more economical to vaccinate against erysipelas than to gamble treating it. If there has been erysipelas in your area, consult your veterinarian about a vaccination program.

Escherichia coli

While *Escherichia coli* is a normal gut bacterium, stressful conditions can cause it to multiply quickly. This usually results in severe diarrhea, weakness, and death. This is a serious problem and causes many sudden deaths in a litter of pigs. Prompt diagnosis by your veterinarian and treatment with antibiotics and electrolytes may save the affected pigs.

Prevention consists of reducing stress on baby pigs. This includes keeping them warm with heat lamps or special pig heating pads, following strict sanitation practices, vaccinating sows before farrowing, and giving baby pigs oral doses of *E. coli* antigen. Talk to your veterinarian, and develop an *E. coli* prevention program tailored to your situation and location.

Failure to Let Down Milk

Some sows fail to let their milk down after farrowing, due either to excitement and stress or to a hormone imbalance. If you do not notice the problem in time, the little pigs will either starve or become so stressed that they develop scours (diarrhea) or other problems. Common signs to look for are pigs that squeal, root the udders, and move about from teat to teat, hunting for better pickings.

When you discover this problem, call your veterinarian at once. Very often an injection of posterior pituitary will cause her to drop her milk down almost immediately. Once the milk flow has started, she will milk normally. If the sow has no milk, however, such an injection will not make her produce milk. In this case you must switch the baby pigs to a foster mother or else bottle-raise them. If you try a foster mother, daubing Vicks VapoRub on the new mother's nose as well as the babies' backs may help her accept the new pigs, but still watch her carefully for several hours to avoid injury to the babies.

Hypocalcemia

Hypocalcemia, also known as posterior paralysis, is seen in heavy milking sows with large, thrifty litters, usually just before or at weaning time. By this time the pigs weigh from 25 to 30 pounds each, and when multiplied by 10 or 12 pigs, you may have the equivalent of a 300-plus-pound pig sucking a 250-pound sow! The sow becomes thin trying to keep milk for her pigs. When most of the calcium has been drawn out of her blood and bone, she will "sit down" and become completely paralyzed in the rear quarters. She will then go off her feed and die.

If you catch the problem early, just weaning the pigs will effect a cure. But once the sow's hind legs become quite weak, she will need treatment by your veterinarian to live. Intravenous or intraperitoneal calcium often works well. Good nursing is also important. If the sow is left in the sun without feed or water, she will just give up and die, regardless of treatment. Special feed additions, such as milk, greens, and bread, will help perk her up as the calcium takes effect. If you let the sow go too long, no amount of treatment will enable her to recover.

To prevent hypocalcemia, make sure the sow receives an adequate diet with a calcium-mineral supplement. Creep-feeding the pigs, especially with large litters, helps keep them from draining her physically. Hungry pigs are always nursing, trying to fill up. But if they have adequate feed available, they will nurse less, which will in turn help the sow. Early weaning of very large, husky litters can also help prevent hypocalcemia.

Lice

Lice sometimes infest pigs. They are most often a problem during the winter, when the pigs do not have access to sunlight. Lice are grayish parasites that you can see with the naked eye if you look closely. Infested pigs will scratch, appear restless, and not do as well as they could. A severe infestation of lice can cause severe anemia and death.

If you find lice on one of your pigs, it is a good idea to thoroughly check any others in the building. There are many effective louse powders on the market. Be sure to read the label before buying, to make sure it is safe for pigs (and you!). Most powders made for dairy cattle are safe enough for swine. I prefer to use a rotenone or pyrethrin powder. Powder the animals weekly for three weeks to kill all the lice as they hatch and before they can reproduce.

Mange

Mange is the most extensive external parasitic condition in swine. It leads to weight loss through irritation and intense itching. Mange is caused by tiny mites—most commonly sarcoptic mites—which burrow into the skin. They are not visible to the naked eye. The first sign that your pigs may have mange is when they constantly rub their ears and then later their sides and body on anything available. If left untreated, the hair may be rubbed off, and red, scabby areas may form. When suspecting mange in your pigs, contact your veterinarian. He can take a skin scraping for positive diagnosis. You'd be surprised at the number of cases of "mange" that turn out to be something else entirely.

If you have recently had a mange problem on your place, treat sows and gilts for mange before breeding them. Ivermectin, a systemic treatment for parasites, is very effective. Also, ask your veterinarian to recommend a spray you can use to treat the pens and the pigs. Spray the farrowing pens, let them dry, and then scrub them with hot water and soap before moving the sows into them. Spray or inject pigs for mange soon after weaning. Then watch them carefully, and repeat the treatment, if necessary.

Mange is very contagious and should be prevented at all costs. Thoroughly examine any new pigs you bring home, and isolate new additions to your herd, including any that have been away for breeding, shows, or sales, for one month. Immediately isolate any pig you suspect has mange, and watch the others closely.

Mastitis

Occasionally a sow will develop mastitis (inflammation of the mammary gland) in one or more of her udders after farrowing. It may be caused by an injury, such as banging the udder on a low doorway, lying on cold cement, or strenuous nursing (especially by young pigs that have not had their sharp teeth clipped at birth). There is usually a bacterial infection present. The udder will become hot and red, and it may be swollen or painful to the sow. She will often run a degree or more of fever, and her milk will often look abnormal. Many sows will go off their feed and act sick.

Systemic treatment with a broad-spectrum antibiotic along with hot packs and warm udder ointment or liniment will help, as will massaging the affected udder and manually removing the milk. Consult with your veterinarian if the mastitis does not improve in two days' time or if the sow gets worse with treatment.

Necrotic Enteritis

Necrotic enteritis, also known as necro, refers to the inflammation and decay of the intestinal tissue. It is caused by bacterial infection or, more often, by dietary deficiency.

Low-protein diets (such as straight corn) are usually the main cause of nonbacterial enteritis. This problem is most common in pigs from weaning to four or five months old. Affected pigs have a lack of appetite, lack of energy, high temperature, and diarrhea. To alleviate this condition, improve the diet, giving a high-protein feed with vitamin B complex supplements. Giving antibiotics or sulfa drugs will help take care of any secondary bacterial infection.

Another type of necrotic enteritis is caused by *Clostridium perfringens* Type C. It affects primarily baby pigs from one day to three weeks old. The first sign is a bloody, profuse diarrhea, followed by sudden death. There is no treatment. Prevention of *C. perfringens* Type C necrotic enteritis consists of vaccinating sows before farrowing and yearly thereafter. Consult with your veterinarian to establish a vaccination program. It is inexpensive and will probably save you many dollars in lost baby pigs if you raise hogs in large numbers.

Pneumonia

Pneumonia can be caused by a bacterial, viral, or fungal infection or simply by inhaling a foreign material, such as dust (commonly sawdust or barn dust). Pneumonia causes many pig deaths—more so, nationwide, than a handful of diseases together. Not all pigs die from pneumonia, especially when they get treatment. But many become like a person with severe emphysema, gasping for breath at the slightest exertion or upon exposure to dust or hot, humid weather. A pig in this condition cannot make decent weight gain or be a productive breeding animal.

A pig with acute pneumonia will act distressed. It may go off its feed suddenly, run a high temperature, and be reluctant to move about. As pneumonia is often very contagious, you should isolate the sick pig in a warm, draft-free pen and call your veterinarian at once. When caught fairly early, there is a good chance of recovery. The longer pneumonia is left untreated, the more scar tissue forms in the lungs and the greater the chances are for death or incomplete recovery. Systemic treatment with a broad-spectrum antibiotic or sulfa combination often works well. If the pig is not coughing enough to raise the congestion in the lungs, an injectable expectorant may be used.

Pleuropneumonia, a very severe and dangerous form of pneumonia, is common in pigs. This pneumonia is caused by *Haemophilus pleuropneumoniae,* and it is very contagious. It often affects young pigs from one week to six months of age. Sometimes the first sign of illness is severe respiratory distress, followed by sudden death. Other times affected pigs develop a high fever, weakness, and lethargy. Call your veterinarian right away. Treatment is difficult as the pigs are often too far gone by the time you notice the problem. Antibiotics and sulfas have been used successfully in combination with good nursing and electrolytes to fight dehydration caused by the high fever. Recovered pigs, however, may remain a source of future contamination in the herd.

Prevention consists of vaccination along with extreme care in isolating any new pigs, including those that have been off your place for shows, sales, or breeding. Ask your veterinarian to suggest a vaccination schedule for your situation and location. Excellent ventilation may help prevent problems, as will avoiding crowding and keeping pigs of different ages separated.

Rhinitis

A pig usually develops rhinitis, or bull nose, following an injury, such as a bite, scrape, or wounds caused by broken needle teeth. Once the bacteria enter the nose, there may be sneezing or a discharge or occasional bleeding from the nose. The pig will often develop a swollen snout or face. Left untreated, the tissue will decay (become necrotic), there will be foul-smelling areas, and the nasal discharge will have a foul odor. Necrotic rhinitis is often confused with another similar condition: atrophic rhinitis. With atrophic rhinitis there are nasal discharge and sneezing, but there is not usually a swelling of the nose and face as seen in necrotic rhinitis. Treatment is similar, although once the condition has become long-standing, no treatment will effect a cure.

Oral or injectable antibiotics will generally help rhinitis, as will sulfa combinations. Keep the affected pig as comfortable as possible, and feed it highly palatable foods that are easy to eat. Slop made of ground feed and sour milk is usually good, as is oatmeal or raw eggs. Keep the nose clean. Swabbing daily with a human nasal spray often helps. If there is a wound, keeping it drained and treated with iodine may increase the success of the treatment.

If several animals in your herd are affected or if the disease seems to be spreading, call your veterinarian. He can take a nasal culture to find out what organism is causing the trouble and determine exactly what antibiotic will be most effective on it.

Spraddled Legs

Spraddled legs is a fairly common condition in baby pigs. Possible causes include a dietary deficiency, disease, or infection in the sow during pregnancy; cortisone given to the sow during pregnancy; or slippery floors at the time the baby pigs are farrowed. It can also be an inherited trait. The newborn pig will be unable to walk normally, and the rear legs will often spraddle apart. With treatment and good care, you can often remedy this condition in a few days. Try taping the hind legs together loosely with a figure eight hobble of adhesive tape, and then make sure the pig gets enough to eat. Keep it warm and on a well-bedded, nonslippery floor, and protect it from being stepped on by the sow.

To prevent spraddled legs, avoid giving cortisone injections during the last half of the pregnancy. Feed the sow an adequate diet, and provide good bedding for the pigs at farrowing. Also, try to give good protection to the little pigs to avoid injury from the mother. Avoidance of breeding stock out of litters where spraddled-leg pigs were present is often a great help.

Transmissible Gastroenteritis

Transmissible gastroenteritis (TGE) is caused by a virus. It is a highly contagious disease that has a very short incubation period. TGE causes diarrhea, vomiting, and severe dehydration. The mortality rate is very high in baby pigs because they cannot withstand the severe diarrhea and subsequent dehydration as well as an older pig can. Older pigs can tolerate the disease better, and the mortality rate drops considerably, although weight loss is common.

Prevention is the best treatment. Isolate any new pigs you bring home for at least a month, especially keeping them away from little pigs and sows due to farrow. Vaccination is a great help in protecting your pigs. Ask your veterinarian for his recommendations for your situation and location.

Worms

Pigs are affected with several species of worms, including three types of stomach worms, ascarids, strongyles, whipworms, tapeworms, and others. Symptoms of worms include a failure to thrive, rough hair coats, coughing, poor appetite, and a thin, potbellied appearance. However, some pigs with a heavy parasite load show very few symptoms. If you suspect worms in your pigs, take a fecal sample to your veterinarian. He can examine it under a microscope for the presence of eggs and minute worm larvae and determine just what parasites your pigs are infested with and which wormer will be most effective.

Due to the life cycle of these parasites, it is nearly impossible to have 100 percent worm-free animals. But if you can keep the number of worms low, there will be no economic loss from them. Good sanitation, pasture rotation, and washing the udders of sows and gilts that are due to farrow soon will do much to help keep your pigs almost worm-free. Worm your pigs routinely: before breeding, after weaning, and before moving to clean pastures or pens. Wormers such as dichlorvos and levamisole—and piperazine for baby pigs—are a great help. Sometimes, where there is an increased worm load, injectable ivermectin will work well, also killing lice and mange mites. Remember that some worms develop a resistance to certain wormers, so it pays to switch from time to time. Always have your veterinarian do a routine yearly fecal exam on at least several pigs in your herd, and ask his advice for developing a worming program based on the types of parasites common in your area.

POULTRY

GENERAL CARE AND MANAGEMENT

Good general care will go a long way toward keeping your flock happy and healthy. In return, you'll get more eggs, meat, and breeding stock for less money than with a poorly managed flock.

Chickens and Guineas

It's worth taking a little effort to meet the minimal housing requirements for chickens and guineas. Ignoring them is asking for health problems, poor production, and large veterinary bills.

Housing

Housing for chickens and guineas can range from a small coop in the backyard, housing 3 or 4 hens, to a huge, automated laying house complex, containing 22,000 birds. For the small farm or homestead flock, though, about the only automatic convenience available is a willing child or spouse doing chores without being nagged! So I'll disregard the large poultry factory here.

A chicken house should be cool and airy in the summer and warm and dry in the winter. In moderate climates these conditions are fairly easy to supply. In cold winter areas, however, it takes a little more work to winterize a shelter. You may need double-walled construction to keep the poultry house warm enough in the severest part of the winter. If possible, build your chicken house into a bank of soil on the north side. (The earth will help to keep the house warm and protect it from winter winds.) Stacking bales of straw against the outside walls will also help block storm winds.

The house should face the south, with windows on the south side. Double-glazed windows on the south side not only will let in sunlight, which is necessary for the health and well-being of the flock during the winter, but also will provide a lot of warmth. Generally, you want the air in the coop to stay above freezing. The birds' body heat will usually keep the coop warm enough to be comfortable, provided the building has double walls and double windows. When chickens are stressed by cold, egg production will drop quickly. In very severe weather, you may need a heat lamp or two during the night to provide adequate warmth. Be careful to hang these heat lamps securely as many fires are caused by heat lamps that have been knocked to the bedding.

PARTS OF A MALE FOWL

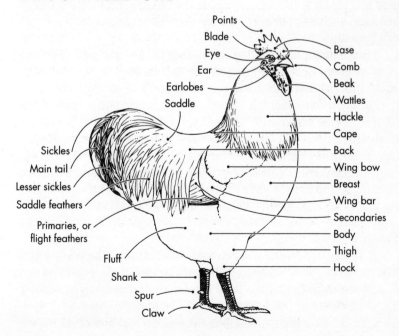

An immense amount of cold air can flow through a keyhole or knothole, not to mention the crack under the door, so be sure to plug all drafts. You will still need to ventilate the house, however, to draw out moist, stuffy air. A simple ventilation shaft through the roof or a small fan through the wall is often necessary.

Generally speaking, you should allow 1 square foot of coop space per bird. Larger birds require more space. Crowding chickens will cause disease and stress, reducing egg production in layers and weight gain in broilers. Build roosts of 2 × 2 lumber, rounded on the edges with a plane or drawknife. Allow at least 8 inches of roost for each bird and more for larger chickens, such as Cochins. Space the roost poles 1 foot apart, and place them so that the birds on the top roosts do not manure on the lower ones.

Layers will need nests: either manufactured nesting batteries made of sheet metal or homemade wooden nests. The dimensions should be about 12 inches long × 12 inches wide × 11 inches high. Place a roosting pole along the front of each row of nests so the hens can fly up, choose their nest, and enter. Without the pole many eggs will be broken as hens must fly right into the nest. Supply one nest box for each five hens. Be sure the boxes contain some sort of bedding, such as shavings, to keep them clean and to help prevent egg breakage.

Use plenty of dry bedding on the floor of the coop; a 4- to 6-inch layer is good. Scatter some chopped hay through it to encourage your chickens and guineas to scratch about and get exercise.

During the summer it is a good idea to have an outside run or pen for the birds to exercise in. If possible, two yards are best. Being able to alternate yards is a large step toward poultry cleanliness and parasite control. Giving the birds a large area to run in will also cut down on your feed costs considerably while providing excellent nutrition. Planting a crop in their yards, such as rape, clover, or millet, will give the chickens some greens and also encourage exercise.

Fencing

A fence around the chicken yard is a must. While poultry can just run loose, your garden and flower beds will suffer, and you can expect losses to predators, such as raccoons, foxes, coyotes, stray dogs, hawks, and owls. The best type of fencing is woven 2 × 4-inch, 12- to 14-gauge wire. Make the fence 6 feet high, and stretch it tight on solid wood posts. Guineas can fly over a 6-foot fence, but usually they won't if they have adequate feed and are not excited. (If they persist in flying out, you can clip the feathers on their wings with a pair of scissors to discourage this.)

Woven wire is more expensive than mesh chicken wire, but it will last a lot longer and will protect the birds from dogs and strong wild predators. It is smart to extend the wire 1 foot below the ground; otherwise, foxes, coyotes, and dogs can dig under the fence. If hawks become a problem, you should cover the yard, as well. Poly or nylon mesh or chicken wire is fine for this, as a fairly lightweight covering will discourage raptors. Some folks have gotten by using nylon fish line woven back and forth across the top of the yard.

It is necessary to lock your birds inside the coop during the night because this is the prime time for predator visits.

Feeding

Chickens and guineas eat the same foods, although guineas are "wilder" and gain a good part of their living on free-range if this is available to them. Both will forage for insects, grubs, and greens when allowed onto a good yard.

You should also provide free-choice scratch feed or a laying ration. A pelleted laying ration is best as there is less waste and also fewer problems with impacted crops. Unless homegrown grains are available, it is usually cheaper to purchase premixed chicken feed owing to the cost of handling and mixing small amounts of grains and concentrates. Chickens make excellent use of many grains. Corn, oats, wheat, milo, barley, rice, millet, and buckwheat are all used in various poultry rations as a major portion of the grain mix. Rye and buckwheat may represent up to 15 percent of the grain ration, with the others making up an even higher percentage. If your chicken house is on the cool side, give chickens and guineas more corn in winter to provide needed carbohydrates for body warmth and energy.

Cooked potatoes, milk, skim milk, buttermilk, sour milk, meat scraps, fish meal, cooked bloody eggs, soybean oil meal, sunflower seeds, and other foods are also used as part of the grain ration in different areas. Any wholesome table scraps and garden waste make an excellent addition to the menu.

Your chickens and guineas will also need minerals added to their ration. Keep oyster shell and limestone grit available for your poultry at all times. This provides not only grit needed for digestion but also calcium carbonate for maintenance and eggshell formation. Many growing rations include bonemeal for calcium, phosphorus, and protein. A 1 percent salt supplement added to the ration improves palatability and digestion. Trace minerals, such as iron, iodine, and manganese, are also added to most commercial mixes.

Chickens and guineas enjoy alfalfa, either green or as chopped hay, and it provides vitamins A, D, and G as well as other vitamins, protein, and minerals. Alfalfa meal is also often included in poultry rations. During the winter, adding alfalfa meal to warm water so that it swells and freshens up makes a special treat for your flock and also helps keep egg production up during the cold months.

Supply the feed ration in feeders that discourage the hens from wasting the feed by scratching it out into the bedding or roosting on it and depositing manure there. Commercial hanging feeders work well, but a carefully constructed homemade feed trough can work fine, also.

Be sure your birds have all the fresh water they will drink, all year-round. If the water freezes during the day, provide at least three refills daily with fresh water, warmed enough to take the chill off. Dehydrated birds soon become stressed and ill.

Breeding

It is not necessary to keep a rooster to have eggs. In fact, many urban homesteaders choose not to have a rooster so early morning crowing won't disturb the neighbors. But if you intend to keep hatching eggs from your flock, you will need to let a rooster run with your hens.

Most poultry raisers choose a rooster of the same breed that the hens are or of a heavy breed for a mixed group of hens. Heavy-breed roosters are not generally mean unless they have been teased. Handle all roosters calmly and gently. If a rooster develops aggressive tendencies toward people, you can clip his spurs with a pair of side cutters or cull him. Never keep an aggressive rooster where there are children, as he can seriously hurt a small child. Fortunately, a rooster like this is in the minority, and the ringing crow of the "master" is beautiful to people—as well as his hens!

Generally 2 or 3 roosters are adequate to ensure fertile eggs in a 50-hen flock.

Incubation

Gather the eggs at least once, and preferably twice, a day unless you are allowing a broody hen (one that wants to sit on her eggs) to build a clutch.

If you plan to raise some chicks from your flock, there are several methods of incubation. First there is the natural method of letting a hen lay a clutch of eggs and then incubate them herself. Then there is the method of letting one or more hens lay the eggs and slipping them under a broody hen to hatch. She will sit on the eggs and then take care of the chicks after they hatch. Or you could buy a small incubator—one that holds 100 eggs or so is more than enough for most folks. In some locales there are people with large incubators who do custom hatching. For a small fee or a share of the chicks, they will take your eggs, incubate them, and then give you back your day-old chicks.

If you plan to have the mother hen or a setting hen hatch the eggs, you just have to let nature take its course, more or less. With the setting hen, you can let her sit on a couple of plastic nest eggs until you collect enough eggs to make a comfortable clutch for her to sit on. Do not overload her as she will be unable to keep the clutch warm if it's too large. (All of the hen's clutch should be under her feathers at all times. If some are peeking out, it's better to remove a few eggs than to risk a poor hatch.) It's best to place eggs under a broody hen at night, very gently, without disturbing her greatly. If a hen is not quite sure she wants to set, placing her in an enclosed box may help her decide to go ahead. When a hen is setting, she should be in a small box attached to a wire run, with plenty of food and water readily available.

When saving eggs to take to an incubator or put into your own incubator, handle them very carefully, without jarring. Store them between 50° and 60°F (10° and 15.6°C). Cooler temperatures sometimes affect the hatchability of the eggs. High temperatures (above 82°F [27.8°C]), such as occur during the summer, will encourage slow development and weaken the embryo during storage. You can hold eggs from 7 to as long as 28 days, depending on the temperature and handling. Varying temperatures will greatly decrease the hatchability after 14 days. For best results incubate the eggs for 21 days at 101°F (38.3°C), with about 60 percent humidity. Turn the eggs at least four times daily. Under normal conditions the eggs will hatch in 20 to 22 days. You can delay the hatching by lowering the incubator temperature slightly.

Caring for Chicks

As the chicks hatch, a hen will take over completely, keeping them warm, showing them how and what to eat, and so on. Be sure the watering pan is not deep, or the baby chicks will get in and drown. Providing the feed in a shallow pan is a great help the first few days, as the baby chicks must get in the pan to eat.

When you buy baby chicks or hatch them yourself, you will have to be their "mother." You'll need to keep the chicks warm and keep them from straying away from the heat. A good solution is to take a large cardboard box, round the inner corners by taping cardboard in them, and hang a heat lamp in the center. The temperature should be about 95°F (35°C), with no hot spots or cold drafts. If the chicks are too cool, they will huddle together and smother. If possible, use a thermostat with the brooder lamp to prevent accidental temperature changes. Be sure the lamp is fastened securely because many fires are started each year by heat lamp accidents.

Chicks need access to fresh water at all times. Whenever they start to empty their waterer before refilling, use more or larger waterers. Be careful not to use a large waterer at first, though, as chicks can drown in water 1½ inches deep.

Sprinkle chick starter on the floor the first day to encourage the chicks to peck. The second day, place the feed in shallow dishes, such as plastic can covers. As soon as the chicks are eating well, you can switch to regular chick feeders. Be sure you get the kind that does not allow them to stand in their feed. If they do stand in it, a lot of feed can be soiled and wasted.

As the chicks grow, reduce the temperature of the brooder by 5°F each week. Also, increase the brooder area to give the chicks more room, which often prevents cannibalism.

Ducks and Geese

Good management will help maintain the health and productivity of your ducks and geese. It will also save you money by reducing their need for special veterinary care.

First Aid Kit for Poultry

Here's a list of the basics anyone who raises poultry should keep on hand. Depending on your situation and how many birds you raise, you may need or desire to add more items. Ask your veterinarian to make recommendations for your particular kit.

Blood stopper

Chick waterer

Dog/cat nail trimmer

Heat lamp with red bulb

Mineral oil

Rotenone powder

Veterinarian's phone number

Housing

Ducks and geese are easier to house than chickens and guineas owing to their built-in down insulation. They do need shade from the summer sun and a warm, dry shelter in the winter. Many ducks are lost or suffer damage from having their breasts or keels freeze to the ground during severely cold weather.

Ducks and geese do not require roosts because both rest lying on the floor. Construct duck nests of 1-inch lumber, and make them 12 inches wide × 18 inches deep. The height is usually 16 to 18 inches, with larger breeds obviously needing larger nests than small breeds like Call ducks. Make the nests like stalls, with a 4- to 5-inch strip nailed across the front to prevent the birds from dragging out the bedding. Tacking canvas across the top will make the nest more desirable to hen ducks, which prefer a secluded nesting spot. Goose nests are similar but larger. The size depends on the breed of goose, but nests about 20 inches wide × 30 inches deep are average. You can also make the nests out of small wooden barrels. Geese seem to prefer single nests rather than community nests.

Since ducks and geese are sloppy with their water, you must always keep adequate bedding in a duck or goose house. Sawdust or wood shavings work best as both are very absorbent and easy to replace when soiled. Be sure the waterers are heavy enough to prevent tipping over and small enough that the birds cannot climb into them. Bathing ducks and geese really soak the bedding, making the house continually damp, ideal for disease to take hold.

Usually 6 inches of bedding is enough, but if it gets wet, you need more and may need to clean it more often.

Fencing

Although you can usually contain geese and ducks in a 24- to 30-inch-high fence, it is wise to use a 6-foot fence made of woven wire with a 2 × 4-inch mesh, as described in "Fencing" on page 252. This will prevent a massacre in the event a stray dog or fox wanders by. If nothing else, contain the birds during the night as this is when most predation takes place.

Feeding

If ducks and geese have access to range or pasture, they will forage most of their food. You should, however, also provide some mixed grain, such as corn, oats, and wheat, daily. They'll get along on an 18 percent protein feed under range conditions. During the laying season, though, feed a higher-protein laying ration. Supply the food free-choice in commercial feeders or in well-constructed homemade troughs that keep the birds from soiling the feed. If your birds are getting too fat (which is seldom the case with birds that get daily exercise), you may need to cut back on their food for a while.

Although ducks and geese like water when they eat, do not place the feed near a stream or pond in the yard as the area will soon become foul and attract flies. Place waterers on higher ground. *Never let the feed get sour or moldy,* as ducks and geese are very prone to botulism, which will quickly kill them.

Oyster shell is necessary at all times, fed free-choice.

Breeding

To obtain fertile eggs for hatching, you need to let a male run with the females. Choose a male of the same breed as your hens or geese unless you have crossbreeds and want to improve your flock; then choose a young, healthy male of a breed with the characteristics you desire (for example, meat, color, or size). While best results are obtained by mating one gander to two geese, a drake can mate with four or five hens.

Incubation

Collect the eggs daily unless you will be allowing the mother to incubate the clutch. Store them safely (as you would chicken eggs), and then place them under a broody hen or in an incubator. A hen can handle from 3 to 5 eggs, a duck 7 to 10, and a goose 10 to 15. If you are using an incubator for duck and goose eggs, handle them as you would chicken eggs, but keep them at a slightly higher humidity at hatching time. Most duck eggs hatch in 28 days, with Muscovy eggs taking 34 days. Goose eggs incubate for 25 to 35 days, depending on the breed. Smaller breeds take less incubation time than do the giant breeds.

Caring for Ducklings and Goslings

Ducklings and goslings do not need heat for as long a period as do baby chicks, but for the first week or two, keep them warm and away from dampness and drafts. Although wild ducks and geese swim with the mother just after birth, domestic ducklings and goslings should not be allowed to swim or get very wet until they have feathers.

Do not feed ducklings and goslings chick starter, because they cannot handle the medication in the feed; give them duck starter. Always make sure the watering containers are full before feeding dry feed so the young birds can drink before they eat. Otherwise, ducklings and goslings may drink quickly after eating and then die from severe impaction.

Turkeys

A flock of turkeys needs rather basic good husbandry and knowledgeable care. But without it, the flock will do poorly, despite adequate feed and veterinary care.

Housing

Turkeys need good shelter in the winter, similar to that of chickens, except their roosts must be larger and heavier. Make roosts with 2 × 4 lumber, rounded on the edges with a plane or drawknife. Similar-sized poles also work well. There should be more than adequate roosting space for each bird to prevent injuries. It's best to allow 2 feet of roost per bird; if your turkeys are a very large breed, though, allow 3 feet for each.

More turkeys in farm flocks are lost to dampness than any other single cause. Turkeys, especially young ones, cannot tolerate damp bedding or dirty pens. For this reason, it's essential to raise young turkeys on wire or in pens with very dry bedding. The turkeys should not have access to their droppings under the roost. Covering the area below the roost with woven wire works well.

Provide one nest for every three hens. This can be a simple wooden box large enough for her to turn around in, depending on her breed. Make it 12 inches tall if open, and higher if enclosed, to prevent damage to eggs. Place some sort of bedding, such as shavings, sawdust, or straw, in the nest to keep it clean and prevent cracked or broken eggs.

Fencing

Turkeys also do well on range conditions, with portable shelters and portable roosts. Enclose the entire pasture with 2 × 4-inch mesh wire fencing at least 5 feet high, both to keep the turkeys contained and to keep coyotes, stray dogs, and foxes from killing them. In areas where raccoons are common, you will still need to house the birds securely at night, or you will suffer great losses. (A raccoon can climb the fence with ease—even with a 20-pound turkey in its mouth.) Some people clip the wings to keep the turkeys from flying over fencing, but I don't recommend it, as it can lead to abscesses and other problems. Clipping the flight feathers of the wings serves the same purpose, but you must repeat the clipping as the feathers grow back.

Feeding

Turkeys eat the same type of ration suitable for breeding chickens, only they consume much more of it because of their greater size. Make sure the feed is clean and free from mold. Special turkey rations are available in most parts of the country. When making your own homegrown feed ration, consult your county Cooperative Extension Agent (usually located in your county seat) for guidelines on creating a balanced ration using concentrates and other grains available readily in your area. Dried skim milk, dried buttermilk, soybean oil meal, and meat scraps are all used as concentrates in turkey rations.

For the first five or six weeks of life, young turkeys require a high-protein ration, up to 24 percent. This diminishes by about 5 percent for the next six weeks and then drops to about 15 or 16 percent protein.

Allow breeder turkeys access to good, clean range for greens, or else place alfalfa meal or freshly cut greens in the yard daily.

Turkeys must have a constant supply of water, especially during the hot summer. A small flock of turkeys can drink a surprising amount of water in a day, so be sure to check their waterers often.

Breeding

One tom can breed 10 to 15 hens, so you'll need only one tom for an average-sized farm flock. More toms will only cause fighting at breeding time and possible injury. Select a male that's as close as possible to the ideal turkey you would like to see. It is best to use a younger tom as large, heavy males can injure the hens during breeding. If you do use a heavy tom, clip his sharp toenails to prevent injury to the hens when he climbs on their backs during breeding. Some people use canvas saddles to protect their hens during breeding, as many hens are lost when injuries from excited, clawing toms become infected.

Incubation

Turkey eggs can be hatched by the hen herself, by a setting hen, or by an incubator. You can get a good start in turkeys by purchasing hatching eggs from a breeder or neighbor and hatching them under a setting hen (chicken). A good, large hen can usually handle eight turkey eggs. When you let a hen or hen turkey incubate the eggs, leave her alone, except for the time it takes to feed and water her. Confine her in a pen and nest box until the poults are able to follow her steadily.

If you are holding eggs for incubation, keep them between 55° and 60°F (12.8° and 15.6°C). You can store them as long as four weeks, although two weeks is more reliable. Careful handling and storage, with the small end down, in a carton improve hatchability.

Turkey eggs take four weeks to hatch, and the best temperatures in the incubator during these four weeks have proved to be 100.5°, 101.5°, 102.5°, and 103°F (38.1°, 38.6°, 39.2°, and 39.4°C), respectively. Make sure the incubator temperatures are accurate, and check them several times daily for best results. Set the humidity level at 60 percent until the last 4 days before hatching; then raise it slightly. Keep the incubator well ventilated. Turn the eggs at least four times daily until the 24th day.

Caring for Poults

If the poults are hatched by a hen, they can stay with her until they are grown. She will teach them to eat, drink, and range. But while the poults are very young, you should restrict them and the hen to a small yard and house. Otherwise, the hen will take them out into the damp grass, which can quickly kill them.

Care of turkey poults in the brooder is similar to chicks. (See "Caring for Chicks" on page 256 for more information.) Poults are a little slow at first about learning to eat. If there is no litter in the brooder but just a thick layer of newspaper and some chick starter sprinkled on the floor, they will usually begin to peck at the food. After the first day, provide the food in shallow pans, such as pie pans. If the poults don't eat well, place a few shining objects in the food dish, such as old jewelry. This will attract their attention and cause them to peck, eventually getting some food. Soon they'll get the hang of it; when they are eating aggressively, you can graduate them to chick feeders.

Also, make sure the poults are drinking water. If they don't learn right away, try dipping each one's beak in the water gently. This usually does the trick. Sometimes, placing a few chicks in with the poults being raised without a mother will help as the poults will attempt to mimic the chicks and will soon learn to eat and drink.

Do not raise young turkeys where chickens or older turkeys have been within several months because of the possibility of picking up diseases, such as blackhead. (For more information, see "Blackhead" on page 263.)

DISEASES AND OTHER PROBLEMS

It's important to be aware of potential diseases and health problems in your flock. Often, simple measures will keep minor problems from becoming a major economic loss. It's also important to know the normal temperatures of your poultry so you can check for fever or other abnormalities. The normal body temperature of chickens and guineas is 106° to 108°F (41.1° to 42.2°C); of ducks and geese, 105° to 106°F (40.6° to 41.1°C); and of turkeys, 105° to 106°F (40.6° to 41.1°C).

Avian Leukosis

Avian leukosis is most often seen in three categories: neural (affecting the nerves), ocular (affecting the eyes), and visceral (affecting the body organs). A bird that is affected can show one type, a combination of any two, or all three. Avian leukosis is a common problem in both large and small poultry operations.

A bird with neural leukosis will show paralysis of the leg, neck, or wing. It can be one or both legs or wings. A bird affected in both legs will often assume a squatting position. When one leg is affected, it will be stretched either backward or forward. If the neck is affected, the head will hang or twist to one side. Ocular leukosis may be suspected in birds with bluish clouding or speckling of the iris and irregularities of the pupil. Visceral leukosis may give indefinite symptoms and be difficult to diagnose unless it is accompanied by ocular or neural leukosis. The comb may shrivel or appear blue, and the bird may lose its appetite, lose weight, and have diarrhea. You may be able to feel an enlarged liver. On autopsy there will often be an enlarged liver, enlarged kidneys, and hundreds of tiny, hard, pearlike tumors in the intestines.

There is no treatment or reliable vaccine for avian leukosis. Fortunately, this is not a terribly contagious viral disease, and you can usually eliminate it with good sanitation practices. Do not save hatching eggs from suspect hens. Cull any affected birds, and do not buy breeding birds from flocks with suspect birds.

Blackhead

Although blackhead most often attacks turkeys, it can be found in chickens, also. It is caused by protozoa (one-celled organisms) carried by the cecal worm, which infests chickens and turkeys. Blackhead organisms can be passed directly from an infected bird to a healthy bird through the droppings. Or they can be encased in the egg of the cecal worm and passed through the droppings in this way. The organism may live for several months like this, contaminating the soil for a long period of time. Poults from hatching to 12 weeks of age are most susceptible to blackhead, but older birds can also be affected by it.

Birds affected with blackhead will show droopiness, sulfur-colored diarrhea, and weight loss. The head may become dark blue from cyanosis, thus the name blackhead.

Several drugs are available and quite effective for blackhead, including furazolinone, obtainable through your veterinarian or poultry supply house. Worming the birds with phenothiazine may help remove the cecal worm (the carrier) but not the organism itself. Strict sanitation will also help. Place the feeders and waterers on platforms in dry areas. Rotate yards or pastures, and keep young turkeys away from ground where chickens or other turkeys have been for two years. Raising young turkey poults on wire so that they don't have access to their droppings helps, as well.

Bluecomb

Bluecomb, also known as corona viral enteritis or transmissible enteritis, occurs almost exclusively in turkeys. Caused by a virus, it hits hard and is very contagious. Stress factors, such as hot weather, inadequate water supply, lack of shade, or a change in feed, seem to predispose a flock to the disease. Affected birds will often have a watery or pasty diarrhea and weight loss. The disease may last two weeks in older birds, but poults often die sooner because they have less resistance.

It's best to consult with your veterinarian for diagnosis and treatment advice, especially if several birds are affected. Treatment consists of good nursing: keeping the birds warm, clean, and well fed. Adding antibiotics to the drinking water, along with electrolytes to combat dehydration, will usually help.

There is no vaccine available. You can usually prevent this disease by providing good general care, allowing ample room for birds to prevent crowding, and disinfecting buildings, brooders, and pens before using them. Take care not to bring the virus home through purchasing or coming in contact with birds with suspicious illnesses.

Cannibalism

Cannibalism most often occurs in young chicks that are overcrowded and bored. It often starts with toenail picking. When a toe becomes bloody, the other chicks will begin to savagely attack the area, and often the injured chick will do nothing to discourage them. The sight and taste of blood will start the chicks pecking at one another until one or more has died and been eaten.

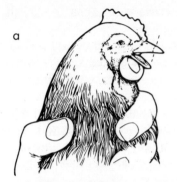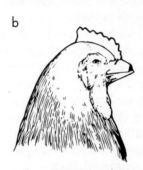

Debeaking chickens. Debeaking is usually a permanent solution to cannibalism. a. Push the tongue back by placing the point of your index finger in the center of the lower beak; then cut off one-third of the upper beak using a dog toenail clipper. b. If necessary, cauterize or use a styptic pencil on the cut end to stop bleeding.

Cannibalism is easier to prevent than to stop. Using a red lamp in the brooder is a big improvement over a clear bulb. Provide good ventilation, avoid crowding the chicks, and make sure they always have enough feed. Watch the temperature in the brooder since chicks peck more often when overheated. Giving them a chunk of sod or handfuls of grass to pick on will often help prevent this habit.

Once started, cannibalism can usually be stopped by removing any injured chick. Also, wash any that have spots of blood spattered on them. Then move the chicks to less crowded quarters, giving them grass to pick on and plenty of feed. Some people have found that applying pine tar to the wound on a chick, as soon as you notice pecking and bleeding, has also controlled the problem. Debeaking chicks will usually offer a permanent solution to habitual offenders. Dog and cat toenail clippers work well to debeak a chick. Move the tongue back by pressing a finger under the lower beak, and then trim off the end third of the upper beak. Control any bleeding by cauterizing the area or by using a styptic pencil.

Coccidiosis

Coccidiosis is caused by protozoa (coccidia). These parasites attack the intestines, causing diarrhea, unthriftiness, and death. This disease usually affects birds that are kept continuously in the same house and the same yard, especially when neither is routinely cleaned well. Although most often seen in chickens, coccidiosis can affect all poultry.

Moving the flock with coccidiosis to a warm, dry, well-lighted coop and beginning treatment with an intestinal sulfa will often help. Some coccidia have become resistant to certain drugs, so it is best to consult your veterinarian right away for advice as well as positive diagnosis through a fecal examination. (Several diseases cause diarrhea, and you need a positive diagnosis to choose an effective cure.) It's important to start any treatment before the birds become weak and before there is too much internal damage done for anything to help.

Prevention consists of good husbandry practices. Rotating yards and keeping pens dry are great helps. Keep young birds separated from older ones. Avoid fecal contamination of feed and water by using feeders and waterers that prevent birds from roosting on and soiling the contents.

Fowl Cholera

Fowl cholera is often a fast-hitting, high-mortality disease. Many times the first sign of trouble is dead birds. Fowl cholera is the first disease you should suspect in seriously ill birds, especially waterfowl. Symptoms include bluish combs and skin, a fever, increased water intake, difficult breathing, drowsiness, emaciation, and a drawn-back head. Fowl cholera may become chronic, remaining hidden in the flock until it becomes acute in a few birds, killing them suddenly. In chronic cases there is often lameness or swollen joints, caused by the bacteria invading and settling in the joints. Positive diagnosis is made on autopsy, by culturing and finding the causative organism, *Pasteurella avicida.*

It's best to consult with your veterinarian for diagnosis and treatment advice, especially if you have a large flock. Treatment is often successful in the early stages. Sulfas, such as sulfamerazine and sulfamethazine, and other antibiotics are frequently used, either in the drinking water or via intramuscular injections.

Prevention consists of vaccination, cleanliness, and reducing crowding and stress. Also, you should isolate any new birds to the place, including those that have been away at shows or sales, for one month.

Gapeworm

Gapeworms are parasites that invade the trachea and lungs of poultry and wild birds. They are carried by earthworms, flies, snails, and slugs. Young birds are most often infected when they swallow contaminated feed; eat earthworms, slugs, snails, or flies; or come in contact with infected wild birds that congregate in yards and feeding areas. The larvae migrate to the lungs within a week and then move into the trachea and become imbedded. Here they cause trouble, blocking the trachea and inhibiting breathing and eating to some extent.

Symptoms of gapeworm infestation include sneezing, coughing, stretching the neck out frequently, yawning, loss of appetite, and dullness. Feeding 0.05 percent thiabendazole in the feed for a period of two weeks will usually eliminate the parasites. (You can purchase this medication from your veterinarian or from a local feed mill or a mail-order farm supply catalog.)

To prevent problems, keep young poultry out of their yard until the dew is off and the earthworms have returned to their burrows. Rotating pastures and tilling the unused yard and planting it with a crop, such as millet, will also help. Control snails, slugs, and flies in the area with baits, traps, and rotenone powder, if necessary.

Laryngotracheitis

Infectious laryngotracheitis is a very contagious viral disease, causing coughing, weakness, lack of appetite, and a decline in egg production. In severe cases the coughing may last up to two weeks or more, while in milder cases the only symptoms may be mild coughing and reddened eyes. After recovery birds may become carriers.

There is no treatment, but good care, such as reducing dust, increasing ventilation, giving expectorants, and providing palatable feed, will help. To prevent this problem, completely isolate any new birds for one month. Always disinfect cages, feeders, and buildings that have previously been used for poultry. If the disease has been a problem, it's smart to vaccinate your flock; ask your veterinarian for his recommendations.

Lice

Over 40 species of lice can affect poultry. These parasites are generally small and grayish. Lice feed on bits of feathers, skin, and blood, causing extreme discomfort to the infested birds. When severe, they can cause death, especially in young birds. Lice are generally more of a problem in the winter months, but you should keep them in mind throughout the year. If you suspect lice are a problem, examine the bird in good light by parting the feathers and looking closely at the skin with a magnifying glass.

Dusting with an effective louse powder, such as rotenone, weekly for three weeks usually gives good control. When treating the birds, remember that the lice may be in the house, roosts, and nest boxes they use, too. It is a good idea to remove the birds, waterers, and feeders and spray the entire house with rotenone or pyrethrin. Pay special attention to nest boxes, roosts, and cracks where the parasites may be hiding; then close up the building for an hour or more. Be sure you allow adequate ventilation for an hour before returning the dusted birds to their house.

Marek's Disease

Marek's disease is caused by a herpesvirus that affects mainly chickens. It is very contagious and can cause symptoms ranging from paralysis to weakness, depression, and death. Recovered birds often remain carriers. On autopsy tumors are usually evident in organs, such as the liver, spleen, lung, and heart. If you suspect this problem, consult with your veterinarian for correct diagnosis.

Marek's disease is a serious problem, and there is no treatment; so it's worth taking steps to prevent it. Vaccination is very important, especially in larger flocks. Provide good general care, with plenty of room to avoid crowding, and make sure your poultry house is well ventilated. Also, be sure to isolate any new additions to the flock for at least a month, and vaccinate the new birds during this time.

Mites

Mites are smaller than lice. They live in cracks and crevices near the roosts, in nest boxes, and in the litter, where they deposit their eggs. They feed on blood. Birds bothered by mites are anemic and appear unthrifty. Wild birds, as well as domestic birds that are moved from place to place, spread the mite infestation. You can see mites with the aid of a magnifying glass: They appear as tiny, crawling "bugs" on the feathers or skin.

To rid your flock of mites, dust the birds well with a rotenone powder. Remove them from their house, along with their waterers and feeders; then completely spray the house with rotenone or pyrethrin, and close it up for two hours. Repeating this treatment weekly for three weeks (treating both the birds and their house) will usually eliminate the pests for a long period of time.

To prevent mite problems, change the litter on the floor and in the nest boxes frequently (at least monthly). Twice a year, take the nest boxes down, clean them out, and scrub them with soap and bleach; repaint wooden boxes. Once a year, completely spray the empty house, paying special attention to the cracks and crevices. Dusting your birds with rotenone powder at the same time will pay in more productive and contented birds. Also, clean roosts, and treat them with varnish or paint yearly. Keeping wild birds out of the coop by screening the windows and doors will also help greatly.

Newcastle Disease

Newcastle disease is caused by a virus. It kills chicks and causes economic losses due to a severe drop in egg production in laying flocks. It strikes suddenly, spreads rapidly, and can affect all poultry. Young birds show respiratory distress, such as gasping, sneezing, and coughing. This is often followed by the development of nervous disorders, such as circling, incoordination, twisting of the neck, drooping wings, and spasms or twitching, and then death. Some birds may recover from the respiratory condition but will often retain the nervous affliction.

Layers will show a sudden attack of respiratory distress, which spreads very rapidly through the flock. The birds will often quit eating, suffer a severe drop in egg production, and begin to show nervous disorders. The eggs they lay are commonly thin shelled or otherwise abnormal. The disease will run its course, often without mortality, and the hens will begin to lay normally in a month or so. Pullets are often thrown into a molt by the disease, which delays normal egg production even further.

There is no treatment for Newcastle disease, but you can vaccinate your poultry against it. Consult with your veterinarian to see if Newcastle disease is a problem in your area and to begin a vaccination program for your flock, if necessary. It is inexpensive and will prevent great losses.

Pullorum

Pullorum, caused by *Salmonella pullorum,* has been a severe problem in poultry farming. It is now more under control as the large commercial hatcheries and flocks are doing more testing and eradication. This is one good reason for buying chicks from a well-known hatchery. Most of them sell pullorum-free chicks, which are from tested flocks.

There is a chance, however, of a farm flock having this disease since few farm flocks are tested for pullorum. Pullorum appears most often in young chicks from one to three weeks of age. There is diarrhea, which often sticks to the vent, or rectal area. The chicks huddle together and act droopy; they often die. Adult birds may not die from the disease; but the hens will quit laying well, and those eggs that are laid will not hatch properly. Several antibacterials can treat pullorum, but they do not eliminate infection in the flock.

It's easy to test for pullorum, so contact your veterinarian to test your flock if you suspect this disease. Actually, it is a very good idea to have your flock tested routinely. Some flocks are tested yearly, others every three years or so, depending on size and the amount of "in and out" in the flock (due to showing, fairs, or sales). Talk to your veterinarian.

Fowl typhoid is a similar disease, caused by *S. gallinarum.* It is now uncommon in the United States and Canada but is still common in other areas. Treatment and testing are the same as for pullorum.

Scaly Legs

Scaly legs is caused by a mite that burrows into the skin under the leg scales. This causes the legs to become thick, ugly, and scaly. It is most often seen in older birds.

Treatment consists of isolating affected birds and treating their house as explained in "Mites" on page 268. You can treat individual birds by dipping their legs in kerosene or mineral oil or by rubbing petroleum jelly into the scales. Repeat this every 10 days, treating three times.

Tuberculosis

Avian tuberculosis (TB) is most common in chickens and pen-raised pheasants, but it has been found in ducks, geese, and turkeys, as well. Avian TB is transmissible to swine and can cause reaction to a bovine TB test, although the cow does not show lesions. For this reason, you should not allow poultry to run freely on your place, and do not keep them in the same building with swine or cattle. TB occurs mainly in older poultry, which is the primary reason for not keeping older birds. It is rarely seen in flocks of birds less than two years old.

Birds affected with this bacterial disease may show weight loss and unthriftiness, or they may show no signs at all until slaughtered and then examined. On butchering you may see tumors in the liver, spleen, and intestines.

There is no effective treatment and no vaccination available. Testing is possible, but it's costly unless your situation warrants it; talk to your veterinarian. To prevent problems, avoid housing your flock where any birds with TB have been housed. Keep your breeding or laying flock young, and cull any birds that are doing poorly. And isolate any new birds for two months before turning them in with the rest of your flock.

Worms

While it's possible for over 50 intestinal parasites to attack poultry, there are only a few kinds that are common problems; the rest are relatively rare. Ascarids, or large roundworms, are one common parasite in poultry. Ascarids are most injurious to young birds owing to their small size and lack of resistance. These worms cause unthriftiness, anemia, and droopiness. Ascarids infect a bird when it eats soil or feed contaminated by worm eggs or contaminated fecal material.

If you suspect that your flock is having trouble with worms, take one bird and a fecal sample to your veterinarian for examination. It's possible to treat many parasites easily and effectively, at little expense, so there is no reason to take an economic loss due to parasitized birds. Worming with piperazine is effective for treatment of many worm infestations. It is a good idea to repeat the worming two weeks after the first treatment to ensure the best possible results.

To minimize worm problems, rotate birds between two yards, tilling the empty yard and allowing it to rest for several months. Good sanitation and keeping young birds separate from older birds will also help.

RABBITS

GENERAL CARE AND MANAGEMENT

*P*roper housing and feeding will go a long way to keeping your rabbits healthy and productive. You'll also want to know how to handle them properly to prevent injuries to yourself as well as to them.

Housing

It is best to keep your rabbits in hutches or individual cages. If you plan to raise more than a few rabbits, it's smart to visit with several rabbit breeders in your area and inspect their cages and facilities. They will usually be glad to tell you what they wish they had done differently as well as the features they like best.

Hutches

Construct outdoor hutches of all wood or a combination of wood sides and a 1 × 2-inch galvanized wire front. (Don't use poultry netting, because the rabbits will chew it and attacking animals can get through it easily.) Medium-sized breeds need a hutch at least 2½ × 4 feet; 3 × 6 feet is fine for larger breeds. The height can be roughly 2 feet; it really depends on how big your rabbits are. Make the bottom of the hutch of hardware cloth, with the bottom of the nest box solid for protection from drafts and winter cold. Bedding in the nest can be straw, hay, or wood shavings.

In northern areas where the winters are quite cold, the sides and back of the hutch should be solid and draft-free. Where temperatures drop below zero and winds blow in the winter, it is a good idea to move the hutches into a barn or shed. Or move them on the south side of a building for shelter, and provide removable panels or canvas flaps to completely shut out the blowing wind and snow on bad days. In the summer make sure the hutches are shaded by a tree, a sunshade, or a trellis covered with vines like grapes, squash, morning glories, or melons.

Cages

Larger rabbitries tend to use all-wire cages with metal nest boxes. Unlike wooden hutches, wire pens are easy to keep clean and fresh smelling. It's also possible to sterilize wire cages, eliminating parasites and disease organisms. In most areas you'll need to house all-wire cages in a building to protect your rabbits against the elements as well as marauding animals.

Nest Boxes

You should provide nest boxes for all rabbits, especially does near kindling and rabbits housed outdoors. A solidly built box will give the rabbit seclusion and protection from the elements. The

PARTS OF A RABBIT

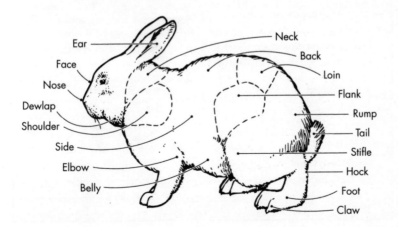

overall size of the box depends on the size of the rabbit. It should be large enough for the rabbit to turn around in comfortably, with an entrance that's large and low enough that a doe with milk-swollen breasts can jump in and out without banging them. If a rabbit repeatedly soils the bedding in its nest box, you may need to remove the box.

Feeding

In most places rabbit pellets, available through feed dealers, constitute the major portion of a rabbit diet. Although rabbits can make use of other feeds, you should use free-choice pellets as a base for the diet, if possible, as they provide a balanced diet with all the nutrients needed. There isn't much waste with pellets, and they won't become foul, as does uneaten green food (such as garden vegetables and weeds). You can feed grains, such as rolled oats, cracked corn, or wheat, but only in very small amounts until the rabbit is used to them. Garden waste, such as crooked carrots, wilted lettuce, sunflower leaves, or beet tops, is okay in limited amounts. Cabbage often causes digestive upsets, so it is best not to feed it to rabbits. It is best to introduce *any* new feed slowly because a too-sudden change in the diet can cause digestive troubles and ill-

First Aid Kit for Rabbits

Here are some suggestions for a basic rabbit first aid and equipment kit. If you have only one rabbit, you should have at least the items marked with an asterisk. A larger rabbitry should keep all of these items on hand. Your veterinarian can recommend other additions to your kit based on your situation and needs.

Antibiotic ointment*
Bottle waterers
Bunny bottle*
Clippers
5-cc syringe*
Nail trimmers*

Rectal veterinary thermometer*
Sifter-type feeders
Three 20-gauge, 1-inch needles*
Veterinarian's phone number*

ness. Young rabbits especially are bothered by digestive problems due to feed changes, so be particularly careful how and what you feed them.

Rabbits also enjoy a rack or manger filled with fresh hay. Keep this full, and don't allow the hay to become moldy or stale. Make sure each rabbit always has a salt spool or block as well as fresh, clean water. Automatic waterers, whether homemade or bought, are the best as they never allow foul water in the hutch. Heavy crockery dishes are often used, but they are easily contaminated by dirt and fecal material.

If rabbits have access to their droppings, they will consume a portion of their night feces. This is not a symptom of a deficiency but a natural occurrence, as they obtain vitamin B in this way.

Restraint

People today are getting away from the idea that rabbits should be picked up and carried by the ears. This is a good thing as handling rabbits this way often injures them.

The easiest way to handle small rabbits is to grasp them firmly over the loins and pick them up. Do not let go if they struggle briefly; you can injure them if you drop them suddenly.

To pick up a medium-sized rabbit, grasp the skin above the shoulders with one hand, and support the hind end with the other hand, as shown in "Picking up Rabbits" on page 276. Do not pick up a rabbit as you might a small dog, by lifting it under the front legs. The rabbit will often respond by kicking and scratching with its hind legs—and a rabbit can inflict some painful scratches this way!

To carry large and giant breeds, grasp the neck skin fold, and support the side of the body with your other arm, with the head tucked under your arm.

Breeding

Wait until your rabbits reach their adult size before breeding them. For example, if the breed of rabbit you raise has an adult weight of 10 pounds, you should wait until the doe reaches that size before breeding her. Those few extra weeks are not too long to wait, when you consider the extra quality you will be putting onto your doe. The doe that is bred too early will never grow to her full potential, and she will often look stunted and weedy. Small breeds

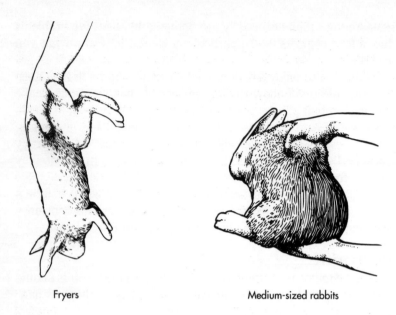

Fryers

Medium-sized rabbits

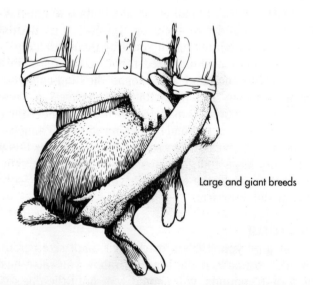

Large and giant breeds

Picking up rabbits. *The easiest way to pick up fryers and small rabbits is to grasp them firmly over the loins. Carry medium-sized rabbits by gripping a good handful of neck skin and supporting the hindquarters with your other hand. For a large or giant breed, grasp the neck skin fold, and support the body with your other arm.*

usually reach breeding size by about 5 months old; larger breeds may take 9 to 10 months.

House the doe fairly close to the buck's pen, but don't keep her with him as she may injure him. When in heat, she will often thump her feet, grunt, and rub her chin on her food dish, the waterer, and the edge of the hutch. Her vulva is usually purplish and moist. When the doe shows these signs that she's ready to breed, put her into the buck's pen. If you do the reverse, there can be fighting instead of breeding.

Following a successful breeding, don't be surprised or alarmed when the buck suddenly falls backward or to the side afterward. This is natural, and the buck is not harmed. A buck can breed 1 doe daily, allowing from 10 to 20 does maximum per buck in the rabbitry. More use may impair his fertility.

Kindling

The gestation period for a doe is about 31 days. Provide her with an adequate nest box at least a week before her due date. Changing her nest box or moving her to another hutch shortly before kindling can cause her to reject or even eat her babies. (For more information on preventing the latter problem, see "Cannibalism" on page 280.) If the rabbits are in an area that is below freezing in the winter and the doe is about to kindle, make sure the box is snug. To help cut down on chills, use double-thickness walls for the box, and place it on a layer of sawdust sandwiched between two heavy layers of cardboard. If necessary, you can tack a flap of canvas over the entrance of the box. Keep in mind that the box shouldn't be *too* warm, however, or you will lose litters due to a damp nest box. In hot weather make the nest box enclosed but airy. Some breeders place a block of ice a short distance from the nest box to help cool the area on very hot days.

Provide the doe with plenty of nest-building material, such as clean straw or even cotton. She will add to this by pulling hair from her belly to use as a lining for the nest. She will usually make her nest three to four days before kindling. Do not bother her during this time or while she is having the young, and do not disturb the nest soon after she kindles. Any such disturbance could be disastrous to the babies.

Some strains of rabbits have periodic problems with kindling. Call your veterinarian if the doe seems to strain a long time between bunnies or if she goes into labor but produces nothing within two hours. Very often an injection of posterior pituitary will cause sufficient uterine contractions to allow natural birth.

Caring for Bunnies

After kindling lure the doe out of the nest with some feed, and quickly but carefully check to be sure there are no dead babies. (If you do find any, remove them, disturbing the nest as little as possible.) Also, make sure the litter is not too large for the doe to handle. A doe with more than seven or eight young may have trouble feeding them all, and it may be necessary to farm some of the young out to another doe with a smaller litter. (Rubbing the doe's nose and the new babies with Vicks VapoRub will usually facilitate the adoption process, as she will not be able to tell the scent of her own young from that of the newcomers.) If all seems well after birth, leave the babies alone, just peeking in now and then to check on them when the doe leaves to drink or eat.

Orphan Bunnies

Occasionally a doe will die or she will have too many babies to raise, and you will not have a foster mother available at home. This leaves you with motherless baby rabbits and two choices: to raise the babies on a bottle or to kill the young. Killing them is much simpler for many people, but then you will not have the rewards of successfully raising a nice litter on a bottle.

Young rabbits must receive a small amount (1 to 2 cc) of milk every two hours for at least the first week. This means day *and* night. They have sensitive digestive systems, and too much milk gulped down at one time will kill them. A doll bottle with a small rubber nipple works well. Better yet are the infant small animal bottles available through rabbit and pet supply catalogs or though your veterinarian. An eyedropper is not good as it can give too much milk at a time, choking the rabbits and getting milk into the lungs, which can cause inhalation pneumonia. Goat milk or regular baby formula, readily available at any grocery or drugstore, will be fine for new rabbits. Be sure each bunny urinates and defecates after eating. If it does not, massage the genital area with a moist, warm cloth to stimulate action; otherwise, the young may become constipated and die.

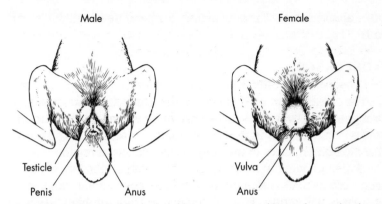

Male   Female

Testicle

Penis   Anus

Vulva

Anus

Sexing a rabbit. *In older male rabbits, you can see the testicles, and with younger rabbits the penis can be gently forced out of its sheath. In females the vulva is more visible when you press it with your hand.*

You must also keep the babies warm. House them in a small box with some nesting material, and set the box on a heating pad. Keep the pad set at a temperature that is just warm and cozy in the box. (Feel the warmth in the box with your hand.) Take care when using the heating pad as fires are always a possibility. Sandwiching the pad between two cookie sheets will help prevent overheating. Lay a towel over the box to prevent drafts.

After the first week, gradually increase the amount of milk you give your bunnies until they are weaned. As soon as they open their eyes, they will begin to nibble on pellets and soft grains. Placing good-quality hay in with them will also encourage them to eat solids. Giving a vitamin-mineral supplement in the milk and later in the water will keep the young growing as well as their brothers and sisters who were raised by a doe. When bottle-raised bunnies are eating pellets and hay quite readily—usually around six weeks of age—you can wean them from the bottle.

DISEASES AND OTHER PROBLEMS

While rabbits are generally disease-free and quite hardy, learning how to prevent their potential health problems is much more economical and reliable than trying to treat them later. It's also important to know the normal temperature of your rabbit so you can check for fever or other abnormalities. The normal body temperature of a rabbit is 101° to 103°F (38.3° to 39.4°C).

Abscesses

Abscesses are often caused by *Pasteurella*, although they may also be caused by other organisms. These infections are commonly brought about by injuries, such as fighting wounds, wire tears, and cuts on sharp objects in the hutch. In many cases there is additional infection other places in the body, such as internal organs.

Although you can try to treat a rabbit with an abscess, the treatment often costs more than a replacement rabbit, and some abscesses will return. Using a broad-spectrum antibiotic, such as oxytetracycline, sometimes is valuable. Applying heat to the abscess to encourage it to come to a head, so it can be lanced, may also help. While many rabbit breeders lance their animals' abscesses themselves, some people feel more comfortable having a veterinarian perform this minor surgery. *Pasteurella* abscesses can be contagious, so keep the rabbit isolated. If you do the lancing yourself, wear rubber gloves, and destroy any materials you used to treat the rabbit because they may be contaminated. (For more information on lancing, see "Abscesses" on page 114.)

Cannibalism

On occasion a doe will eat her babies after kindling. There is no one cause for cannibalism in rabbits, but certainly a nervous doe will be more apt to eat her young. It is believed that cannibalism is often a warped desire to protect the young. Stresses that can lead to cannibalism include people disturbing the nest, neighboring rabbits stamping or grunting, and skunks, raccoons, or dogs hanging around the rabbitry. It can also be caused by a vitamin or mineral deficiency. Heredity may also be a factor.

To prevent problems, avoid disturbing the nest, work quietly around the doe, and remove any dead bunnies right away. If a doe eats her young more than once and there is no stress to explain it, you should cull her; some does refuse to stop this habit.

Coccidiosis

Liver coccidiosis and intestinal coccidiosis are both found in rabbits. Coccidia, which cause coccidiosis, are protozoa (one-celled organisms) and are parasites of birds and animals. Animals that are stressed or living in poor sanitary conditions are most vulnerable.

Symptoms of coccidiosis can include weight loss, unthriftiness, diarrhea, and weakness, although infected rabbits often show no external symptoms.

It is a good idea to have your veterinarian do a routine fecal examination yearly to detect coccidia before they become a problem in your rabbits. Treatment with intestinal sulfas, such as sulfaquinoxaline, will usually clear up all but severe cases, where much irreversible damage has been done. Improving sanitation and reducing any stress will also help to both treat and prevent coccidiosis.

Conjunctivitis

Rabbits raised in dusty quarters or in pens where sawdust is used regularly are especially prone to eye irritations and infections. Conjunctivitis, also known as weepy eye, is due to irritating foreign material scratching the eye or the conjunctiva, the mucous membrane on the inner side of the eyelid. Affected rabbits will rub their eyes with their front feet and have mattered or runny eyes.

You can usually treat conjunctivitis yourself with a good ophthalmic ointment. Look for one containing an anesthetic to cut down the itching and burning, which encourages rubbing and further irritation. It is important to treat this condition as soon as it shows up because early treatment can prevent infections or irreversible damage to the eye.

Ear Mites

A rabbit with a severe ear mite infestation will shake its head, flopping its ears. It will scratch its ears and the backs of its ears until large scratches and scabs appear. Inside the ear there is usually a brownish, foulsmelling discharge. When secondary infections attack the

Attitude of a rabbit with ear mites.
The affected ear will often be held flopped over. If a secondary infection moves into the inner ear, the rabbit may have a twisted neck or hold its head to one side.

irritated area, they can quickly move into the inner ear, damaging the central nervous system. Here the rabbit may have a twisted neck or hold its head to one side, being unable to turn it to a normal position.

Treat the rabbit for ear mites at the first signs of ear scratching. Clean away the brownish discharge with a ball of cotton soaked in alcohol or peroxide. Dry the ear, and then apply drops like those used for mites in cats. Massage the base of the ear to allow maximum coverage inside the ear; wipe off the excess. It is a good idea to completely clean the rabbit's pen and to dust the rabbit with a low-toxicity insecticide, such as rotenone, at the same time.

Enteritis

The term enteritis actually includes several conditions that have separate causes but similar symptoms. Frequently, there is severe diarrhea, weakness, and death. Possible causes include impaction, enterotoxemia, salmonellosis, mucoid enteropathy, and Tyzzer's disease. These diseases are often initiated by stress from simple impaction due to chewing on the wood of the hutch, a diet of pellets not agreeing with the rabbit, or a low-fiber diet. When you notice the problem early, you may be able to prevent further problems by adding electrolytes to the water and increasing the fiber (by feeding hay and a different pelleted feed). When constipation is present, giving 2 to 8 cc of mineral oil orally may help. Other than simple good husbandry and nursing practices, there is no effective treatment for these bacterial diseases.

It's important to isolate any rabbits with diarrhea because many of these bacterial diseases are contagious. Contact your veterinarian for a diagnosis.

Heat Exhaustion

Rabbits are very sensitive to overheating. Enclosing them in a wooden hutch, a closed-in building, or a shipping crate during hot weather can cause extreme stress and collapse. A rabbit with heat exhaustion will breathe very rapidly, and it will die unless you quickly place it in cool water until recovery is quite complete.

To prevent heat stress, provide shade and ventilation in the summer, and keep fresh, cool drinking water available at all times. (Placing a few ice cubes in the drinking water in the early afternoon is often a great help.) A block of ice near the nest box will help keep baby rabbits from dying from heat exhaustion. Using all-wire cages in hot-summer areas is beneficial, as is placing a box fan near the cages.

Hutch Burn

Rabbits kept in wooden hutches sometimes are troubled with hutch burn. This condition is caused when rabbits sit in urine, in a wet, unclean hutch. The irritated rectal area and genitals will be red and chapped looking, and there may be brownish crusts over the area.

Proper sanitation, along with washing the area, drying it, and applying a bland ointment (such as petroleum jelly), will hasten recovery. Dusting the surrounding area with cornstarch will also help. In some instances a bacterial infection will follow the initial irritation. In this case systemic or topical treatment with an antibiotic is recommended.

Sometimes the infection will spread to the nose, producing the same type of lesions and giving the condition the name scab nose. Scab nose usually involves a bacterial infection, so provide systemic treatment with an antibiotic (ask your veterinarian to recommend one) along with improved sanitation.

Lice

Although it's rather uncommon for lice to infest rabbits, it's wise to keep the possibility in mind. Lice most often attack rabbits in wooden hutches, especially during the winter months. They can get quite a start before the rabbit gives warning of their presence by beginning to scratch. Lice can make the rabbit anemic and cause death if left untreated. Scratching, patchy-looking hair coats, and constant rubbing and digging are signs of these pests. If you suspect lice, part the hair, and examine the skin in good light with a magnifying glass. Lice are tiny gray creatures on the skin.

To control lice, dust the rabbit and nest box with a good louse powder. A rotenone or pyrethrin powder works well and is less toxic than many other products. Treat both the rabbit and its nest box weekly for three weeks to kill any newly hatched lice before they can reproduce.

Mange

Mange is a serious problem when it occurs in rabbits as it spreads rapidly and is difficult to treat successfully. Unless the rabbit is very valuable, it is often wisest to cull it rather than keep it in the rabbitry, where it will be a potential source of infestation for the others.

All mangelike lesions are not mange; some bald, red spots are caused by a bacterial infection, fungal infection, or allergy. If you suspect mange, contact your veterinarian. A skin scraping is the only means of positive diagnosis since you cannot see the mites with the naked eye.

When treating mange, it is best to clip all the hair off the rabbit; it is hard to effectively treat mange mites with the hair on. Isolate any rabbit you are treating until it is fully recovered for at least one month. Also, disinfect your clipper blades after using them to clip a mangy rabbit, as you do not want to pass this problem around.

Mastitis

Mastitis, also known as blue breast, is an inflammation of the mammary gland or glands. It is usually caused by a bacterial infection. Stress, such as a doe banging her breasts getting in and out of the nest box or scraping them on rough cage bottoms, will often cause a flare-up of mastitis just following kindling, when there is added stress on the udder due to increases in milk production. An affected doe will act listless, will have hot, swollen, red mammary glands, and may run a fever.

To catch mastitis early, check each recently kindled doe at feeding time for any sign of abnormal breasts. Quickly finding you have trouble and treating it will save many does' productivity and many baby rabbits. Another precaution that is well worth your time is to sanitize the nest box before each kindling as bacteria may lurk there.

Treating an affected doe immediately with a broad-spectrum antibiotic combination will usually bring about a quick recovery. Sometimes the young are affected owing to the severe changes in the acidity of the milk and the presence of the many bacteria in it, so it is wise to watch them carefully. If the babies have trouble with diarrhea, remove them and bottle-feed them until the doe is back to normal. The doe may also exhibit diarrhea due to the antibiotics, so you may want to take her off pellets and give her good hay until she is over the mastitis and no longer being treated with antibiotics.

Pneumonia

Pneumonia is quite common in rabbits. It often follows a period of severe stress, such as overcrowding, overheating, cold snaps, or another respiratory problem like snuffles. Affected rabbits will puff, go off their feed, act listless, run a fever (often 2° or more over normal), and then die.

Isolate any rabbit that you suspect or know has pneumonia, as it is very contagious, and consult with your veterinarian for correct diagnosis. Treatment with a broad-spectrum antibiotic will usually work well if you catch the infection soon. Otherwise, too much lung tissue will have been involved, and the rabbit cannot be saved. Steaming with a human vaporizer and Vicks VapoRub will often bring relief to a rabbit with pneumonia, in conjunction with the antibiotics.

Ringworm

Ringworm is not a worm, nor is it caused by a worm. It is caused by a fungus. The disease gets its name from the round, bald, or crusty areas it causes on the rabbit's skin. Although fairly uncommon, ringworm can be highly contagious, causing serious economic losses due to the pelt damage and damage done to salable breeding stock. (Also, who wants to buy a rabbit from you to eat if all the other rabbits in the building look scaly?)

Immediately isolate or destroy an infected rabbit, and always wear rubber gloves when handling it. Besides spreading easily to other rabbits, some species of ringworm are contagious to people.

If you decide to treat the rabbit for ringworm, call your veterinarian, and describe the trouble. He may wish to see the rabbit to confirm your diagnosis. There are many antifungal drugs on the market, and your veterinarian will recommend one best suited to your situation. When applying a topical drug, be sure there is no hair in or around the lesion; clip it very short. Work from the outside of the area to the center as you administer the medication. (If you work from the inner area out, you may spread the infection.) Weather permitting, move the cage outdoors into a sunny area, as sunshine will often aid in getting rid of the infection. Be sure, however, that there is some shade available to the rabbit. Strict sanitation and cleanliness in the future should prevent the recurrence of ringworm in your rabbits.

Snuffles

Snuffles, also known as pasteurellosis, is a common rabbit disease. Its symptoms are like those of the common cold in a human: The rabbit sneezes, wheezes, and coughs, and its eyes will often run. The rabbit will try to wipe its nose and eyes clean, getting nasal mucus on its front feet and legs. Snuffles is caused by *Pasteurella* and is highly contagious. It most often occurs after a period of stress. A cold, damp day followed by a hot day, changes in feed, moving, kindling, and so forth can all bring about enough stress in a rabbit to allow the disease to begin. Rabbits that recover from snuffles are often carriers.

If you suspect snuffles, consult with your veterinarian. Treatment with antibiotics sometimes works, but the disease will often break out again in animals that were previously sick. You may need to cull an affected animal or isolate it permanently.

Prevention consists of proper nutrition and good general husbandry, including adequate ventilation, ample space to prevent crowding, and a dust-free area. (Use pellet feeders with wire bottoms to allow the dust in the feed to pass through.) Isolate all new rabbits for a month.

Sore Hocks

Injured, chaffed, or bruised feet—not actually the hocks—often give way to a bacterial infection in that area. If left untreated, the rabbit can develop a bloodstream or bone infection and die.

To reduce the chance of infection, give prompt attention to any bald, red, scabby, or swollen hind feet. Treating the area with an antibiotic or sulfa ointment (if the area is dry and chapped) or powder (if the area is moist) works well in many cases. Systemic treatment with sulfa combinations or a broad-spectrum antibiotic will help to control an infection.

Part of successful treatment is correcting the conditions that caused the trouble in the first place. Thoroughly scrub and disinfect damp hutches, and leave them empty for a day in the sun to dry out well. Placing wooden slats across wire cage bottoms or providing a smooth board or piece of metal for the rabbit to sit on will often help the condition by relieving the pressure of a heavy rabbit sitting on wire. Thumping the hind feet (often caused by excitement, fear, or aggression) will sometimes bruise the feet enough to cause trouble, so avoid exciting the rabbits; also, keep dogs, cats, and playing children away from the rabbitry. If your bucks stamp at each other, separate them further. Sore hocks can be hereditary in heavy breeds and in the Rex, so do not breed rabbits that have sore hocks.

Wet Dewlap

This condition usually occurs with heavy rabbits that have a large dewlap. When the rabbit drinks out of a low crock dish or is forced to live in damp quarters, the dewlap gets wet and never completely dries. The skin becomes inflamed and later may become infected.

If you catch the problem early, it's fairly easy to treat. Clip the wet area, dust it with an antibiotic powder, and correct the causative condition. Sometimes all you need to do is raise the crock by placing it on a brick or replace the crock with a bottle-type waterer. Once the dewlap becomes severely infected, systemic antibiotics or sulfas are necessary, and the chances for a complete recovery are less than excellent.

Prevention through good husbandry is the best cure for wet dewlap. With a very large doe, it may also help to dust the dewlap periodically with cornstarch to help the skin remain dry.

Worms

Many species of internal parasites can infect rabbits. However, because most domestic rabbits are raised on wire and are kept in individual cages or hutches, worms are seldom much of a problem.

Signs of worms include unthriftiness, dull fur, diarrhea, cysts, and mucus or blood in the droppings. If you suspect a rabbit has worms, take it and a small sample of its droppings to your veterinarian. On microscopic examination the presence or absence of worm eggs or minute larvae will be evident. If necessary, your veterinarian will recommend the appropriate treatment.

Most worm contamination occurs via fecal matter in the feed or water. Thus, keeping feed bins tightly closed and watering with fresh water, using enclosed watering devices, will do much to prevent a worm problem in your rabbits. Many species of worms can be transmitted from one animal to another, so keep dogs, cats, poultry, rats, mice, and wild rabbits away from the rabbitry.

DOGS

GENERAL CARE AND MANAGEMENT

Although sometimes disregarded as too basic, good knowledgeable care and management will greatly lengthen your dog's life and make it healthy and full of enjoyment. A dog's basic needs are few, but if ignored, health problems and disease will follow. Likewise, a few dollars spent on vaccinations and routine veterinary care can pay big dividends throughout your dog's life.

Housing

A dog's housing requirements are few. While many adapt well to life indoors, they still appreciate attention to these minimal needs. And dogs required to live outdoors, such as guard and stock dogs, need additional housing attention as they are more exposed to the elements.

Bedding

Even if your house dog sleeps on the couch or on your bed, it should have a bed or a spot of its own. Here it can escape children, catch quick naps, and keep its bones and toys. The bed should be slightly bigger than the dog is when the animal is curled up. A larger bed is not as comfortable to the dog, because a dog likes to feel something around it while napping.

Doghouses

The outside dog needs a snug doghouse as protection from the elements. It should be solidly constructed, with a windbreak at the door. Except in very cold climates, it should not be insulated. Insulation sometimes allows the humidity to build up, causing condensation to form. This thoroughly chills the dog and makes it very susceptible to illness.

The house should face the south and be just a bit larger than the dog is when the animal is curled up. This will let the dog's body heat warm the house in cold weather. The roof should be only an inch or two higher than the standing dog's back, for the same reason. Make the roof flat with a mild slope to it. Many dogs like to lie on top of their houses to sun themselves and get a better view.

There should be plenty of fresh bedding in the house in the winter as a dog likes to curl up in a "den." Even during the summer, some bedding is necessary to provide comfort during cool or rainy spells. Keep the bedding fresh and dry. After a rainy spell, change or dry the bedding, as necessary. Old blankets, deep cedar shavings, or a nice dog bed are all good, provided you keep them clean and dry.

PARTS OF A DOG

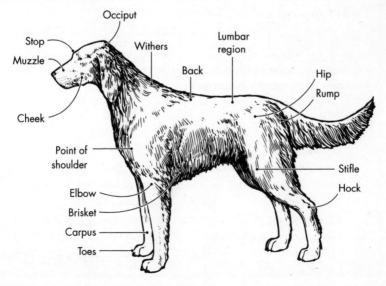

Move the doghouse from place to place periodically. This not only keeps the area cleaner and allows the grass to regrow but also aids in parasite control.

Dog Runs

A dog kept outside, such as a farm dog or hunting dog, also may need restraint, be it an enclosed dog run, a chain, or a fenced yard or pen. Unless you live in an isolated area, any dog must be kept restrained when unsupervised. Even farm dogs need restraint unless they are thoroughly trained to stay at home. Thousands of deer and other animals, including sheep, are killed by someone's pet out "having fun." Your dog doesn't have to be kept shut up all the time, just when there is no one around to keep an eye on it.

If you're building a closed-in run with a doghouse, use chain link or welded wire fence at least 6 feet high, and make the enclosure 4 × 12 feet. If your dog is a jumper, you may have to add a top. A cement floor is easiest to clean and keep parasite-free; it will also prevent the dog from digging. Pea gravel and crushed rock are other popular flooring materials. They are better on the dog's feet than cement but

First Aid Kit for Dogs

Here's a list of first aid items and supplies you'll want to keep around—just in case! Every dog owner should have at least the items marked with an asterisk. The other items can be useful if you own several dogs or if you are a breeder. Your veterinarian can make more suggestions based on your location and situation.

Betadine
Collar*
Cotton*
Ear mite remedy*
French feeding tube
Leash*
Pet nail clippers*
Puppy nursing bottle

Rectal veterinary
    thermometer*
Styptic pencil or blood
    stopper*
Tweezers/forceps*
2-inch gauze*
Veterinarian's phone
    number*
Whelping nest heating pad

harder to keep clean. And a dog will often dig holes in the run, which makes it appear dirty. Place the doghouse at the end of the run, outside the enclosed area. Otherwise, the dog can climb up on the house and use it to jump over the fence.

If you must chain your dog, use a chain heavy enough so that it will not break when the dog gets excited. Many dogs have been hung while dragging a length of chain after breaking loose. The chain should be 10 to 15 feet long, with a strong swivel at each end. Very strong dogs, such as Huskies, should have shorter chains. Otherwise, the dog may get a foot or its head in a loop of chain and then get excited and run off, breaking a leg or even choking itself. A dog that hits the end of its chain may have trouble with hematomas (large bruises) or throat injuries. Fastening the end of the chain to an old inner tube can provide enough "give" to prevent many of these injuries.

Feeding

Mature dogs in good health should be fed one meal a day or have free access to dry food at all times. The average dog, given food free-choice, will not overeat and will stay in just the right shape, provided it gets some regular exercise.

Whether fed free-choice or once daily, dry dog food of good quality is generally the best choice. It is better for the teeth than moist food since its abrasive quality keeps them clean and free of tartar buildup. Most well-known brands of dry food are a completely balanced diet, whereas many canned foods are not. An all-meat diet is not a balanced diet for a dog. In the wild, canines eat not only meat but also stomach contents, bones, and wild fruits and grasses. Whatever food you choose, read the list of ingredients. A lot of cheap dog foods have a very high cereal content, with very little meat or meat by-products. If cereal grains are listed first, one after another, chances are very high that the food is composed largely of cereal. Look elsewhere for a good food.

To increase consumption of dry food, you can add chopped or ground raw meat to the dry food and mix it in well. (Some dogs need a bit more weight than they normally carry, and the added consumption of dry food will aid in this needed weight gain.)

In addition to dry food, your dog can also have meat scraps, cooked eggs, stale bread, cottage cheese, milk (in limited quantities), and table scraps as side dishes. Dogs should never receive more "goodies" than they do dry food, however, as this is what makes a picky eater. It is like feeding children chocolate cake and then asking them to eat their sandwich and vegetables.

Do not feed your dog highly spiced, fried, or greasy foods or foods with sharp bones, such as fish, poultry, or pork chops. Cooked bones are brittle, sharp, and dangerous, able to penetrate the bowels and stomach. Feeding potato chips to a dog can also be dangerous. Some dogs do not chew their food; and when unchewed potato chips reach the stomach, the sharp edges and points can cause so much pain that the dog can actually be thrown into convulsions. In fact, any indigestible food can produce gas or stomach pain, which in turn can cause convulsions.

Unless you are feeding plain dry food free-choice, throw away any food that's left by the next feeding, and give a little less at that feeding. You don't want the dog to always be hungry, but you do want it to finish its food between feedings. Never leave moist food, such as dry food mixed with liquid or canned food, in the dish all day. It can become sour or have high bacterial growth, and your dog may get sick if it gets hungry enough to eat the food later.

Like people, some dogs have certain foods that disagree with them and cause digestive upsets, from flatulence to diarrhea. Foods that occasionally cause problems include eggs, milk, soy products, and corn products. If your dog experiences digestive upsets, try changing its food to see if that helps.

Exercise

A house dog should receive exercise of some type every day. A tiny dog can get exercise by chasing a ball, playing tug-of-war, or just being naturally active. A larger dog should either be allowed to run in a fenced yard or be taken for a walk every day. A dog that receives insufficient exercise is apt to become fat and develop more physical defects, and it often becomes neurotic. Letting a dog roam freely for its exercise is not a good idea. Not only is it dangerous for the dog, but it can cause trouble for you, as well. An unsupervised dog is like an unsupervised child: It can get into too much trouble without half trying! Tearing open garbage bags, digging in neighbors' flower beds, chasing bicycles, and bothering neighbors' pets are all common problems with unsupervised dogs.

A dog that is tied or kept in a run should have regular periods of free time or exercise out of confinement. Whether it is work, such as hunting or herding stock, or just a good run in the woods with its owner, the dog will appreciate it and will not become bored. A bored dog is often a barking dog.

Restraint

Most dogs are easy to restrain for examination and treatment as they are trusting of people and seem to know that they are trying to help. But sometimes a dog becomes frightened or is in severe pain, which transcends reason. In such cases safe and effective restraint is necessary.

First of all, a strong and safe collar is a must, if only to lead the dog into a veterinarian's office—where even a brave, calm dog fears to go. The collar should fit snugly enough that the dog cannot slip its head free by twisting and pulling back, and it should be loose enough for comfort. A flat nylon or leather collar is best. A choke collar can be used for everyday, but it is best to use it only as a training collar because a frightened dog can choke itself trying to escape in an emergency.

A strong, dependable leash is also necessary, if only from time to time, as in going to the veterinarian's clinic. The leash should be nylon or leather, and the snap should be heavy enough to hold the dog, whatever it decides to do.

No matter how well trained your dog is, use the leash and collar any time you have it in strange surroundings or if it has been injured. A frightened or injured dog may panic and run off, totally unaware of its owner's repeated calls.

To effectively restrain a small dog, place one hand on the back of its neck, over the collar (which can be grabbed, if needed). Place the other under its chin, and tip the head up slightly. Massaging the neck a bit and speaking reassuringly to it will also help.

To restrain a large dog, straddle its neck, and tip its head up with one hand while you hold its collar with the other. In this way, you can hold it while a helper takes its temperature, removes a burr from its tail, or performs whatever minor treatment is necessary.

If additional restraint is necessary, such as when a smaller dog tries to nip the person holding or treating it, simply tie a length of 1-inch gauze snugly around the muzzle and then behind its ears in a bow. This works great for treating a small dog with a broken toenail, a minor cut that needs examination, or other minor problem.

Breeding

A female dog will come into heat roughly every 6 months. Smaller breeds usually begin cycling at 6 months of age, with larger breeds coming into their first heat between 8 and 12 months. Any female that you do not specifically plan to breed should be spayed before her first heat period. There are too many unwanted puppies out there to allow a chance breeding and therefore contribute to the immense problem already present. Spaying will not alter a female's personality or make her fat and inactive, and it will help prevent such things as uterine infections and breast tumors. And never breed a bitch unless you have the time, space, and money necessary to raise the puppies until you can find homes for them. It is no solution to say, "I'll just sell the extra ones to a pet shop." A high percentage of pet shop puppies never reach adulthood.

If you have a purebred female with a good disposition, conformation, and pedigree, wait until after her second heat period, at least, to breed her. It is not advisable to breed the bitch on her first heat as she is still a puppy herself then; she will not be able to handle the nutritional requirements of her unborn puppies and the nutrients necessary for her own growth at the same time. Thus, she may never reach the size and conformation she would have attained if you had waited until at least her second, or preferably her third, heat to breed her.

Choose the male, and make arrangements with the owner well in advance of the date your bitch is due to come into heat. Don't choose the male on bloodlines or looks alone; also consider his temperament. The most beautiful dog in the world is of no use if it is neurotic or mean. Also, take special care to avoid genetic or hereditary problems. Most breeds of dogs have an undesirable characteristic that dedicated breeders are trying to weed out, such as deafness in Dalmatians and hip dysplasia in German Shepherds. Never breed a dog with any hereditary defect or that has parents with a defect, as there is too much of a chance that the puppies will either pick it up, too, or pass it on to *their* puppies. Study your breed well, and make a good choice based on soundness, good disposition, and good conformation—not the popularity, length of hair, color, or some such trait.

Before breeding, the female should be in good physical condition and free of worms, skin parasites, and vaginal or uterine infections. She should also be up-to-date on all her vaccinations. She will be in heat for approximately three weeks but will generally accept the male only from the 10th to the 14th day. Take her to the male early so that she can become accustomed to him and his surroundings. A frightened bitch may not accept the male and may even injure him.

After a successful breeding, resulting in a tie (where the male and female are joined for a period of time following ejaculation), the female can usually be taken home, although many breeders prefer to continue breeding the female until she rejects the male. Do not allow any other males near her while she may still be in heat, as a bitch can have puppies by two or more fathers in the same litter. This can be a disaster with a purebred bitch. After all, who will pay a good price for a registered Collie pup when two of the littermates have curly black hair like the male poodle next door?

The bitch will have her puppies after a gestation period of 58 to 62 days. As the pups grow larger inside her, she will begin to develop a ravenous appetite, and she will often eat twice the amount she ate before she was pregnant. She will need this food as well as an extra protein source, such as lean meat, cooked liver, or hard-boiled eggs. She should also receive adequate exercise. A too-fat or too-soft bitch will often have whelping trouble. She should not, however, have rough exercise, as it could cause abortion.

Whelping

Give your bitch a whelping box a week before she is due so she can get used to it. Some bitches will insist upon having their pups in a closet, in the barn, or on your bed anyway, but you can try to persuade her to use the box you provide for her. Place the box in a warm, hidden location where she will not be bothered. The sides should be high enough to prevent drafts and to keep the puppies in the nest. And they should be low enough that she can escape the pups to get exercise and take care of her own needs. Some breeders, especially those having large, heavy breeds such as the St. Bernard, like to use a whelping box with a rail to give added protection against the mother lying on the pups.

You can be quite sure when your bitch will have her pups by taking her temperature. It will drop from her normal temperature of 101° or 102°F (38.3° or 38.9° C) to 100° or 99°F (37.8° or 37.2°C). When it falls below 99°F (37.2°C), she will whelp within 12 hours. When beginning labor, she will pant, dig, push her nest material around, and act restless. If she does not produce a puppy within 3 hours, call your veterinarian.

Most bitches will have their pups and take care of them without any assistance from you. But it does pay to keep watch on her from a distance to make sure all is well. If a pup is born and is still in the sac, break the membrane, and rub the pup dry with a clean towel; otherwise, the pup may drown in the fluid.

If the bitch goes longer than 30 to 45 minutes between pups and you feel she is not finished, take her out, and force her to take some mild exercise. If she does not produce another pup within 30 minutes after returning to the whelping box, call your veterinarian. She may have an obstruction, or her uterus may be tired and require an injection of posterior pituitary to get things started again.

After whelping she will relax and begin caring for the pups. Unless the bitch has a very large litter, she should be allowed to eat the placentas. Eating too many can cause digestive upsets and diarrhea, but eating them stimulates uterine contractions and helps to let the milk down. If it appears that she doesn't have milk, call your veterinarian immediately. If given an injection right away, she may be forced to let her milk down. Such an injection will not, however, produce milk in a bitch that does not have milk in the first place. (See "Orphan and Rejected Puppies" on the opposite page for guidance on dealing with this problem.)

The bitch will have a normal discharge from the vagina for several days or a week after whelping. This is most often bloody and dark and is nothing to worry about. If it becomes foul smelling or looks yellowish, however, call your veterinarian.

Allow your bitch free-choice dry dog food during the nursing period so she can more easily keep up with the terrific drain on her body that nursing a litter of pups causes. She should also receive a good vitamin-mineral supplement. If she appears to lose weight, adding chopped or ground meat to her dry food may help. (For information on other possible problems with whelping, see "Eclampsia" on page 316 and "Metritis" on page 325.)

Caring for Puppies

The puppies will open their eyes at about two weeks. Soon after that time, you can begin to introduce them to semisolid foods. At three weeks most puppies will lick a bit of cooked mashed liver from your fingers. At four weeks you can usually put a shallow pan of baby cereal mixed with cooked liver and milk in with the pups. The first few times you feed them this way, they will get most of it on them instead of in them; but they will soon learn to lap up the gruel with relish. Don't make the food too thin, or they may get some of the fluid into their lungs.

At eight weeks the pups will be eating considerable amounts of food. In the weeks that follow, you can slowly switch to dry food, ideally fed free-choice. The pups also need a calcium-vitamin D supplement for proper bone growth and the prevention of rickets. If not fed free-choice, the pups should be fed four times daily at eight weeks of age, three times daily at three to four months, and two times daily until nine months.

At eight weeks the pups should have their first adult distemper-hepatitis-parvo combination vaccination and also be checked for worms. Ninety percent of puppies have some type of worms; even if the bitch was wormed, it is a good idea to have the puppies checked before they go to their new homes.

Orphan and Rejected Puppies

Sometimes it becomes necessary to raise a litter of puppies by hand. A bitch with mastitis, no milk, or a too-large litter; a rejected pup; or a bitch that dies may leave you with this tiring, but rewarding, job.

The puppies must be fed small amounts of goat milk or puppy formula (available at your veterinarian's clinic or larger pet shops) every two hours, day and night. This has to continue for at least one week. After the week you may drop to every three hours during the night, but keep with every two hours during the day. The following amounts are about right for the average pup:

- Large breeds (50 to 75 pounds, adult weight): 2 to 4 cc milk
- Medium breeds (25 to 50 pounds): 2 to 3 cc milk
- Small breeds (10 to 25 pounds):1 to 2 cc milk

Start with these amounts, adjusting as necessary by the look and feel of the pups. After two or three days, increase the milk gradually until it is doubled in quantity. If the pups seem very hungry after feeding, you may increase the amount of milk enough to almost satisfy them. Keep increasing as the pups grow and require more food. Do not overfeed, however, as this will cause digestive upsets and possibly death.

The easiest way to feed pups their milk is with a feeding tube. This is a flexible rubber or plastic tube that fits on the end of a syringe. Draw the milk up into the syringe and tube, where it is measured, and then slowly push it down the pup's throat. As the tube goes down, the pup will swallow it. Be sure it does swallow, or the tube could go into the lungs. When the feeding tube is down the esophagus (judge by the length of the neck), slowly inject the milk. If you do it too fast, the milk will be sprayed and cause cramps. This method requires little experience and is fast and easy. Total time required for feeding and cleaning each pup is about two minutes.

Make sure each pup urinates and defecates after each feeding. If it does not, massage the genital area with a moist cloth or cotton to stimulate action. This is the way the mother teaches her young to defecate. If it is not done, the pups may become constipated and die.

Introduce the pups to semisolid food when they are about three weeks old, as with mother-raised pups. Hand-raised pups often take readily to semisolid food a bit earlier than pups raised by their mother. By four weeks the pups will usually lap gruel made of milk mixed with good-quality canned food and a bit of baby cereal. They can be completely weaned from milk when they eat well on their own—usually by six weeks of age.

When raising very young pups by hand, you must make sure they stay warm enough. One way is to use a whelping nest heating pad, available through many kennel supply houses. Placed in the box that houses the pups, it supplies necessary supplementary heat (as their mother's body would do naturally). Without extra heat, pups often chill and soon die. Of course, you should use caution with any electrical heating device to prevent fires.

Neutering

The decision whether or not to neuter your dog is one of the major decisions that you must face in pet ownership.

Spaying

Neutering is especially a concern if you own a bitch. An unspayed bitch comes into heat every six months and is in heat for three weeks' time. During this period she may spot blood on the furniture, rugs, and floor, and her scent will attract male dogs of all descriptions from near and far. There is often fighting among these males as they vie for her attention.

Friends and relatives may offer "helpful" advice on neutering, such as "Don't spay her until she has had a litter, or she'll (pick one) (1) get fat, (2) be unfulfilled by missing motherhood, (3) get lazy, (4) get mean, (5) act like a male," and so on. There are lots more "helpful" hints—as many hints as people that give them. But the truth is this: It's easiest and safest to spay a female before she has her first heat period. Spayed at this time, the young bitch will come through the surgery with little setback and be ready to hunt, play, or work in a few weeks. Also, spayed dogs get fat for the same reason that unspayed dogs do—people feed them too much! And spayed females do not get mean because they are "unfulfilled in motherhood." They become mean because of ill treatment or poor inborn temperament.

Spaying saves the female from the stress of raising countless puppies and possibly helps her avoid uterine infections and breast tumors. It also saves generations of unwanted puppies from being born, which would lead short, miserable lives in most cases. Animal shelters and dog pounds are full of such unfortunates, killed by the hundreds every day for lack of homes.

Spaying consists of complete removal of the uterus and ovaries. The dog is given a general anesthetic and prepared for surgery. (There are several methods of surgery, so keep in mind that the method used by your veterinarian may differ from this one in some aspects.) The hair is clipped from the belly. The line of incision is scrubbed and then painted with an antiseptic. While the dog is resting on her back, the incision is made a short distance behind the umbilical scar. The incision is carried through the skin, through the muscle, and into the abdominal cavity. The ovaries are brought up one at a time by means of a hook. Each ovary is clamped off from the ligament and tied off to prevent bleeding. Then the uterus is clamped off, just toward the vagina from where the two horns of the uterus join (the bifurcation). This is tied off securely. The uterus and ovaries are removed from the body. The peritoneum and muscle layer are sutured closed, followed by the skin incision. The dog is then moved to a recovery cage to come out from under the anesthetic.

Of course, this surgery is something you'd have your veterinarian do. But I've included this description because the average person does not have the slightest idea of what is involved in a spay and is often afraid to ask the veterinarian about it at the risk of appearing stupid. The spay, or ovariohysterectomy, is a major surgery, but when done on a young female in good health, there is little risk of complication.

Castration

A male dog does not present as great a problem in the home as the female. He is most often castrated because of his wandering instincts. As with the neutered female, a castrated male does not change his appearance, temperament, or working abilities. A male dog is usually castrated at about eight months to one year of age, before he starts wandering about, searching for females in heat. As castration is not abdominal surgery, it is usually less expensive than spaying the female.

Grooming

In certain areas a dog kept in the house needs some special attention to maintain a healthy coat. As our homes are often warm and dry in the winter, many dogs shed a little (or a lot) all winter, and the coat may become dull and stiff. Even a short-haired dog needs regular grooming, not only to keep it looking good but also to keep oil in its hair and to remove dead hairs. Another benefit of regular grooming is that you'll discover any injuries or skin problems quickly, before they cause trouble.

The best way to groom short-haired dogs is with a stiff brush and chamois cloth. Be careful not to have too stiff a brush, or you may scratch a thin-skinned dog during grooming. After brushing the coat thoroughly in the direction in which the hair grows, rub the chamois a few times over it to add extra sheen to the coat. Thorough grooming of a short-haired dog, other than an occasional bath, takes only 15 minutes at most and will greatly improve the health of the dog's coat.

On a medium-coated dog, such as a Chesapeake Retriever, go over the coat first with a slicker. (This is a flat brush with bent metal pins.) A slicker is very effective for removing dead hair and stimulating the skin. Then use the regular brush and chamois.

Long-coated dogs, such as Old English Sheepdogs and Afghan Hounds, need more frequent, thorough grooming. Use a pin brush first and then a comb. (Using a slicker will tear hair out, and using the

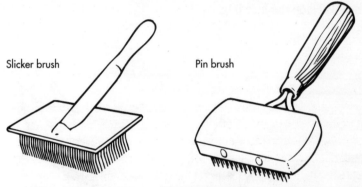

Slicker brush

Pin brush

Brushes for grooming. *A slicker brush, with bent metal pins, is useful for grooming a medium-haired dog. On long-haired dogs, use a pin brush (with straight metal pins) instead because a slicker can damage the hair.*

comb first will cause severe pulling if you run into mats.) On long-coated breeds, always groom from the bottom of the legs upward to be sure that the coat is mat-free all the way through, not just on the top layer.

While grooming, watch carefully for any fleas, ticks, or red, irritated areas. Taking prompt care of such problems will bring a faster cure and prevent further trouble.

Trimming Nails

Check your dog's nails periodically. Some dogs, especially house dogs that live on carpeted floors, fail to wear down their nails naturally, and the nails can grow so long that they spiral until they stick into the pad. Such a condition is very painful and can bring permanent lameness if not taken care of quickly. Normal, well-worn nails are about even with the bottom of the pad of the foot, so that when the dog walks, the nails just brush the ground. Nails should also have a blunt appearance. When they begin to develop a hook, they are too long. When your dog walks across the linoleum or wood floor, you should not hear "click, click, click."

A pet nail trimmer is inexpensive and a handy thing to have on hand. With a little practice, almost anyone can keep his or her dog's nails trimmed and neat. When beginning, take only a little bit from each nail. There is a vein that runs down inside the nail; if the nail is clipped too short, it will bleed. Should this occur, a daub with a styptic pencil will stop the bleeding.

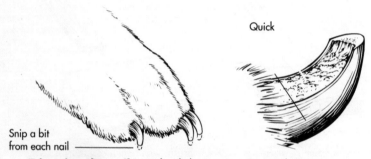

Quick

Snip a bit from each nail

Trimming the nails. *With a little practice, you can keep your dog's nails trimmed. Just take a little bit with each snip. Avoid cutting into the quick, the fleshy portion of the claw.*

Caring for Ears

Checking your dog's ears regularly is an important part of good care. Not only do they frequently need cleaning, especially on long-eared dogs, but they are also a favorite hiding place for ticks.

If you see any brown discharge and wax, clean the ears. Using a ball of cotton moistened with alcohol or peroxide, remove the wax from as deep in the ear as your finger will reach. Using a cotton swab can be dangerous if you are inexperienced or if the dog jumps, for it can puncture the eardrum. If the wax in the ear seems very dry, putting a few drops of vegetable oil in the ear and then massaging the base well will often soften the wax. In a few hours, clean the ear as usual, and the wax will be easy to remove. The oil will also serve to soothe any itching and may smother ear mites, as well.

Keep a close watch on an ear that has shown a discharge. If the discharge continues or the dog shakes its head and digs at its ear, take the animal to your veterinarian as there may be an infection or ear mites present. (For more information on these problems, see "Ear Infection" on page 316.)

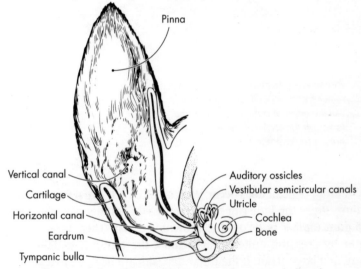

Pinna

Vertical canal

Cartilage

Horizontal canal

Eardrum

Tympanic bulla

Auditory ossicles

Vestibular semicircular canals

Utricle

Cochlea

Bone

The ear. *When cleaning the ear, use only a cotton ball and your finger. Inserting a narrow object could easily injure the delicate structures inside the ear.*

Caring for Teeth

Dogs very seldom have any dental problems, unless caused by disease or old age. The main trouble with dogs' teeth is the diet they are fed. A soft diet, such as one consisting mainly of canned food or table scraps, does not keep the tartar cleaned from the teeth. As tartar builds up, it works down into the gum, often causing infection and soreness. Regularly giving a few hard dog biscuits or large bones to gnaw on will often prevent this trouble, as will keeping your dog on a diet of dry dog food.

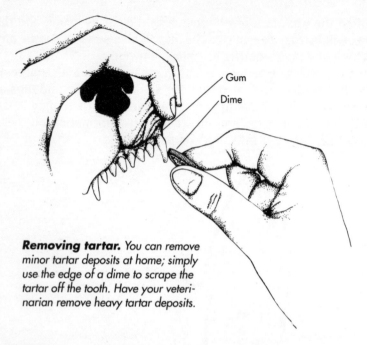

Gum

Dime

Removing tartar. *You can remove minor tartar deposits at home; simply use the edge of a dime to scrape the tartar off the tooth. Have your veterinarian remove heavy tartar deposits.*

If tartar deposit does occur, you can often remove it yourself using a dime. Press the little rim of the coin down just beneath the edge of the gum until it is below the brownish tartar. Then scrape off the tartar by pressing quite firmly against the tooth. It usually comes away in a large flake. If the tartar deposits are heavy, have your veterinarian remove them. You should also have him examine your dog if you notice any foul odor or redness in the mouth.

If your dog has had dental problems in the past, using a canine toothbrush and dental cleanser can help minimize further problems. Some folks feel silly brushing their dogs' teeth, but it is no more foolish than brushing your own—and your pet dog cannot do it for itself! (Wild canines "brush their teeth" by daily chewing and gnawing bones, hide with the hair on, roots, and other hard objects.)

Checking Anal Glands

Every dog naturally has two scent glands, called anal glands, one on either side of the rectum. Most dogs should have these checked at least twice a year; smaller dogs, monthly. Your veterinarian can show you where these glands are and how to express the accumulation in them to prevent problems. Plugged anal glands can abscess and cause lameness and even hindquarter paralysis. An easy procedure is to routinely express the anal glands while bathing your dog, as any odor is then easily washed away. And there *is* a foul odor from scent material in those glands!

Expressing the anal glands is easy to learn to do. With a wad of cotton or tissue in your hand, raise the dog's tail. Place your thumb on one side of the rectum, *beyond* the location of the anal gland, and your second finger beyond the other anal gland on the other side of the rectum. Gently but firmly press in, as though you were trying to get behind the glands, and squeeze firmly. This will force any accumulation in the anal sac into the rectum and out onto your cotton. If the procedure was a success, you will notice an odor and be able to see a brownish gray liquid on your cotton or tissue. When you do this routinely, there is seldom any problem with the anal glands. (For more information on preventing problems, see "Anal Gland Impaction and Infection" on page 308.)

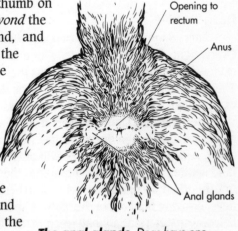

The anal glands. *Dogs have one anal gland on each side of the rectum. Checking your dog's anal glands regularly can help prevent impaction and infection.*

Caring for Aged Dogs

Older dogs often need special care to live out their lives in the best possible health. They may, for instance, need extra dental attention as their teeth wear down. Older dogs are often fed canned food, which does not remove the deposits of tartar that accumulate on the remaining teeth. These tartar deposits work into the gums, causing sore and inflamed gums, and then infection sets in. The teeth loosen, and the dog is unable to eat. Usually this infection finally claims the life of the unfortunate pet.

Check the teeth of your older dog regularly for irritation and tartar. If there is any redness, foul odor, or sign of loose teeth, take the dog to your veterinarian for treatment before the situation becomes worse. Remove tartar accumulations as they form so they don't build up into thick, irritating scales. When your aged dog's teeth receive periodic examination and treatment, there is little cost to you, and your dog will live a longer, much happier life.

Heart Trouble

Older dogs, like older people, often develop heart trouble. Overweight dogs are especially prone to this condition. Dogs need exercise and a good diet, especially as they age, to stay in good shape. There are now special diets for geriatric dogs, which tend to put on extra weight as their activity slows down.

Often the first signs of heart trouble are coughing and enlargement of the abdomen due to ascites (fluid accumulation in the abdomen). A dog with heart trouble will often have poor circulation, with fluid settling out of the blood and into the tissue. You can often control this fluid accumulation with diuretics, which stimulate the kidneys, drawing fluid out of the body. A special diet, low in salt, usually helps. Your veterinarian may recommend oral drugs to strengthen the heart; follow his instructions carefully. He can also advise you on a correct diet, which will greatly aid in maintaining the heart patient.

Urinary Incontinence

Aged dogs sometimes have trouble with urinary incontinence. This means the dog cannot control urination completely and may dribble urine unknowingly or be unable to hold the urine all night. It is most often seen in spayed, aged females.

Check with your veterinarian for advice, as most dogs can be helped with this problem. Diethylstilbestrol is often given daily, usually in oral form. The dosage is gradually reduced as the dog responds, until it is kept on a low-level maintenance dosage. Geriatric tablets containing vitamins and minerals often help in mild cases. Making sure the dog is allowed outside often to remind it to relieve itself will also help. *Do not restrict the dog's water, because you could cause kidney problems.* If the dog dribbles urine, using "bitch in heat" panties with a sanitary napkin, changed regularly, in between trips outdoors will eliminate household problems.

Breast Tumors

Breast tumors are quite often seen on unspayed, aged females. They may or may not be malignant. Have your veterinarian check any breast lumps as soon as you find them. With some tumors injections of testosterone will result in regression of the growths. Spaying the female and removing the tumors will also help in some cases. Surgery is recommended for patients in good health, while the tumors are still small in size. Once they are large, the chances for successful surgery are greatly reduced.

Arthritis

Arthritis is a common problem with older dogs, again most commonly in heavy, obese dogs. It is important to keep your old dog from getting fat. There is a tendency toward stiffness in old age, and extra weight only intensifies the problem, making it crippling in many cases. Treatment with drugs, such as cortisone, aspirin, and phenylbutazone, will often help dogs with periodic pain. Keeping the dog in warm, dry quarters and off cement will aid in preventing stiffness. Make sure your older dog has extra bedding to protect its joints.

Often confused with arthritis, especially in older dogs, is lameness due to long toenails or ingrown nails. Because older dogs exercise less, their nails do not wear down normally, and they require periodic trimming. Otherwise, the nails will grow long, putting strain on the tendons and muscles of the leg. If allowed to grow even longer, they will curl, twist, and even grow into the pad of the toe. This causes terrific pain, and the dog will be very reluctant to move about; when it does, it will limp badly. You can very easily learn to trim the nails from your veterinarian or local dog groomer. (Also see "Trimming Nails" on page 301.)

DISEASES AND OTHER PROBLEMS

While most dogs are very healthy, it's worth your while to learn about the diseases and problems that can occur. This way, you'll know how to prevent them and how to handle them if they do happen. It's also important to know the normal temperature of your dog so you can check for fever or other abnormalities. The normal body temperature of a dog is 101° to 102°F (38.3° to 38.9°C).

Sample Vaccination Schedule for Dogs

Use this suggested vaccination schedule as a basis for getting your dog the shots it needs. But be sure to consult your veterinarian for his specific recom- mendations based on your locality, the prevalence of particular diseases in your area, and the particular products he uses.

	DISEASE	WHEN TO VACCINATE
PUPPIES	Distemper, hepatitis, parvovirus (combination)	8 weeks
	Distemper, hepatitis, parvovirus, leptospirosis (combination)	12 and 16 weeks
	Rabies	3 months or older
DOGS	Distemper, hepatitis, parvovirus, and leptospirosis (where Lepto is a problem or your dog will be travelling where it may occur)	Yearly
	Rabies (booster)	Every 3 years

According to the American Veterinary Medical Association, dogs at low risk of disease exposure may not need to be given a booster yearly for most diseases. Consult with your local veterinarian to determine the appropriate vaccination schedule for your dog. Remember, recommendations vary depending on the age, breed, and health status of the dog, the potential of the dog to be exposed to the disease, the type of vaccine, whether the dog is used for breeding, and the geographical area where the dog lives or may visit.

Anal Gland Impaction and Infection

On either side of the rectum, your dog has a small gland, which serves mainly as a scent gland. You'll notice that when strange dogs meet, they smell each other's rectum. This is to identify each other by means of the scent particular to each dog. These glands empty into the rectum during a bowel movement or at times of fright. The opening into the rectum is narrow, however, and sometimes it becomes plugged with fecal material, so the gland cannot empty. Thus, the gland fills and can become infected.

A dog with a full anal gland will drag its rear end on the ground or carpet in an attempt to squeeze this accumulation out of the gland, as it is becoming uncomfortable. People sometimes think that this means the dog has worms since itching of the rectal area is a symptom of pinworms in humans. Dogs do not have pinworms. Worming a dog with infected anal glands can be dangerous: Many times constipation goes along with the condition, and if the dog cannot get rid of the wormer, it may make the dog sick or even kill it.

Your veterinarian can show you where the anal glands are and how to express them yourself. (Also see "Checking Anal Glands" on page 304.) Doing this regularly will help reduce the chance of infection. Feeding a diet of dry dog food or giving several hard dog biscuits daily can also help prevent the condition as soft stool cannot express the glands. Feeding a diet that will give a firm stool will aid the dog in expressing the glands naturally. Exercise will usually help, as well.

Infected anal glands can cause several problems, such as lameness (due to pressure against the spine), itching, and tonsillitis, when the dog licks at infected anal glands in an attempt to relieve and soothe the area. In fact, most dogs that have tonsillitis also have infected anal glands! If your dog has recurrent trouble with the anal glands, your veterinarian can remove them.

Back Problems

Some breeds of dogs are quite prone to back problems, arising from the protrusion of a spinal disc. Long-backed breeds, such as the Dachshund and Pekingese, are prime candidates due to their conformation. For discussion of this condition, see "Intervertebral Disc Lesions" on page 322.

Breaks

The bones most often broken on dogs are the legs, perhaps because of their long length and relative vulnerability. Car accidents, traps, blows, and gunshot wounds all often result in broken limbs.

The broken leg will usually dangle in an unnatural manner. The dog is not able to place weight on it. There are extreme pain and lameness. With a compound fracture (break in skin and bone), the end of the bone will be seen sticking through a break in the skin.

Keep a dog with a broken leg quiet, and handle it gently. If the dog is in pain, slip a gauze muzzle around its muzzle and behind its ears to prevent any accidental bites. Where a human might groan or scream in pain, the dog will bite, no matter how much it loves you—it just can't help it.

Be careful not to cause trauma to the leg by roughness. Blood vessels can be torn by the sharp end of the bone. However, do not try to splint the leg, even for temporary protection. Many incorrectly placed splints have caused more damage to a break than the dangling leg. Using care, get the dog to your veterinarian as soon as possible.

The break can be set with a plaster cast, splint, or intramedullary pin, which goes up through the bone marrow (best in many breaks). Most broken legs mend completely, with no difficulties, if you give the dog nursing at home.

Car Accidents

When a dog has been struck by a car, the first two things you should worry about are shock and internal bleeding. A broken leg or gash is a minor worry compared with these problems. Check the dog's color (see if the gums are pink or pale white, indicating shock), and get the animal to your veterinarian immediately. The best way to move a small- or medium-sized dog is to first muzzle it and then grasp the skin behind the neck and on the back, gently lifting the dog to a blanket or rug. Grabbing the dog around the waist or chest can stick a broken rib through a lung.

Do not try to give the dog any food or water. An injured dog is usually in shock and is not in any condition to take food or water, even if panting. Severe vomiting can result, which could start internal bleeding. And should the dog need immediate surgery, food or water in the stomach could make the surgery dangerous. Let me repeat here: Take the dog to a veterinarian immediately. Often an injection of a clotting drug, a stimulant, or immediate surgery can save a dog that would die otherwise.

After the first 24 hours, there is another danger period that can last for about four days. It is in this time that occasionally a dog is lost from a blood clot. The dog may be acting fine—it is active and eating—then suddenly die. (This also happens in humans.) You can guard against this somewhat by restricting the exercise the dog takes and feeding small amounts of easily digested foods several times daily. Your veterinarian may also prescribe drugs, taken orally, in some cases. There is *no* "sure cure" preventive.

Coccidiosis

Coccidiosis is caused by coccidia, parasitic protozoa (one-celled animals). It most often affects puppies, although adult dogs are often carriers and can infect younger dogs or become affected themselves when under stress. Coccidiosis causes diarrhea, coughing, and dehydration. There are often secondary infections, such as pneumonia and distemper. Damp, unsanitary conditions and overcrowding help to spread coccidiosis, as it is passed by contact with fecal material containing eggs or oocysts. A fecal examination is necessary both in diagnosing and in treating coccidiosis as many other things can cause diarrhea, especially in puppies.

Combination intestinal sulfas will usually work in treating coccidiosis. I have also had good success using cottage cheese. This seems to change the pH of the intestine, killing the coccidia. I have had pups that did not respond to sulfa clear up immediately when fed cottage cheese as a sole diet. I know it sounds like a quack remedy—I chuckled the first time a veterinarian friend told me about it—but it does usually work and causes no side effects, as sulfa drugs sometimes do in cases of dehydration.

Pups with diarrhea also benefit from receiving electrolytes in their water, until the stool is firm again, to combat dehydration that can kill them.

Conjunctivitis

Conjunctivitis is inflammation of the conjunctival sac next to the eye. The area will be red and swollen and appear bloodshot. The eye may run or stick shut. There may be pain or itching. Often there is a bacterial infection following the initial irritation. Conjunctivitis commonly starts with a foreign body, such as dust, pollen, or weed seeds, blowing into the eyes. A good way to have eye problems with a dog is to let it hang its head out the car window while you are driving. The speed of the moving car adds great force to any grit or dust blowing in the wind, driving it into the eye or conjunctiva. If left untreated, the condition can get bad enough to cause blindness.

Often, treatment consists of flushing the eye with a mild solution and applying an ointment containing an antibiotic or a sulfa and an anti-septic to ease the pain and itching. Rubbing the eye only increases the injury. Also, tape the dog's dewclaws to its legs to prevent the dog from scratching its eye. If it paws at the infected eye, it can hook the eye or the rim of it and cause serious damage.

Conjunctivitis is usually a simple condition but can be a symptom of certain diseases, such as distemper; so it is best to take the dog to your veterinarian, just to be safe.

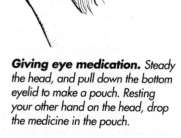

Giving eye medication. *Steady the head, and pull down the bottom eyelid to make a pouch. Resting your other hand on the head, drop the medicine in the pouch.*

Cuts, Bites, and Other Wounds

Dogs suffer the same types of injuries humans do, including cuts, bites, and scrapes, and the same types of basic first aid work for both. First, stop the bleeding by applying pressure to the wound with a gauze pack. Call your veterinarian at once unless the injury is minor. If it *is* minor, you can treat the wound yourself. Clip the hair from the edges, and clean the wound gently with warm, soapy water. Do not use Lysol or any such strong disinfectant, as you may be killing more cells than you are cleaning. Also, do not bandage the wound. Bandages retard healing and often cause infection by providing a warm, pro-tected, moist area for bacteria to breed. And do not put ointment onto a wound, as it usually attracts dirt, hair, and other irritants. A liquid antiseptic, such as Betadine, is much better because it dries quickly.

Few wounds on a dog actually require sutures. People usually prefer to have a wound sewn closed, often just so they do not have to look at the ugliness. But wounds usually heal quicker and without scarring if they remain open, healing from the inside. Keep an open mind when asking your veterinarian if he thinks a wound should be sutured. Some should be, of course, but certainly not all of them.

If your dog gets bitten, use special caution as it is always possible that the animal that inflicted the bite was rabid. If you know what animal bit your dog, cage the animal, if wild or stray, taking extreme care *not* to get bitten yourself. If the animal belongs to a neighbor, make *sure* that it has been vaccinated against rabies. Also, ask your neighbor to watch it for two weeks and let you know if it should get sick or die. (Generally, after two weeks' isolation, an aggressive animal will show definite symptoms of rabies or die.) When washing your dog's bite, use rubber gloves and plenty of soapy water to thoroughly flush out all bacteria, possible viruses (such as rabies), and dirt. Do *not* get in contact with saliva from the bite wound.

If you suspect your dog may have been bitten by a rabid animal and your dog is current with its rabies vaccination, revaccinate it immediately, and confine it, using extreme care, for 90 days. Should your dog be bitten by a stray or wild animal, the safest route is to have the offending animal destroyed immediately, taking care to save the entire head, and have the brain tested for rabies. If your dog is unfortunate enough to be bitten by a suspected rabid animal and is not current in its rabies vaccination, the animal should either be destroyed or be completely confined for six months and be vaccinated against rabies four weeks before being freed from total confinement. During the confinement *extreme* care must be taken to prevent possible human infection as rabies may be spread before the dog shows any sign of having the disease. (For more information on this disease, see "Rabies" on page 327.)

Cystitis

Cystitis is an inflammation of the bladder. It is quite common in dogs but not always diagnosed, as many times there is just a mild inflammation that causes no visible problems. Cystitis is most frequently caused by bacterial infections and calculi (stones).

A dog with cystitis often urinates frequently, vomits, dribbles urine unconsciously, and acts restless. There may be a fever. Lifting the dog may bring yelps of pain. There is often blood in the urine. Where the cystitis is caused by a stone (a bit more common in males), there may be a complete blockage in the urethra. When the dog is not able to urinate, it absorbs the wastes and soon becomes toxic. Within a short time, the dog is in real (and possibly irreversible) trouble.

As you can see, prompt discovery of the problem and quick diagnosis and treatment are very important. With an infection in the bladder, antibiotics usually bring about prompt relief. Surgery is generally the best treatment for a dog with stones, as they are usually quite large when causing the dog problems and they are nearly impossible to dissolve. Following surgery your veterinarian may put your dog on a special diet or advise putting a tablespoonful of vinegar in the drinking water to acidify the urine, which often helps prevent the formation of calculi in the future.

Diabetes

Diabetes is a disease that strikes dogs as well as people. It most often occurs in fat dogs over four years of age. The first signs are an increased thirst and frequent urination. Then there is a dramatic weight loss, quickly getting to the point of emaciation. The dog begins to act weak. In severe cases there is uncontrollable vomiting.

When caught fairly early and when there are no complicating factors, diabetes can be controlled quite easily if you are willing to spend a little extra time with your dog daily. Diet and exercise alone can control some mild cases. Reduce the carbohydrate intake severely, and give the dog foods like lean meat, boiled eggs, and boiled fish. Other cases respond well to oral medication. Still other dogs need insulin injections daily, given before regulated meals. If you give the injections religiously, you can maintain a diabetic dog quite well with the insulin. The needle used is very small, and the injection is practically painless. The dog soon associates the injection with eating and often begs for the injection so it can eat! Treatment and maintenance are inexpensive and can do much to prolong the life and health of a diabetic dog. Preventative measures include maintaining an active lifestyle in your dog, including regular exercise and keeping your dog within a good weight (not overweight!).

Distemper

Distemper is a disease of the central nervous system caused by a virus. It is usually severe, and there is no certain treatment. Distemper is very contagious among all canines, not only dogs. The common signs are mattered, running eyes, a plugged, crusty nose, diarrhea, and vomiting. Chorea—twitching of a leg, one side of the body, or tail—usually develops when the disease is nearing its worst.

Distemper is often confused with rabies, also caused by a virus. There is no similarity between them. You *cannot* get distemper if bitten by a dog ill with distemper; you *will* get rabies after being bitten by a rabid dog unless you get treatment. A dog sick with distemper may be crabby, but biting is not a symptom of distemper.

Distemper may occur year-round, and it is so highly contagious that it does not even need close contact to spread. You can bring it home on your clothes, or a dog with distemper can just pass through your yard and spread the virus to your unvaccinated dog.

Treatment, once the disease has started, is often frustrating for both the owner and the veterinarian. The sick dog may look better and have signs of recovery one day but then get worse the next. Antibiotics will not cure the disease, as it is a virus, but they can prevent secondary infections, such as pneumonia, in a very stressed dog. Injections of antiserum or globulin can help some dogs.

Good nursing is very important in treating this disease. Without it most dogs will die. A dog sick with distemper will not want to eat, so it must be coaxed to eat, force-fed, or tube-fed. Also, keep the dog warm and clean. Clean the eyes and nose several times daily, treat the eyes with ophthalmic ointment, and moisten the nose with mild petroleum jelly. A dog having convulsions must sometimes be given drugs to combat them so that it does not become overtired.

As with many other diseases, distemper is easier to prevent than treat. A puppy born from a dam that is immune to distemper through vaccination will have a certain level of immunity from its dam's milk. This immunity wears off at about eight weeks, however, so the pup must be vaccinated to remain protected. This first vaccination is usually done at eight weeks of age. It is often given in a combination shot containing distemper, hepatitis, and parvovirus. Leptospirosis used to be included in this first injection. But as it is quite rare now and because it is believed that early lepto vaccination can tie up a pup's immune system, making it less responsive to the distemper, hepatitis, and parvo portion of the vaccination, it is now usually deleted until a booster vaccination, given several weeks later.

If necessary, puppies may be vaccinated earlier, at three weeks of age, with a "puppy shot," or temporary vaccination. Puppies not receiving their vaccinated dam's milk or those under stress or in a high distemper area often do well with this added protection. As opposed to the older belief, there is not a "permanent" distemper vaccination. To keep active immunity, the dog should receive a yearly booster, once it has received its initial series of vaccinations.

Ear Infection

Dogs, especially long-eared dogs, are prone to several types of ear infections. The most common is due to ear mites. Ear mites burrow into the ear, creating places for bacteria and fungi to enter. The moist, dirty ear that often accompanies the mites makes a perfect breeding place for these infections. Bacterial and fungal infections can also get a start from irritation due to dirt and wax buildup, water or shampoo in the ear, foreign bodies, or injuries.

The dog will usually scratch at its ears with its hind feet and rub its head on the floor or against a chair. It may also shake its head, hold it to one side, and appear uncomfortable. When you look in the ear, it will often appear red and swollen, have a brownish, foul-smelling accumulation inside, and feel hot.

Mild cases, caused by accumulations of wax and dirt, may be taken care of at home. Dip a ball of cotton into alcohol or peroxide, and gently but firmly swab out the ear by using your finger and the cotton ball. Repeat the next day. There should be a great improvement, but if not, take your dog to the veterinarian. Fungal and bacterial infections do not respond to simple treatment and can get worse if not treated properly, possibly damaging your dog's hearing. Any extreme itching or aggravation should be taken care of at once before other problems develop, such as a hematoma (a large, blood-filled bruise of the ear, usually caused by flopping the ears back and forth, due to irritation).

Ear mites are treated like wax and dirt accumulations, with a cotton ball dipped in alcohol or peroxide, along with adding a few drops of vegetable oil to the ear every day. (The oil smothers the mites and soothes the irritation). If there is not much improvement after two days, call your veterinarian. It is sometimes necessary to use an ear mite remedy containing an insecticide, such as rotenone or pyrethrin.

Eclampsia

Caused by a low blood calcium level, this condition in many respects resembles one called milk fever in cows and goats. It can occur before whelping, but it is generally seen in bitches after giving birth, when the puppies are a few days old. It is often a small female with a fairly large litter that is affected. She will begin to pant, walk with a stiff gait, stumble, fall, and be unable to rise. She may have convulsions later on, stiffening out rigidly. If not treated, she will likely die.

Take the bitch to your veterinarian, who will give her an intravenous injection of calcium. Most females will instantly respond and rapidly become normal in their actions. It is possible that she may need a repeat injection, sometimes in a day or so, so be watchful for the first signs of trouble. When the litter is large and several weeks old, it is best to wean some or all of them at once. If they are allowed to continue nursing, the condition will recur.

Epilepsy

Epilepsy is quite common in dogs, especially in some breeds like Cocker Spaniels, Miniature and Toy Poodles, German Shepherds, and some of the smaller house dogs. This is not to say many of these dogs have epilepsy but that it is more common in these breeds.

A dog with epilepsy will have recurrent "fits," or convulsions. The dog shakes, stiffens out, falls, and jerks its legs; its head often tips backward. Often the dog will lose control and empty the bowel and bladder. After the seizure the dog usually recovers and acts dazed. Excitement may trigger these seizures. They may occur only once a year or several times daily in severe cases. They don't last long each time they occur.

There are several oral drugs that can be given when epilepsy has been diagnosed. Primidone and Dilantin, which are used with human epilepsy patients, will usually keep the dog from having seizures if given regularly. After a few months of treatment, you can gradually cut down the dosage until you reach a level that will just prevent the seizures. (One German Shepherd in our clinic required Dilantin only during periods where thunderstorms threatened, as these—and nothing else—set off his seizures!)

Do not use dogs with epilepsy for breeding, because it has been proved to be a genetic trait in canines.

Fleas

When a dog parasite is mentioned, everyone immediately thinks of fleas. But as long as you take a few preventive measures, fleas usually aren't much of a problem for most dogs. However, there are some dogs that develop an allergy to fleas. An allergic dog will break out with a rash, scratch, and be miserable if even one flea takes up residence in its coat.

Fleas are little, quick-moving, flat, brown insects that suck blood and annoy dogs and people. And dog fleas will bite people! Sandy, dry areas are favorite spots for fleas, and there are geographic locations where fleas are very prevalent. Fleas do not spend their life on the dog but hop off and on. This is why, when treating the dog with a flea powder or spray, you should also treat its bedding, rug, or sleeping area—even the house and carpet if the fleas are numerous.

An herbal flea deterrent, such as a pennyroyal mixture, either powdered on the dog or in a flea collar, often works when fleas are not numerous on the dog. If this is not successful, you can use a powder or spray containing rotenone, which is generally safe and effective. Dust or spray weekly for three weeks for surest results. Even more effective, but slightly more work, is using a shampoo containing rotenone. There are topical flea killers which also work on mites and ticks. These, such as Frontline, available through your veterinarian, are applied in a strip down the back, on the skin. They are then absorbed into the body and bloodstream making the dog's blood toxic to biting insects. Your dog may get fleas on him but when they bite, they will then die. I only recommend these when fleas are a problem on your dog.

If your home gets infested with fleas (which can happen even with no animals in the house), it is best to call an exterminator. Most flea sprays on the market will kill fleas, but the exterminator will be experienced in knowing the favorite hiding places and will know how to get maximum kill with a minimum of spray. It is a good idea to tell your exterminator that you are concerned about using undue toxic chemicals in your home, as there are certainly alternatives!

Flies

Biting flies are often a problem for an outdoor dog. Dogs with erect ears, in particular, are often attacked so badly on the ear tips that they bleed and scab over. These scabs in turn attract more flies. A daily application of a wipe-on insect repellent, such as that used for horses, will prevent this. If the dog has already been bitten, daubing scarlet oil on the raw spots will help heal them and repel flies at the same time.

Besides biting, flies also cause trouble by laying eggs on "woolly" areas of the dog, especially if they are soiled by diarrhea or blood from an injury. The rear parts of such breeds as Cockapoos, Collies, Cocker Spaniels, and Old English Sheepdogs are common sites of fly strikes. Soon after the eggs are laid, they hatch out into maggots, which not only eat the filth but quickly begin to destroy living flesh, as well.

Immediately examine any dark, foul-smelling areas, and wash them thoroughly if there are no maggots present. Clipping the area will also be a help. If you do see or suspect maggots, call your veterinarian at once (within a day or two) as the maggots may eat their way into the dog's abdominal cavity. Common treatments include clipping all the hair off in the area, washing the maggots out, flushing the open wound with an insecticidal antiseptic, and giving antibiotics to prevent infection.

Fungal Infection

Many types of fungal infections can attack dogs, but perhaps the most common is the fungus that causes "hot spots." Hot spots often appear very suddenly during the summer and fall. They are bald, angry red spots that have a moist, whitish look in the center. They either itch intensely or are very tender, causing pain if touched lightly. They usually occur on the neck and back, and they spread outward, generally keeping a roundish shape.

Have your veterinarian examine your dog when you suspect this problem. He can prescribe an antifungal, which quickly clears up the trouble. You'll need to clip the hair away from the entire red area so you can be sure the medication will reach the skin and to keep the hair from causing further irritation.

Other types of fungal infections affect the skin in less dramatic ways, but they still produce red, scabby, itchy lesions that irritate the dog greatly. When you suspect any fungal infection, take your dog to the veterinarian to have the problem correctly diagnosed and begin a treatment program. Many times the only treatment needed is a medicated bath. Other times you'll need to use local treatments after the bath or give antibiotics when a secondary bacterial infection is also present.

Gunshot Wounds

For some reason, dogs receive more gunshot wounds than any other animal. Perhaps it is because they do more "roaming" into other people's yards and are "chased off" at gunpoint—a very good reason to be *sure* your dog stays home, under supervision. Also, during hunting season some hunters will shoot at anything, be it a sparrow or dog. Knowing where your dog is at all times will protect it from such wounds.

Being shot with birdshot (many small pellets) is often more dangerous than being hit with a single rifle bullet. This is because rifle wounds are more noticeable and tend to get treated right away, while pellets from birdshot often leave very little outward sign when they penetrate the body.

If you suspect your dog has been shot, examine it carefully. Really pick and feel. With birdshot you will want to know where the majority of the shot struck. With a rifle wound, look for an entrance wound and exit wound. The exit wound may not be in line with the entrance wound, as the bullet often deflects off a bone.

Keep the injured dog warm and calm. Stop any bleeding that is present using a pressure pack. Then call your veterinarian at once.

Hematomas

Dogs sometimes get bruises, as people do. However, a dog's skin is looser, allowing more bleeding under the skin (a *bruise* is bleeding under the skin). These bruises fill the area with blood, making a lump called a hematoma. Hematomas are often found on ears, due to flopping the ears in attempts to get rid of itching ear mites or dirt accumulation. They're also commonly found on the neck from collar injuries, such as those that occur when a dog lunges on a chain, or on the elbow of a large dog that lies on concrete or other hard surfaces.

With an ear hematoma, the layers of skin pull away from the ear cartilage, and this can cause severe thickening and deforming of the ear flap. Ear hematomas can sometimes be eliminated without surgery if caught early, but often surgery is required to save the normal appearance of the ear. With other kinds of hematomas, it's best to leave them alone unless they are large or in a place where they might cause trouble, such as near the mouth or genitals; then take your dog to your veterinarian for an examination and treatment suggestions.

Many animals have bled to death when owners have lanced a hematoma, thinking they were lancing an abscess. But once relieved of the pressure that stopped the bleeding under the skin, the animal continues to bleed, sometimes so much that it is fatal. Never lance any bump before drawing some of the fluid out of it with a syringe and 18-gauge needle. The fluid in an abscess is yellowish or whitish. If the fluid is dark in color, suspect a hematoma: Do *not* lance it.

Hepatitis

Hepatitis is caused by a virus and very contagious, often spread by the urine of infected dogs. Its symptoms resemble those of distemper. There is usually a fever, inflamed eyes, vomiting, no appetite, and diarrhea. Hemorrhages and hematomas sometimes occur.

If you suspect your dog has hepatitis, call your veterinarian. Treatment for hepatitis consists of blood transfusions, intravenous fluids, and broad-spectrum antibiotics to prevent secondary infections. Since distemper often follows or accompanies hepatitis, it is usually a good idea to give globulin to prevent it, especially in a unvaccinated dog or a dog with a distemper vaccination that is not current.

A dog with hepatitis may also develop white eyes, which can cause temporary blindness. This usually follows the acute period of the disease, in which the dog is the sickest. If not treated, it will usually disappear in a week or two. This condition is called blue eye. The same condition can follow vaccination. It, as well, usually clears without treatment. Do not put cortisone ointments into the eye or give injections of cortisone, as this sometimes causes scar tissue to form, making the eye permanently blind.

As with many canine diseases, vaccination is much more satisfactory than treatment—and cheaper, as well. Most times hepatitis (canine adenovirus 1 [CAV 1] and related CAV 2, one of the causes of canine tracheobronchitis, or kennel cough) is included in the distemper vaccination combination; ask your veterinarian.

Hip Dysplasia

Hip dysplasia is a problem of the hips. It is often not noticeable without an X ray, except when the dog is severely affected, often in later years. It is a hereditary condition, and as with most hereditary problems, it is found most often in purebred dogs of certain breeds. German Shepherds, Old English Sheepdogs, and St. Bernards are a few of the breeds with a high incidence of hip dysplasia. Inbreeding or linebreeding on lines with even a scattered incidence of the condition can produce a litter with several pups affected with various grades of hip dysplasia, and the rest of the pups can be carriers of the condition.

It is recommended that every bitch and male used for breeding be X-rayed at 24 months of age—before being bred. An earlier X ray can provide false readings. It is not enough to say that the animal appears sound. These X rays may be taken at your local veterinarian's office or a state veterinary school. They can then be sent into the Orthopedic Foundation for Animals (OFA), where the dog is issued an OFA number, provided it is found sound. If all breeding animals were examined in this way, hip dysplasia would gradually be weeded out. But this is a utopian dream as it is nearly impossible to get all breeders (or all people, for that matter) to cooperate.

Your veterinarian can treat hip dysplasia once it is diagnosed. Dogs with this condition are often maintained for years on periodic doses of buffered aspirin and anti-inflammatory drugs such as phenylbutazolidin, combined with a strict diet to limit body fat, as the added weight puts extra stress on the hip joint.

When the pain and anti-inflammatory drugs no longer seem to be working, surgery is recommended in many cases. Complete removal of the femoral head sounds very radical, but in most cases the dog continues to walk nearly as well as it did before the surgery.

Intervertebral Disc Lesions

Certain breeds, usually long-backed breeds, are quite prone to back problems arising from protrusion of a spinal disc, which puts pressure on the spinal cord. It can arise from an injury and is hereditary in a certain sense, as Cockers, Pekingese, and most often Dachshunds—all having long backs—are affected.

Jumping on and off furniture, climbing up and down stairs, and leaping in and out of cars often cause sudden, acute pain and sometimes paralysis of the hind legs. Sometimes you'll first notice severe lameness and an unwillingness to stand or to move about. The problem quickly progresses. In a few days, the dog will often assume a froglike position, with the hind legs out behind the body.

Surgery is often used, but as with humans, not all back surgery is successful. Very often, though, these back injuries can be healed to the point that the dog can walk and lead a normal life with the help of drugs, good nursing, and physical therapy.

Leptospirosis

Leptospirosis is caused by a bacterium and can be passed to humans. There are many locales where there is a high incidence of this disease, higher than most people realize. It can be passed through dogs, rats, or wildlife, depending on the type of lepto organism considered.

The first signs may be fever, diarrhea, increased urination, bloody or discolored urine, vomiting, and weakness. There is often permanent kidney damage, even if the sick dog survives the disease. The mucous membranes in the mouth may become inflamed and sore and later slough off.

If you suspect your dog has leptospirosis, call your veterinarian at once, and use good personal hygiene when handling the dog. Antibiotics, such as streptomycin or tetracycline, are often used for treatment as well as intravenous electrolyte therapy to combat dehydration and help stressed kidneys.

Prevention consists of vaccination and of keeping your dog away from places rats are known or suspected to frequent, for rats are often the carriers of this disease, spreading it through contamination with their urine. Cattle and other dogs may also spread the disease, so it's important to control your dog to keep it away from potential carriers.

Lice

Lice are small, slow-moving, grayish parasites that occasionally infest dogs, usually outdoor farm dogs. They are most often seen on medium- or long-coated breeds as the long hair enables them to hide from the light. When lice are bothering a dog, the animal will usually begin scratching excessively. On parting the hair, you will see the tiny lice and the little specks that are their eggs. A severe infestation of lice can kill a dog through severe anemia.

When you discover lice on your dog, clip the entire dog short. With no hair to shelter and protect the lice, it's usually easy to take care of these pests, often with a medicated shampoo. Repeat treatment every week for three weeks to kill any new lice that have hatched out. Remove the doghouse bedding and burn it, and dust the dog's bed with a safe louse powder.

Lyme Disease

Lyme disease is becoming more and more of a problem in dogs as well as in people. Most frequently spread by deer ticks, Lyme disease has been found in dogs in nearly every state of the United States as well as in Canada, Europe, and Australia.

The symptoms of Lyme disease can be vague, but a fever, lameness, weakness, and swollen lymph glands are commonly seen. Diagnosis is difficult as even blood tests on humans are often incorrect and misleading. Most veterinarians will test a dog suspected of having Lyme disease, but they treat depending on the symptoms, especially in high-Lyme areas. Treatment usually consists of long-term therapy with antibiotics, such as penicillin, tetracycline, or doxycycline.

To minimize the chance of Lyme disease, remove all ticks very promptly (daily at least), taking special care not to handle or "squash" the tick with your bare fingers. Dispose of any ticks by burning; then wash your hands well. A vaccination is now available for dogs and should be given in any area where Lyme disease has been diagnosed. Consult with your veterinarian.

Mange

Mange is quite common in dogs. Perhaps this is because they have such close contact with people! You see, people can often carry the mange mites on their skin and don't realize it because the mites don't bother people. Once, a vet school class took skin scrapings from the whole class—and over 90 percent were found to have mange mites! And this was before they had any actual contact with animals. (They also weren't a dirty, scruffy bunch!)

These mites are so tiny you cannot see them with the naked eye. They burrow into the skin, causing intense itching. A mange infestation often follows a period of severe stress. Malnutrition, followed by poor skin health, often lets the mites get a head start and cause problems for the dog. Any skin eruptions, especially those about the face, legs, and belly, should be regarded as suspicious. Pustules, scabby areas, thickened grayish areas, and baldness are all symptoms of mange.

Mange is very contagious to other dogs, so it is best to isolate the suspect until your veterinarian makes a proper diagnosis. Do not just let a neighbor tell you that your dog has mange, as there are several other skin troubles that look like mange. (See "Fungal Infection" on page 319 for more information on other skin problems.) The only way to make a correct diagnosis is by examining a skin scraping under a microscope.

A dog affected by mange should be clipped entirely. This is often hard to agree to, especially if your dog has a long, beautiful coat, but it is the only way to stop the mange at once. You can't treat spots for mange if you can't find them, and you can't treat through hair and do a decent job. Many times there are mites present in areas that do not yet show lesions.

Using medicated shampoos, along with ointments containing rotenone, lime-sulfur, or pyrethrin, will usually effect a cure. Many times you must repeat treatment two or three times, at weekly intervals, even if the skin seems much better. There are several newer treatments, including dips, such as Amitraz and Paramite and topical solutions applied once a month, such as Selamectrin, that offer quite reliable results. Ivermectin has also been used on some dogs with good results. Always consult your veterinarian, as some breeds of dogs require different treatments as some have undesirable side effects from some of these drugs.

Metritis

Metritis is inflammation of the uterus. There are two types: acute and chronic. With acute metritis the bitch is very sick. She has often retained a placenta or fetus and absorbed the foul uterine discharge, making her extremely toxic. She will vomit, have diarrhea, run a high fever, and act listless. If your bitch has recently whelped and acts dull or has abnormal uterine discharges with a foul odor, have your veterinarian examine her at once. It could save her life.

With chronic metritis there is often a low-grade infection. The bitch can often go a long time with a mild infection without acting sick. Sometimes the only sign of trouble is breeding difficulties. The bitch may be bred once or several times and not conceive. If she does conceive, the puppies may either be stillborn or die shortly after birth. Although antibiotic therapy can be used, the best course of action in many cases is to remove the uterus. Sometimes the low-grade infection can "blow up" into an acute attack, and the bitch will be lost. It is very hard to get rid of chronic metritis without removing the uterus. With a very valuable breeding female, your veterinarian may try infusing the uterus periodically with antibiotics and using injections of prostaglandin to help push any foul matter out of the uterus.

Parvovirus

Parvoviral infection, often referred to just as parvo, is a relatively "new" disease, first recognized only in the late 1970s. There are two different forms of the disease: myocarditis, causing sudden death, often in young puppies, and enteritis, causing diarrhea, often severe and streaked with fresh blood. Parvovirus is very contagious, chiefly through exposure and ingestion of feces-contaminated food or water. Death is not always the result, but it is common with young, unprotected puppies.

If you suspect your dog has parvo, call your veterinarian at once. Treatment often consists of intravenous fluids and antibiotics to prevent or treat bacterial infections that accompany or follow the parvovirus infection. You'll also want to isolate the dog promptly and give careful attention to cleanliness.

Prevention consists chiefly of vaccination, beginning at a young age, with revaccination yearly.

Porcupine Quills

Sooner or later, nearly every farm, ranch, or hunting dog runs into a porcupine (provided, of course, that it lives in an area where there are porcupines). These slow-moving animals prefer to just go about their business; but when harassed by a dog, they can quickly slap a lot of quills into the dog's nose.

Many dogs have the sense to quit after they've gotten four or five quills stuck into their noses. But once in a while, a dog really gets mad and tries to tear the porcupine up. The usual result is a dog with a mouth, nose, and throat full of quills. When this happens, take the dog to the veterinarian for quill pulling. Any attempt to remove the quills at home will be futile.

Porcupine quills have tiny barbs that, when imbedded in the flesh, make them hard to pull. These same barbs cause the quill to work deeper and deeper in time. If the quills are grasped firmly and pulled very slowly, usually with forceps or pliers, the barbs will release. But if yanked, which is not uncommon if the dog is struggling, the quills will snap off, leaving a large amount of quill beneath the skin. These quills often become infected, causing swelling and pain. There are also tiny quills that get into the skin when the dog bites at the porcupine. These are little bigger than a hair, but if left in or broken off, they can cause as much trouble as the 3-inch-long quills. This is why it is usually best to take the dog to your veterinarian, where it will receive a general anesthetic so it can be relaxed while the painful operation of quill pulling is done.

Once in a while, a dog gets into quills so badly that it goes into shock. In this case it must be treated at once, or it will die. If the dog seems suddenly shaky, looks pale, and acts strangely, get it to your veterinarian immediately, while keeping it quiet and calm. Do *not* attempt to feed or water a dog suspected of being in shock. This could kill it.

Rabies

Rabies is caused by a virus that is very highly concentrated in the saliva of infected animals. It used to be called hydrophobia (fear of water) because the paralysis of the throat made it hard or impossible for a rabid dog to drink.

There are two types of rabies: dumb rabies (the dog just sits, with its mouth often hanging open, and has a peculiar look in its eyes, later frequently howling strangely) and furious rabies (the dog hallucinates, snaps at imaginary objects, wanders, and becomes increasingly irritable). Often the dumb rabies is the most dangerous as many people pry into the mouth, thinking the dog has something stuck in its throat or mouth. Getting the dog's saliva into a small cut or scratch can give you rabies, so *never* stick your hand into such an animal's mouth.

Not all rabid dogs attack people and have frothy mouths. A rabid dog often has a personality change. A timid, fearful dog will get brave and friendly. A normally friendly dog will get surly and timid. A rabid dog will often leave home and wander until exhausted.

Skunks, raccoons, foxes, and bats are frequently carriers of rabies, so never try to pick up or catch a "friendly" wild animal. Keep your dog away from such animals, as well. Rabid skunks frequently bite, not spray.

If your dog is bitten by a stray or wild animal, carefully cage or kill the suspect, leaving the entire head intact. Taking great care not to become infected yourself, transport the suspect to your veterinarian for rabies testing. Immediately place your dog in strict quarantine while you are waiting for the test results. If the test proves positive (the animal that bit your dog *was* rabid) and your dog was not vaccinated against rabies, it is recommended that your dog be destroyed at once. If you cannot bring yourself to do this, it must be kept in *strict* isolation for six months—which is very hard to do, especially if there are children at home—and vaccinated against rabies a month before release.

If your vaccinated dog was bitten by a known rabid animal, it is recommended that you revaccinate it and then place it in strict quarantine for 90 days.

It is recommended that any dog bitten by an unknown wild or domestic animal be regarded as having been bitten by a rabid animal and treated as such.

As you can see, vaccinating your dog against rabies and keeping its vaccination schedule current protect not only your animal but your family, as well.

Snakebites

Many dogs are bitten by poisonous snakes every year. However, don't assume that because your dog was bitten by a snake, it will certainly die. First of all, many snake bites are by nonpoisonous snakes, such as the bull snake, garter snake, and king snake, all of which bite as part of their aggressive display, meant to frighten away attackers.

Poisonous snakes in the United States encompass the pit viper family, including rattlesnakes, copperheads, and water moccasins, whose bite causes pain and swelling and will cause the area to become necrotic and slough off in time. Another poisonous snake is the coral snake, found chiefly in the southeastern United States. It is known by the old rhyme "Red touch yellow, kill the fellow," referring to the red, yellow, and black banding of its coloring. The coral snake's short-fanged bite paralyzes the victim's respiratory center, frequently causing death in a short time.

If your dog is bitten and you see the snake but are unsure if it is poisonous, kill the snake, and take it and your dog to the veterinarian at once. Do *not* get bitten yourself; "dead" snakes are perfectly capable of inflicting poison via a bite, even when the head is off the body.

It is important to know that not all bites by poisonous snakes result in injection of poison. It has been proved that over 50 percent of all bites by venomous snakes do *not* contain poison, for one reason or another. But if your dog is bitten, assume that the bite contained poison, and get your dog to a veterinarian at once. *Do not attempt first aid.* Just keep the dog calm and quiet. Carry it, if you are able, to your car, and drive immediately to the nearest veterinarian.

Treatment consists of giving injections of antivenin, often intravenous fluids, and frequently cortisone. Antibiotics and tetanus antitoxin are also frequently given to prevent further problems once the bite has been treated.

Strychnine Poisoning

In the past strychnine poison was used to control rats and mice. While it has been replaced with such products as warfarin, it is still found in many rural areas for use on gophers and prairie dogs. And there are some malicious people in the world that use strychnine to poison neighborhood dogs.

A poisoned dog will usually begin to show symptoms an hour or so after having eaten the tainted food. It will begin to tremble, pant, and act nervous. As the symptoms progress, it will respond to any loud noise, such as a car horn beeping, by having convulsions. As the condition worsens, even clapping of the hands can produce a severe convulsion.

If you take the dog to a veterinarian immediately, it can be given emergency treatment. This consists of emptying the stomach to prevent further absorption of the strychnine, intravenous injection of sodium pentobarbital to control seizures, and often an intravenous dextrose solution to provide fluids and improve kidney action.

When left untreated, the dog will suffer one convulsion after another until it dies from exhaustion. It is a cruel death that not even a rat should suffer.

Ticks

Ticks are quite a problem for dogs in many areas. There are several types of ticks that infest dogs; all are basically the same. They are blood-sucking parasites that attach themselves to an animal until full of blood. In small numbers they generally cause no trouble except irritation. In large numbers, however, they can produce anemia and extreme agitation. Scratching and digging at the tick bites break off the tick heads, irritate the skin, and aggravate the situation. Secondary infections often follow. Unfortunately, in increasingly large areas of the country, ticks can carry Lyme disease, which is contagious to humans. This disease is often carried by the brown deer tick, which can be very tiny. (For more information, see "Lyme Disease" on page 324.)

It is wise to examine your dog daily for ticks. Remove these pests with a gloved hand and a ball of cotton or tissue. Pull slowly but firmly until they release, and then burn them to be sure they are completely destroyed. If you just yank a tick off, the mouth may remain attached, causing infection and soreness.

Where ticks are a problem, there are topical flea and tick killers that are very effective. These, such as Frontline, available through your veterinarian, are applied in a strip down the back, on the skin. They are then absorbed into the body and bloodstream making the dog's blood toxic to biting insects. Your dog may get ticks on him but when they bite, they will then die and fall off when quite small. It is still a good idea to check your pet daily for ticks.

Tonsillitis

Tonsillitis occurs often in dogs. It is usually caused by a bacterial infection. I have seen many dogs having a simultaneous anal gland infection caused by the same bacteria infecting the tonsils. I believe these dogs had their anal gland infection first, licked the anal area in an attempt to alleviate the condition, and picked up the infection in the tonsils. In chronic cases, once the anal glands were removed, the dogs never had tonsillitis again. Coincidence? I hardly think so.

A dog affected with tonsillitis will usually cough, gag, and vomit. It may paw at its throat. Often there will be a fever, lack of appetite, dullness, and lack of energy. Many times you can feel one or both tonsils, just below the jaw, when they are swollen.

If you suspect tonsillitis, consult with your veterinarian. When taken care of promptly, most cases of tonsillitis clear up in three to four days. Using a broad-spectrum antibiotic, plus cortisone to take the swelling out of the tonsil and throat, works in most cases. Good nursing also plays an important part. You can often coax your dog to eat by giving it ice cream, cold milk, and cold broth. These foods are soothing on the sore throat and will encourage the dog to take more nourishment.

With cases of recurrent tonsillitis where anal infection has *not* been present, it is often advisable to remove the tonsils surgically.

Worms

Every year your dog should receive a regular fecal examination as well as a heartworm check, done via blood sample, by a veterinarian. If there are worms present, your veterinarian can then suggest the right wormer for the job. True, there are "shotgun" prescriptions available at many stores that claim to kill all worms. Unfortunately, they either do not kill the worms or, worse, can kill the dog if misused. Each worm requires different drugs to kill it. Some drugs kill several species, some only one. Few wormers do a good job on more than three types. Therefore, examination and treatment by your veterinarian are essential to keeping your dog worm-free.

Heartworm

Heartworms infest the heart. Once mainly a problem in southern areas, heartworm has become widespread. It is spread by mosquitoes, which suck the blood of an infected dog and transmit the microfilariae (prelarvae) to another healthy dog. Here they develop into mature heartworms. These in turn reproduce, and there are more microfilariae to infect another dog. Heartworms are large worms and can completely block the heart. When a badly infested dog is exercised, it may show shortness of breath, coughing, and lack of stamina, and it may be easily tired. Sudden death can result.

Every dog should have a yearly check for heartworm. If found free of them, it can be put on an oral heartworm preventive. This is given throughout the mosquito season.

Treatment for heartworm can be tricky but is usually successful. The drug that kills the adult heartworms must be used with extreme care: If too many worms are killed quickly, they leave the heart, causing blockages in the bloodstream, like a spring logjam. This can result in death. Often, repeated treatments are necessary. Following treatment the dog must receive very restricted exercise until your veterinarian feels the adult worms have all been killed and passed out of the heart and lungs.

Hookworm

Hookworms are one of the most severe intestinal parasites. They cause unthriftiness, diarrhea, blood in the stool, and death in young puppies due to anemia. Puppies can be infected before being born and become reinfested very early. Death may result at an early age. Hookworms enter the body by penetrating the skin. In this way they can also infect people, especially those who prefer to walk barefoot.

All puppies should receive a fecal examination for worms at weaning; but if there has been trouble with hookworm in the past or if the pups are not doing as well as they should, they should receive an examination at two to three weeks of age. If you wait until eight weeks, there may not be any puppies left.

Strict sanitation measures are necessary when hookworm has shown up. As the larvae are in the soil, you should move the dogs to a new, clean area after worming them. Have regular stool checks done after that to ensure that the parasite is really gone, not just in hiding. There are chemicals that kill hookworm larvae on concrete runs and in the soil, to some extent; ask your veterinarian for his advice.

Roundworm

Roundworm is the most common parasite affecting dogs. Most puppies are born with roundworms, even when the dam was faithfully wormed before she was bred. These worms are quite large, white, and tapered at both ends, resembling a bean sprout. They are often coughed up or seen in the stool, especially in puppies. A small puppy can harbor huge amounts of these parasites, which harm the digestive tract and cause malnutrition. (After all, you can't feed a puppy what it needs if the worms beat it to the food!)

The worms migrate through the bloodstream and thus can be difficult to treat. One worming is not enough. That kills only the worms present in the stomach and intestine, but it does not kill the larvae in other places or destroy the eggs that will hatch and soon reinfest the dog. Worming a second time, two weeks after the first treatment, will often provide best results. Ask your veterinarian for his suggestions.

Tapeworm

Tapeworms are carried to the dog by fleas. A flea larva ingests tapeworm eggs, becomes an adult, and is ingested by the dog; then the eggs hatch, starting the cycle again. The adult tapeworm is large and flat and can grow to a length of several feet. It is made up of segments, each containing eggs. These sections are passed in the stool; they are whitish pieces that look like inchworms when first passed and quickly dry to look like grains of rice. They are often found in the hair around the dog's rectum and tail or in its bedding.

Your veterinarian can prescribe a drug that will effectively rid your dog of tapeworm. Along with fleas, rabbits also serve as an intermediate host of the tapeworm, so never feed rabbit entrails to your dog. Reducing the flea population on the dog and restricting its diet to domestic foods, such as dry dog food, as opposed to "what it catches," will help keep it tapeworm-free.

Whipworm

Whipworm is less common than the other worms. It can be hard to get rid of, though, because it lives in the colon and cecum (a blind pouch resembling the appendix in a human). Often the most common sign of whipworm is the liquid, foul-smelling stool. Unthriftiness and anemia follow.

Consult your veterinarian for diagnosis and a treatment program based on your dog's needs. Treatment consists of giving oral drugs or occasionally, where warranted, injectables. Strict sanitation will do much to cut down on whipworm infestations, as well.

C<small>ATS</small>

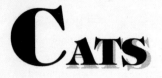

G<small>ENERAL</small> C<small>ARE AND</small> M<small>ANAGEMENT</small>

*A*lthough the average cat is very independent, it does require care to remain happy and healthy. Daily feeding isn't enough; all too many cats die at an early age owing to their owners paying no attention to their other needs or cat comforts.

Housing

The house cat should have a clean litter box available or have use of a pet door (in safe rural areas) to go outdoors when necessary. A scratching post, for the natural process of cleaning the claws and for exercise, is appreciated both by the cat and its owner; without it, the cat will often use the furniture or carpet. Likewise, a few toys, such as a sock stuffed with another one, a catnip mouse, a ball, or some of the more sophisticated and expensive toys, will make your cat happier and healthier as it will get more safe exercise.

Although a cat may nap on the sofa or chair, most appreciate their own beds. A simple cardboard box with a couple of old towels in it will work well, or the owner may opt for a more elaborate "kitty condo," carpeted and made fun with cutout windows throughout.

Feeding

Generally, cats do well with a good-quality dry food available at all times, with perhaps a small can of food given daily as a treat. I stress "good-quality" here. Several brands of cat food are cheaper than others, but they are also lower in quality, having lesser ingredients than the better foods. You can usually trust your cat to tell you. If it likes the food, it is often of higher quality than one the cat turns its nose up at. Shop around, buying small bags at first, until both you and your cat are satisfied. Reading product labels is a help, but it is getting increasingly hard for the layperson to understand terms such as "poultry digest" and "meat and bone byproducts." Again, trust your cat. If it appears sleek, active, and happy, you've made the right choice. If it is rough coated and sluggish, has bouts of diarrhea, or vomits its food, make a switch.

Do not feed cats any cooked fish or poultry containing the bones. Small, sharp bones can cause not only stomach pain but also impaction of the intestine and death. Also, avoid feeding highly seasoned foods to cats. Remember, nature did not intend cats to eat hot peppers, bologna, or sausage. Gastric upsets often result, which can lead to more serious troubles. Keep in mind, too, that cats do not like

PARTS OF A CAT

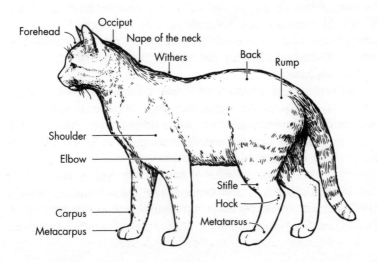

335

First Aid Kit for Cats

Here's a list of suggested supplies for your feline first aid kit. Every home with a cat should have at least the items marked with an asterisk. If you have several cats, all of the items in this list may come in handy at some time. Ask your veterinarian for his recommendations for your particular locale and situation.

Antiseptic wound liquid*

Cat carrier*

Cotton*

5-cc syringe

Forceps*

French feeding tube

Pet nail clippers*

Pet nursing bottle

Rectal veterinary
    thermometer*

Veterinarian's phone
    number*

sour or moldy food. Never leave moist food, such as canned cat food, in a bowl for longer than six hours. If it is too much for the cat to eat in that period, feed less food. Sour or moldy food can be filled with bacteria that will make the cat sick or even kill it.

If you keep cats to control mice, don't depend on their hunting to supply the food they need. The old idea that a hungry cat is a better mouser is untrue. The well-fed, but not fat, cat gives the best in its hunting. A female cat, hunting instinctively for her kittens, will hunt all day. She should have adequate nourishment to do this. Her kittens should also receive additional food as often one aggressive kitten will grab all the prey the mother brings, leaving its brothers and sisters hungry.

All cats should always have access to fresh, clean water. If they do not receive adequate water, they may become dehydrated and susceptible to illness. Inadequate water consumption, especially with a diet high in minerals and ash, can lead to a problem known as urinary calculi. Dry cat food can also cause trouble in this way. If the cat does not drink adequate water to compensate for the lack of moisture in the dry food, it is more likely that urinary calculi will form. (For more on preventing and controlling this problem, see "Urinary Calculi" on page 362).

Do not let your cat drink out of the bathtub or toilet bowl, because many cats are poisoned by drinking toilet bowl fresheners, Lysol, and cleaners.

Restraint

Occasionally it will be necessary to restrain your cat. This is much more difficult than restraining a dog as cats are generally more "wiggly" and aggressive in fighting restraint. Using tried-and-true methods of restraint will make it much easier for you or your veterinarian to examine, treat, or groom your cat.

Sometimes there is a certain knack to just holding onto a cat. When it has decided that it would rather be elsewhere, a cat can turn into a slippery, twisting bundle with claws. Being a naturally nervous animal, a cat can be upset by many things, even if it normally has a calm disposition. A loud noise, a moving car, barking dogs, and strange surroundings can all bring on the desire to "escape" and hide. The best way to hold a cat that wants to wiggle away is to grasp the forefeet with one hand and the hind legs and tail with the other hand. The cat uses the tail for balance when jumping and the hind legs for ripping and clawing when frightened or angry. Restraining both front and hind legs, plus the tail, will enable the average person to hold on to all but the most frightened or vicious cat.

This hold, however, gives no protection to you against bites. Most cats will not bite unless hurt first. When given an injection, though, some will try to claw or bite. The easiest way to hold the cat for a procedure such as this is to grasp the skin firmly behind the neck and just in front of the tail, placing the cat on a slippery table or other surface. Use care not to pinch the skin, and hold the cat's body close to your own for security and added restraint.

Wrapping the cat in a towel sometimes aids in minor treatment but will not work with a very frightened cat. When you need more restraint, slip the cat into a canvas bag with a drawstring at the top, allowing the head to come out. Then gently close the bag snugly (but not too tightly) so there isn't enough room for the front legs to work free. This restraint works well for medicating ears, cleaning teeth, giving oral medicines, and examining the head of an excitable cat.

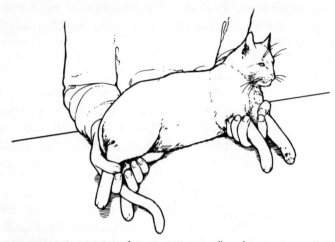

Restraining a cat. *If your cat is generally calm, you can restrain it by grasping the forefeet with one hand and the hind legs and tail with the other. This method will not prevent bites, however.*

Once in a while, it may be necessary to prevent your cat from scratching at its ears, rubbing its eyes, or licking medication off its body. Although tranquilizers can sometimes prevent this, many a cat will continue to scratch or lick, even though really drugged. It might not hit the right place, but it will continue to try, sometimes causing damage. The easiest way to keep the cat from bothering medication or to prevent self-mutilation due to an itching problem (such as ear mites) is to make an Elizabethan collar. A variety of materials will work, but the most common are plastic, such as that cut from plastic pails, and heavy cardboard. Make the collar in the shape of a circle, perhaps 12 inches in diameter, with a hole in the center that fits snugly around the cat's neck. Then make a cut in the collar, from the neck hole to the outside rim. Fit the collar on the cat, overlapping the cut edges and taping them together to form a cone-shaped arrangement. When a collar is the right size and well fitted, only the most determined cat will be able to get it off or get around it with feet or mouth.

Breeding

The queen, or female cat, will come into heat every two to three weeks, most often in the winter, spring, and summer. She is in heat

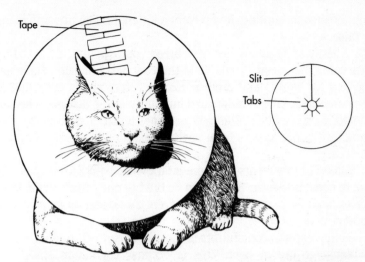

Labels: Tape, Slit, Tabs

Elizabethan collar. *To prevent a cat from licking a wound or medication, create an Elizabethan collar out of plastic or heavy cardboard. Make a slit in one side, and then cut out a smaller circle in the center. Cutting and bending back tabs around the center circle will make it harder for the cat to remove the collar.*

for a period of three to six days. Signs of heat are an arched back, with hindquarters high in the air, a throaty, yowling call, rolling about on the floor, holding the tail upward, and treading the hind legs.

Before allowing your cat to be bred, consider that multitudes of unwanted, mistreated stray cats are already on the streets and being destroyed by the hundreds every day at animal shelters for lack of homes. Do you really want to contribute to that problem by allowing your queen to have a litter of perhaps eight kittens? It is extremely hard to find good homes for kittens, even well-bred pure-bred kittens. It is not good enough to say, "I'll give them to a farmer." Most farmers have too many cats already! Really think it out, and be *sure* you have available homes for all kittens, even ones you can't find other owners for. (This means you'll probably be stuck with one or more female kittens, who will come into heat in a few months and possibly become bred themselves.) It is much better to spay your female pet than to allow her to raise a litter. Spaying will not change her disposition, make her fat, or make her uninterested in hunting. If you want a kitten, find an unwanted one to raise.

When you definitely desire to breed your cat, plan the breeding with care. The queen should be in the very best of health. Have her checked for worms and other parasites before she is even due to come into heat. She should carry immunity to the diseases she can be vaccinated against. This will not only protect her but also give immunity to her kittens from birth to about eight weeks of age in most cases.

Make arrangements with the stud owner before your queen is due to come into heat. If she is to be bred to one certain male, keep her isolated in a secure room to prevent an accidental mating with another male cat.

Following a successful breeding, the queen will often seem to suddenly go out of heat. This is because copulation stimulates ovulation.

Pregnancy can often be detected at about three weeks by an experienced person. Your veterinarian can perform this examination for you. When the abdomen is gently palpated, marble-sized lumps in the uterus can be felt. Do not squeeze the abdomen roughly or very hard as damage to the queen or the kittens can result.

The pregnant queen should receive a balanced diet and be encouraged to eat high-protein foods, such as liver. Also, give a good vitamin-mineral supplement to aid the developing kittens and the queen. The mother's appetite will increase with the size of her abdomen, and she should receive plenty of quality food. It is natural for her to slow down and not play or run about as she may have done prior to feeling her pregnancy.

Birthing

As the queen's time draws nearer, she will seek out a quiet, secluded "nest," such as a dresser drawer, a hole in the hay, or a place in the closet. Fifty-eight to 68 days after breeding, she will be ready to give birth to her kittens. Her temperature will drop sharply 12 to 24 hours preceding birth. The kittens are usually born with no trouble, owing to their sausage shape and small size, but sometimes a physical defect in the queen or other problem will hinder birth. If she labors for longer than half an hour with a kitten, producing nothing, call your veterinarian. He may advise a little more time, an injection to help uterine contractions, or possibly a cesarean if it is impossible for her to make a natural delivery.

Because of the very small size of the vagina and the pelvic opening in the queen, it is best to take her to the veterinarian at once when there are birth difficulties. A queen tires quickly in a difficult birth and can be easily injured by inexperienced attempts to help her. Many a uterus has been ripped by too forceful an extraction of a fetus, and many a queen has been lost due to shock and exhaustion.

If the difficulty is just a larger kitten becoming stuck at the vaginal opening, this is generally no problem. Grasp the head or legs with a dry towel, and pull gently but firmly as the queen strains. The kitten usually is then quickly expelled. Do not just yank the kitten out. This will cause damage and bleeding.

In most cases, however, the kittens are born easily. It is a good idea to keep an eye on the queen while she is having them, for you can often help save a kitten. Once in a while, a queen may be busy cleaning one kitten, ignoring the fact that she just had another one. If the membrane is not removed from the kitten's head after the umbilical cord breaks, the kitten will often smother or drown in fluid. If the queen does not remove the sac, you should do it for her, drying the head (especially the nose and mouth) well.

Each kitten is followed by a placenta (afterbirth). Count these to make sure there is one for each kitten. Once in a great while, a queen will retain one or more placentas, causing an inflammation and infection of the uterus. If you are sure there is a retained placenta, call your veterinarian. Often an injection of hormones is all that's needed to encourage the uterus to release the placenta. Don't, by the way, be alarmed at the color of these placentas: They are often a horrible greenish black. Also, don't be alarmed when the queen eats them; this is normal. Eating the placentas stimulates her milk letdown.

Caring for Kittens

The kittens will be born with their eyes shut tightly. These will open in about two weeks, and the kittens will begin to move about.

It is easiest to sex your litter of new kittens just after birth, if desired. Right after birth, the testicles of the male kittens are readily apparent. In a day or so, it can be very hard to sex the kittens unless you are experienced. Hold the newborn kitten on its back. In the males you will see the testicles as tiny bulges just below the anus, on either side of the penis.

The kittens will nurse for six to eight weeks of age, but as soon as they will eat semisolid food—at about four weeks— you should give them several small feedings daily to relieve the queen of the strain of producing milk.

Kittens can be weaned at eight weeks of age if you are prepared to give them adequate care. (Otherwise, leave them with the mother until she weans them herself or her milk dries up naturally.) Small kittens should be fed four or five times daily. When

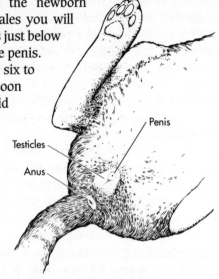

Penis

Testicles

Anus

Sexing a kitten. *It's easiest to determine a kitten's sex right after birth. On males the testicles will be readily apparent as tiny bulges just below the anus, on either side of the penis.*

they are about three months old, cut down to three meals a day, and at six months, feed them twice daily in addition to providing free-choice dry food of a good quality. Kittens need a 30 percent protein diet, so feeding a dry food with 14 percent protein will not maintain a kitten or allow it to grow. Inadequate protein intake will usually result in death. Feeding such foods as liver, kidney, raw ground beef, and small amounts of milk will boost the protein intake, as will feeding a good canned cat food made up of such things as beef and liver. Too much milk or cereals (as found in cheap cat foods) will cause indigestion and diarrhea.

Orphan Kittens

Once in a while, either due to lack of milk on the queen's part or due to her untimely death, you may need to raise the litter by hand. This is quite a job, so be prepared! Fortunately, it is also very rewarding.

The kittens should get about 2 cc of milk (preferably goat milk) every two hours, day and night, for the first week. If the kittens seem very hungry after feeding, increase the amount slowly until they are a little hungry, but not mewing continually, after feeding. It's easy to give the milk, either by tube-feeding (see "Orphan and Rejected Puppies" on page 297) or by using a pet or doll bottle with a soft rubber nipple. An eyedropper is not as good, because it gives the milk too fast, causing inhalation pneumonia as the milk droplets enter the lungs.

After the first week, increase the milk to about 4 cc, depending on the size and health of the kittens. Kittens being fed the right amount of milk will feel full and round, with tight skin. They will squirm and mew angrily when hungry. Too much milk will cause diarrhea, which is often fatal.

As the kittens' eyes open, gradually increase the amount of milk while decreasing the number of feedings per day. At three to four weeks, add semisolid food to their diet in the form of mashed liver.

One caution here: If the queen cannot be around to take care of cleaning the kittens, you are elected—not just for pretty kittens but for their very life. Kittens need to be stimulated to urinate and defecate for a week or more after birth. The mother does this by licking the genital areas. You will have to use a slightly damp wash cloth or tissue after each feeding. If this is not done, there will be serious gastric troubles, and often the kittens will die.

Neutering

Any pet cats, especially those kept in the house, should be neutered—unless, of course, you plan to use them for breeding.

Castration

An uncastrated male will begin to spray urine (which doesn't smell like cologne!) about the house, marking his "territory," at about 9 to 12 months of age. It is the rare male that does not do this. The odor is lingering and hard to remove from fabric, such as rugs and drapes. The unneutered male will also begin roaming, seeking romance. Unfortunately, other toms will have the same idea about the same females, and fighting results. The pet male often returns from these brawls scratched, bitten, and torn. Infections are common.

On a male about 8 months old, this quite inexpensive and safe operation will end these problems before they begin. Castrating an older male who is set in his ways may slow him down quite a bit but may not completely alter his spraying and fighting habits.

Spaying

With an unneutered female, there are other problems. Once every two to three weeks, she will be in heat, rolling about and yowling constantly. Trying to find a place to put her out of hearing, but still away from the visiting males, is a very real problem. If you leave the door open, she will be out like a flash, presenting you with a litter of two to eight kittens in about two months.

The spaying procedure is briefly outlined in "Spaying" on page 299. The same procedure used for dogs is generally used on cats. The operation is usually safer with a cat, however, due to the smaller size of the cat's uterus and blood vessels. If possible, have your cat spayed between 5 and 10 months of age. It is not necessary or desirable for her to have been in heat or to have had a litter before spaying her. She will not suffer from being deprived of motherhood but will be spared the chance of having uterine infections, undergoing birth difficulties, and experiencing the stress of bearing and raising a litter.

Grooming

Regular grooming is very enjoyable to your cat. It will also help prevent such health problems as hair balls, caused by the cat ingesting hair while grooming itself. For short-haired cats, all you need is a soft brush. A pin brush (with straight metal pins) or slicker (with bent metal pins) is usually necessary for longhairs. Brush gently, with the lay of the hair. A finishing rub with an old towel feels good to the cat and will make the coat shine.

Trimming Claws and Declawing

Due to the extreme sharpness of a cat's claws and the tendency for some cats to use those claws on people or furniture, owners often want them dulled or removed. There are two choices here: declawing, which is the surgical removal of the claw and first joint of each toe, or trimming the nails on a regular basis. I would recommend trying to trim the claws before deciding to declaw the cat.

Declawing is permanent and does remove the cat's prime defense. A declawed cat can hunt and climb trees but is hampered compared with its clawed counterpart.

A cat is usually easy to work on when trimming the claws as it causes no discomfort, and you can do a few at a time. The cat's claws are retractable, so you have to press upward between the toes to unsheathe the claws. Most cats have light-colored claws, making it easy to see the pink blood vessel that runs partway down inside the claw. Using a pet nail trimmer, clip off the hook on the end of the claw, staying away

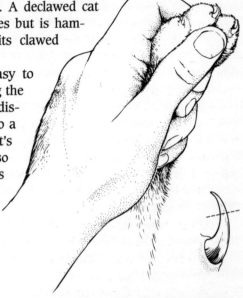

Trimming a cat's claws. *Press upward between the toes to unsheathe the claws. Using a pet nail trimmer, clip off the hook at the end of the claw. Avoid cutting into the pink blood vessel that runs partway down into the claw.*

from the blood vessel. If you do nick the vessel, touching a styptic pencil to the end will stop the bleeding. But cutting so deeply hurts the cat, and it will not be so trusting in the future. Clip one claw at a time until all four feet are finished. The hind claws are not as long or as sharp as the front claws, so do the claws on the front paws first.

If you feel it is necessary, your veterinarian can declaw your cat. But with regular trimming, most cats do not require this surgery to cease clawing their owners and the furniture.

Caring for Teeth

Cats are often prone to dental problems, especially in their later years. A soft diet, such as canned cat food, does not massage the gums or clean tartar deposits from them. These tartar deposits build up and irritate the gums. Swelling, bacterial infections, and abscesses are often a result.

A cat that drools, either when eating or just resting, should be examined for tooth and gum problems. Foul breath is also a sign of dental trouble. Often a cat with bad teeth will eat hard food (such as dry cat food) with its head cocked sideways as it tries to avoid chewing on the sore tooth. Likewise, a cat with an abscessed tooth will often paw at its mouth and shake its head.

To catch problems early, check your cat's mouth periodically, and take it to the veterinarian if you notice any redness of the gums, foul breath, or teeth with brown tartar deposits. If the teeth are brownish or yellow, they should be cleaned. If there are only a few spots of tartar, you can remove them at home by scraping the tooth with the edge of a dime. Few cats will allow a thorough cleaning at home, however. It's easiest to have your veterinarian do this, using a general anesthetic.

Giving your cat dry food from time to time will aid in preventing tartar buildups and gum troubles because it keeps the teeth scraped clean. Likewise, there are special kitty treats formulated to help keep tartar to a minimum.

Transporting

It is sometimes necessary to take your cat some distance by car. By nature, few cats enjoy riding in a car, and the motion and noise make them nervous and possibly even sick. (Of course, if a kitten is taken for rides from an early age, it is *much* more apt to enjoy riding in a car when it is older!) The first reaction of the cat is to try to escape; if this fails, the cat will usually hide under the seat, becoming almost impossible to extract when you want to get it out. And a frightened cat is apt to dash out the door the instant it is opened, never to be seen again.

For this reason, the safest means of car travel for a cat is inside a sturdy cat carrier. It is a great convenience and a great protection to a cat, making accidental escapes nearly impossible. A cat likes to feel hidden and secure, so it will frequently ride happily when snuggled in a cat carrier. Carriers are getting very inexpensive to buy, and I feel every cat owner should own at least one.

For longer trips than to your veterinarian, a larger carrier is necessary. It should allow room for a small litter box besides the cat and its curl-up bed.

Sample Vaccination Schedule for Cats

Keep in mind that this is a suggested vaccination schedule. Your veterinarian may use different products or suggest a different schedule based on your location and situation.

	DISEASE	WHEN TO VACCINATE
KITTENS	Feline distemper, feline leukemia, pneumonitis, rhinotracheitis, and feline calicivirus (combination)	9 weeks; booster at 12 weeks
	Rabies	6 months
CATS	Feline distemper, feline leukemia, pneumonitis, rhinotracheitis, and feline calicivirus (combination)	Yearly
	Rabies	Yearly

DISEASES AND OTHER PROBLEMS

Although cats are generally very healthy and disease-free, it is wise to learn all you can about common diseases and health problems. This way, you'll recognize symptoms of possible trouble before the problem gets serious. It's also important to know the normal temperature of your cat so you can check for fever or other abnormalities. The normal body temperature of a cat is 101° to 102°F (38.3° to 38.9°C).

Abscesses

Abscesses are common on cats, particularly males. Fight wounds, such as bites and scratches that puncture the skin but do not tear, often become infected and then close up, sealing bacteria under the skin. Such punctures will later abscess. With the normal loose skin of the cat, the abscess can spread under the skin and fur until all of a sudden a large bulge becomes noticeable. The abscess

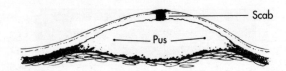

Cross section of an abscess. *Before lancing a suspected abscess, your veterinarian will withdraw some of the fluid. An abscess contains yellowish or whitish pus.*

may break and drain, but often it will ooze through perforations in the skin and not drain adequately.

This abscess should be lanced near the bottom with a sterile instrument. It is safest to have your veterinarian do this, with the cat under an anesthetic, so the area can be thoroughly flushed and cleaned. The abscess should be kept clean and open until it is healed from the inside. Antibiotic therapy is usually advised to prevent a bloodstream infection.

Never be tempted to lance a bump yourself unless you are positive it is an abscess. Hematomas (blood-filled bruises) look like abscesses, but if they are lanced, the cat may bleed to death. Therefore, it is not wise to attempt home treatment of an unopened abscess. Your veterinarian will first withdraw some of the lump's fluid with a needle and syringe to make sure it is yellowish or white (indicating an abscess) instead of dark or bloody (indicating a hematoma).

Breaks

Legs are the most often broken bones in the cat. Maybe this is because they are long and thin and they are positioned in such an unprotected way that they tend to get caught and wrenched. The tail is another area that frequently suffers breaks, usually due to having been slammed in a door.

A cat with a broken leg will commonly limp very badly, holding the leg off the ground. The leg will usually dangle unnaturally. If you suspect a broken leg, quietly get hold of the cat, and carefully place it in a secure cat carrier padded with an old towel. Many injured cats desire privacy and a hiding place when the initial shock wears off. Call your veterinarian at once. A broken leg is most successfully set the day it is broken—not a week later. Cats that are seriously injured and left untreated can develop complications and possibly die.

Do not attempt to put a splint, even just temporarily, on the cat. Many serious complications have arisen following improper placing of a home splint. It is better just to allow the cat to remain quietly in a carrier than to place a splint that may cause more damage and upset the cat.

Most broken legs are easy to set on a cat, with an intramedullary pin, a light aluminum or plastic splint, or a light plaster cast. Cats are generally good patients and heal quickly with good nursing.

Some broken tails can be set easily at home by bringing the tail into a normal position and taping strips of stiff cardboard along the tail to hold it in place. Avoid taping tightly, or you could cut off circulation to the area; the tail will become necrotic and fall off. If the break is near the tip of the tail or if you are nervous about treating the break, take the cat to your veterinarian. He can often splint the tail successfully. Otherwise, a broken tail will often heal by itself, but the cat will permanently carry a kink or two in its tail.

Car Accidents

More cats are injured by cars than any other way. Because cats are hunters, it is natural for them to seek out the grassy roadsides to hunt on, often at night. Unfortunately, many times they are frightened by traffic and then panic, run onto the road, and are hit. If you notice that an outdoor cat suddenly acts as if it is in pain or if it is lame or listless, suspect that it has been hit by a motor vehicle. Inspect the body closely for abrasions, bald spots, bruises, or swellings and sore spots. Look at the gums, as pale gums indicate either shock or internal bleeding. Also, check the eyes to see if one pupil is more dilated than the other, indicating a concussion. Where both are dilated, there may be only shock, or possibly there is a head injury. If you see any signs of possible injury, take the cat to your veterinarian for a thorough examination and perhaps observation for a day or so. Sometimes seemingly minor injuries can worsen over time, with bad results.

Should you see your cat struck by a vehicle, quietly capture the cat, gently place it in a cat carrier, and immediately take it to your veterinarian. Waiting even a few hours could cause death.

Cats also seem to have a problem with fans under the hoods of cars. They like to get up under the hood, especially in cold weather, and when the motor is started, they get caught in the fan belt. If this happens, do not panic. Place the cat in a quiet, dark carrier with some light bedding, and drive to your veterinarian at once. A seemingly horribly torn-up cat may live and make a complete recovery with veterinary help. Don't listen to well-meant advice to "put the cat to sleep" unless it comes from your veterinarian. I've seen some really cut-up cats recover in a short time—no scars even! Cats have a good healing ability when given a chance and good nursing.

Car Sickness

Cats, on the whole, are not good travelers in the family car. They often are not introduced to traveling in a vehicle until they are adults, and the motion frightens them. They may get extremely nervous at the sight and feeling of the movement of the car. They can get so frightened they can go berserk, clawing and yowling. More frequently, they become carsick, hiding under the seat, yowling, drooling, and sometimes becoming nauseated.

Often car sickness can be avoided by placing the cat in a dark cat carrier. Feeling hidden and more secure, the cat will not be as nervous or get carsick. You can also give the cat a light tranquilizer a while before the trip, but sometimes the drug has the opposite effect than you had hoped for. If you plan to tranquilize your cat, it is best to try out the tranquilizer on the animal while at home, before the trip.

If your cat is going to have to ride periodically, it is a good idea to get it slowly used to riding. Short trips, such as going to the corner store, school, or park, are easier on the cat's nervous system, and soon it will nearly relax in the car. Be sure to use a cat carrier as having a cat loose in a vehicle is dangerous: Cats, especially frightened cats, can dash out an opened car door in a flash, often never to be seen again. Slowly increase the time your cat spends riding, until it pays no attention to a trip. Beginning this at a young age makes even a long trip a relaxing, everyday happening.

Conjunctivitis

Conjunctivitis is the inflammation and often reddening of the conjunctiva (the light pink lining around the eyeball). Simple conjunctivitis is often caused by dust, weeds, pollen, or other foreign bodies irritating the area, causing inflammation. Tearing and squinting are commonly found in this problem. Bacterial infections often follow the initial irritation, causing even further irritation and swelling. The cat may rub its eye with a paw or rub its head on the floor. This serves only to irritate the area further.

Most cases of simple conjunctivitis or conjunctivitis complicated with a bacterial infection will clear up when you use an antibiotic ointment for a day or two. There are some inexpensive but excellent ointments on the market now. Besides containing an antibiotic, they also include a local anesthetic to deaden the pain and itching.

You should be aware, however, that conjunctivitis is often a symptom of a disease, such as feline calicivirus or rhinotracheitis. So, if it does not clear up with minimum home treatment or if the cat acts sick or runs a fever, take your cat to your veterinarian at once.

Constipation

Constipation is often associated with improper diet. Eating small bones or eating dry food without drinking enough water will often cause constipation. Never feed any small bones, such as fish, chop, or chicken bones, to your cat. Besides causing constipation, they can also puncture the intestines and kill the animal. When feeding a dry cat food, alternate it at least twice a week with good-quality canned food. If the cat is frequently bothered by hard stools, it may be wise to put about 1 teaspoon of vegetable oil in its food daily or to feed more canned food. Adding milk to a dry diet will help prevent constipation, too.

Adequate exercise is also very important in keeping the cat regular. A cat that just sits in one place all day is prone to constipation. Two other possible causes of constipation are hair balls and a fever, which often partially dries out the intestine, making hard stools appear.

If your cat frequently suffers from constipation, have your veterinarian give the animal a checkup. If there is no health problem, he can prescribe a simple stool softener to be added daily or periodically to the cat's food. These are quite effective and provide great relief to the cat.

Cuts

Any cat can get a cut, but it is especially likely with outdoor cats owing to fights, contact with machinery, and other hazards. First, stop any bleeding that may be present. This is usually quite easy to do with a pressure bandage, which is simply a pad of gauze held firmly against the cut with your hand. Severe bleeding can usually be controlled in the same way, while another person drives you and the injured cat to your veterinarian.

If the cut is a fairly fresh one—not more than a day old—it may heal best if stitched up. Many cuts, however, should not be stitched. This includes cuts that are dirty, cuts over joints, and cuts over heavily muscled areas. Often a bad-looking cut will heal completely in a month without suturing and without a scar. When the same wound is sewn up, healing takes about six weeks and often leaves a scar. One reason for this is that the outside of the cut heals before the inside, sealing in a few bacteria. These bacteria soon multiply and cause an infection. A very mild infection can retard healing for a lengthy period. So let your veterinarian make the decision about whether to suture that cut or not. Many veterinarians are nearly ordered to sew up a cut that they know will heal much better left open. People think the wound looks better if it is not gaping open, I guess. What they don't realize is that it would be around a shorter period of time if left open and treated with an antibiotic.

Bandages are another no-no in most cases. A bandage *can* be useful to hold a pressure pack in place or to protect the animal from self-mutilation. Generally, though, a bandage retards healing by not allowing air to circulate freely around the wound.

Diarrhea

Diarrhea can be a disease or a *symptom* of a disease. Like humans, cats occasionally are bothered by diarrhea. Pampered house cats are most susceptible to this problem. Improper feeding is the most common cause of simple diarrhea. Feeding such things as greasy, spiced foods or excess milk or cream to a cat is just asking for gastric upsets.

When a cat is bothered by diarrhea, take away all of its food, but be sure to leave out a full water dish. Insufficient water intake along with diarrhea can cause dehydration. Give 1 teaspoonful of kaolin-pectin every 3 hours. If this does not stop the diarrhea in 12 hours or if the cat is running a fever or acting listless, call your veterinarian. Diarrhea can be a symptom of many illnesses, some serious. Feline distemper and severe parasitic infestations, for instance, often have an accompanying diarrhea.

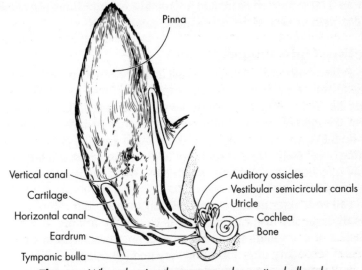

The ear. *When cleaning the ear, use only a cotton ball and your finger. Inserting a narrow object could easily injure the delicate structures inside the ear.*

Ear Infection

Ear infections in cats are often brought about by ear mites. They burrow into the ear and provide places for bacteria and fungi to enter. This is often enhanced by the dirty, waxy accumulation present in the ear.

When the cat shakes its head, scratches at its ears with its hind feet, and yowls, it pays to check the ears. Sometimes there is just an accumulation of wax and dirt in the ear canal. This is easy to remedy by swabbing the ear, first with a ball of cotton moistened with alcohol or peroxide and then with a dry ball. Go down into the ear as far as you can reach with your finger. If you aren't too forceful and don't use anything smaller than a cotton ball and your finger, there's little chance you'll do any damage to the ear while cleaning it. This cleaning may need to be repeated daily for two or three days.

If just cleaning the ear does not bring relief promptly, take your cat to the veterinarian for closer examination and proper diagnosis. Treating the ear for ear mites will not help a cat with a fungal or bacterial infection, which can be correctly diagnosed only by a veterinarian. Left untreated or treated improperly, ear infections can result in deafness or central nervous system conditions.

Feline Calicivirus

Feline calicivirus, often just called calicivirus, is a quite contagious respiratory disease of cats, especially kittens and debilitated cats. Its first symptoms include fever, nasal discharge, discharge from the eyes, ulcers of the tongue or nose, and lack of appetite. While the kitten or cat may be sick for quite a while, only the very young or severely stressed cat is apt to die. However, secondary bacterial infections are common, which may cause pneumonia or other serious problems.

Call your veterinarian as soon as you suspect your cat may have this disease. Because this problem is caused by a virus, treatment consists of controlling the symptoms, giving antibiotics to treat or prevent secondary infections, and very good nursing.

Prevention is always the best "treatment." Have your cat vaccinated regularly, and reduce stress by providing good ventilation and keeping it away from dusty environments. Also, keep your cat away from sick cats that may be roaming around.

Feline Distemper

Feline distemper, or panleukopenia, is a very contagious viral disease. It may strike very suddenly, killing cats, especially kittens, before you notice any sign of illness. When symptoms are present, they include a fever, lack of appetite, diarrhea, vomiting, weakness, depression, and dehydration. This disease is often confused with poisoning as it strikes so quickly and has such a high mortality rate, sometimes wiping out an entire farm's unvaccinated cat population in less than a week.

Treatment consists of administering antibiotics to prevent secondary infection, treating the diarrhea, giving intravenous electrolytes to treat and prevent further dehydration, and general good nursing. If the cat is running a subnormal temperature, placing it in a box on a heating pad often helps maintain a normal temperature. Without the extra heat, the cat will usually die.

When the cat survives panleukopenia, gradually introduce it to mild foods in small amounts until it is eating normally. Isolate it from unvaccinated cats for two months because it may remain a carrier for that period. While treatment can be discouraging and sometimes expensive, vaccination is inexpensive and quite reliable.

Feline Infectious Peritonitis

Feline infectious peritonitis is a contagious feline disease caused by a virus, often resulting in death, even with treatment. Symptoms may be vague and can include a fever, diarrhea, respiratory distress, and sometimes conjunctivitis. Weakness and death usually follow.

Fortunately, this disease is not common; but with new vaccines available, your veterinarian may suggest vaccinating your cat, especially in areas where feline infectious peritonitis has been known to occur. If you suspect that your cat has this problem, contact your veterinarian right away.

Feline Leukemia

Feline leukemia is a serious viral disease, usually spread by contact with infected cats. The virus does not survive outside of the cat. Some cats may develop resistance to the virus after exposure, but some remain carriers, showing no sign of having the disease. Symptoms may include a lack of activity, thinness, anemia, and weakness. There may be tumors of many of the body organs, including the liver, lungs, and kidneys.

If you suspect feline leukemia, your veterinarian can test your cat to find out. There is no successful treatment, but knowing for sure and taking your veterinarian's advice may help protect any other cats you have at home.

It is safest to have your cat vaccinated against this killer. The cost is low, and it is worth the money.

Fishhooks in the Mouth

Cats, being naturally curious and also hunters, often get tangled up in fishing tackle. It's very easy for a sharp, barbed hook to get imbedded in the lips, but it is very hard to remove, particularly from the mouth of a frightened cat.

If only one hook is into the skin, it is sometimes possible to wrap the cat in a sturdy towel and clip the barbed point off with a pair of side cutters. An alternative is to squeeze the barb flat with pliers and then gently but firmly pull the hook.

If the cat is too frantic or there is more than one hook in the skin, it is best to take the cat to a veterinarian for the hook removal. He can give the cat an injection of quick-acting anesthetic that will immobilize it temporarily while the hooks are taken out. Often he will also give an injection of antibiotics and tetanus antitoxin to prevent later problems.

Fleas

Fleas are the main external parasites that bother cats. Lice are uncommon under most circumstances, and ticks are rarely a problem. (For more information on these latter two parasites, see "Lice" on page 323 and "Ticks" on page 329.)

Fleas on cats are quite easy to control if you find them before they infest your cat in large numbers. Dusting or spraying with a rotenone compound is safe and quite effective. Keep in mind that fleas do not stay on the cat—they can be outside in the sand, in your rugs, or in the cat's bedding—so be sure to treat any suspect places at the same time you treat the cat. Remember that cats are extremely sensitive to many toxic insecticides; so read all labels very well, or you may poison your cat!

There are very effective topical products for cats, such as Frontline Plus and Bio Spot Spot On, which are applied to the skin of a cat, drawing a line from the shoulders to the tail. This drug is absorbed into the body and by biting the cat, the flea will be killed. It is also effective on any eggs. Be sure NOT to use a product labeled for use in dogs as cats are highly sensitive to many drugs and it could kill them or make them exhibit severe allergic reactions.

Also available are herbal flea collars, which repel fleas rather than killing them. There are seldom any adverse reactions, and the cat remains flea-free in most cases.

Fly Larvae

A cuterebra is a fly larva that is sometimes seen in cats, especially kittens. There is often only a tiny hole, in the neck area or under the chin. There may be a slight wetness in the area. The larva is large, sometimes nearly an inch long. On close examination you can see the larva in a lump under the skin or moving around in the opening in the skin.

Never squeeze the larva as this can cause anaphylactic shock and kill the cat. Your veterinarian can carefully enlarge the opening slightly and remove the larva slowly with forceps. He will then flush out the wound and treat it with an antibiotic ointment or powder. Once the larva is removed, there are seldom any complications.

Hair Balls

Hair balls are a common problem in cats, especially long-haired cats. As the cat cleans itself, it often swallows loose hairs. In the stomach these hairs can mass together and form a wad, which may be as large as 6 to 8 inches long × 2 to 3 inches in diameter. The cat may vomit these wads or show gastric distress from their presence. When passed further down the digestive tract, they can cause constipation or even complete intestinal blockage in some instances.

Commercial hair ball preparations with a palatable base are useful in helping your cat expel hair balls before they become a serious problem. Mineral oil, milk of magnesia, and castor oil may also bring relief, but they are hard to administer. Giving an oily canned food, such as tuna or salmon, at least twice a week helps some cats.

The best remedy for hair balls is prevention. Daily brushing, which removes a good portion of shed hairs as they occur, will do a lot in relieving hair ball problems in your cat.

Hypocalcemia

Hypocalcemia occurs in mother cats following the birth of kittens, usually when they are from one to three weeks of age. It is most common where there is a very large litter of healthy, hungry kittens and the mother is a good milk producer. The queen needs to produce immense quantities of milk to supply these kittens, and she draws the calcium from her blood. As her blood calcium level falls, she becomes uncoordinated, stiff, shaky, and nervous. She may have seizures or go into a coma.

Fortunately, hypocalcemia isn't common in cats. But when this problem does occur, your cat must get veterinary treatment soon after symptoms appear, or she will die. The veterinarian will give an intravenous injection of calcium to replace the depleted calcium in her blood. Recovery is dramatic and fast. The kittens should be weaned or bottle-raised as allowing them to continue nursing will usually cause the same condition to recur, and the next time it may kill her.

Mange

Mange is not often seen in cats, but it does occur. Mange is caused by several different types of mites that burrow under the skin, but the results are about the same. The first signs of mange are usually scabby spots, often around the face, where the hair suddenly has fallen off. There may be a foul discharge, intense itching, thickened skin, large crusty areas, and large areas of hair loss.

If you suspect your cat has mange, have your veterinarian do an examination. Several other problems can resemble mange, and you'll need a correct diagnosis to choose the right treatment. Also, the earlier you discover and treat the condition, the quicker and more effective the treatment will be.

Clipping the hair short over the entire affected area will help improve the effectiveness of the treatment. Since the mites burrow under the skin, they are difficult to treat with common insecticides, such as those used for fleas. And cats are especially sensitive to toxic compounds, so it is sometimes difficult to treat them effectively. Your veterinarian may use a shampoo containing lime-sulfur or rotenone as well as lotions or ointments containing these ingredients. *Do not use a mange remedy formulated for dogs, because cats are very susceptible to many chemicals.* Many veterinarians have had good luck using Ivermectin or Revolution in treating cats for mange. However, neither product is labeled for use in cats. But under close veterinary supervision, they can sometimes work wonders when other treatments fail. Also, take great care to prevent the cat from licking off the mange remedy; use an Elizabethan collar. (See "Restraint" on page 337 and the illustration on page 339 for instructions on making and using a collar.) Often, repeated treatments are needed to completely rid the cat of mange mites.

Mastitis

Mastitis is an inflammation of one or more of the queen's mammary glands. It is often caused by a bacterial infection that invades the gland due to stress. Some common types of stress include injuries (such as bruises, falls, being stepped on, cat bites, or getting banged in a door), copious milk supply not taken by kittens, and wounds to the teats.

When you first notice the problem, the cat may act sick or in pain, and she may have a fever. The affected gland is often swollen and hard, and there is usually heat in the area of infection. The kittens may also be affected by abnormal milk, acting listless or mewing. Remove them to a warm nest right away, and keep them off the mother until she is better. (You can bottle-feed them, if necessary. For more information on this technique, see "Orphan Kittens" on page 342.)

Consult your veterinarian as soon as you suspect mastitis. Treatment often consists of giving injections of a broad-spectrum antibiotic, applying hot packs on the affected area, massaging the area, and gently squeezing as much milk as possible from the affected glands several times during the day.

Phenol Poisoning

Cats are highly susceptible to phenol and phenol compounds as well as to iodine. Many household cleaners contain phenol, and many cats are poisoned unintentionally when drinking out of a toilet bowl containing Lysol or another cleaner. Never use a phenol shampoo, such as those often used on dogs, on a cat. If you mop your floor with a cleaner that contains phenol, rinse it well and dry it before allowing the cat into the room. Licking wet paws containing a heavy phenol concentration can cause serious, and sometimes irreversible, gastric upsets.

A cat that has ingested large amounts of phenol will often sustain extensive damage before you discover the illness. Successful treatment is very difficult in these cases. When smaller amounts are ingested, inducing vomiting, providing intravenous fluids and preparations to soothe the stomach, and good aftercare will often save the cat. If you suspect phenol poisoning, take your cat to the veterinarian at once. A few hours may make the difference between successful treatment and disappointment.

Pneumonitis

Pneumonitis is caused by a highly contagious virus. It is spread by direct contact between infected cats and unvaccinated healthy cats. The first signs you'll notice are usually sneezing and coughing.

There is often a discharge from the eyes and nose. The cat generally runs a fever. Kittens often have a weight loss as they lose their appetite. They are generally more severely affected by the disease than are older cats.

It is important to remember that there are other feline diseases that have similar symptoms, so be sure to contact your veterinarian at once for a correct diagnosis. Treatment includes intravenous electrolytes, a broad-spectrum antibiotic to prevent secondary infections, such as pneumonia, and good general nursing. Treated fairly early in the course of the disease, most cats recover with little trouble, although they may retain the infection and become sick again later in life if stressed.

Vaccination is very effective and inexpensive protection for your cats. (Your veterinarian may use the term *chlamydia,* which is often a causative agent.)

Rabies

Rabies is not as common in cats as it is in bats, skunks, raccoons, foxes, and dogs, perhaps owing to the cautious nature of cats. But, unfortunately, it can and does occur. It is always fatal once signs of the disease appear. And, of course, it can be spread to humans with fatal results unless treatment is given immediately, before symptoms occur.

Rabies is spread most often by a bite contaminated by saliva, which carries the virus. Exposure is possible from other routes, but it is uncommon. Cats frequently get rabies by catching or being bitten by rabid bats.

Many rabid animals develop a complete personality change. A quiet, loving cat will become shy or vicious. A nasty cat will suddenly become loving and want to be cuddled. There is often a change in the voice due to paralysis of the throat. The rabid cat will often either quit eating or develop a depraved appetite (eating dirt, stick, rocks, or other abnormal items). There may be stiffness in the hind limbs.

There are two types of rabies: furious rabies and dumb rabies. With furious rabies fewer people are actually endangered because they naturally avoid an aggressive, biting, scratching cat. But a cat that has dumb rabies just sits around with its lower jaw hanging down, usually with saliva running out of its mouth. Owners often think that the cat just has a bone stuck in its mouth, and they become infected when they get scratched on the teeth and get the disease-spreading saliva rubbed into the abrasion.

If you see a cat with these symptoms, treat it with caution. Isolate it in an escape-proof carrier, and take it to your veterinarian at once. (Don't, however, think a female in heat has rabies because of her "change in voice" and strange behavior!) For more information on handling rabies, see "Rabies" on page 327.

There is no treatment for rabies in animals, but there is a very effective vaccine available to protect both your cat and your family. (Remember that often a cat is the link between possibly rabid wildlife and your family.) Be sure to keep your cat's vaccination current.

Rhinotracheitis

Rhinotracheitis resembles pneumonitis as the cat has mattered eyes and a copious discharge from both nose and eyes. It coughs, sneezes, and runs a fever. Like pneumonitis, rhinotracheitis is caused by a very contagious virus, frequently complicated by an additional secondary bacterial infection. Except in kittens, the disease is serious but seldom fatal.

Consult your veterinarian right away if you suspect your cat has this problem. Treatment consists of treating the symptoms, giving antibiotics to treat or prevent secondary infections, fluids, and good nursing.

As with most viral infections, vaccination is much more satisfactory than trying to treat the disease. Good combination vaccinations are now available for the major respiratory infections of cats, so it's easy to prevent problems.

Ringworm

Ringworm is caused by a fungus, often *Microsporum canis*. It is not a worm, nor is it caused by a worm. It is a circular lesion, often appearing quite suddenly. The skin is commonly rough, with the hair gone from the spot. If left untreated, the lesion gets larger and larger, usually retaining the circular pattern.

Some forms of ringworm are contagious to humans. All can be passed back and forth among animals of a like species. So if you suspect ringworm, isolate the affected cat immediately, and then check all the other cats or kittens right away. Take any affected cat to your veterinarian for examination. It is a good idea to wear gloves when handling a cat with ringworm.

Treatments vary from soaking the cat in a medicated shampoo to treating just the spots with a low-toxicity fungicide. (Iodine preparations are often used in treating ringworm in cattle and dogs, but most cats are highly sensitive to iodine, and they have *severe* trouble if you use it on them.) If you treat the spots at home, be sure to use rubber gloves and apply the medication from the outside of the spot to the inside of the spot; working outward may spread the fungus.

If you own a number of cats and want to prevent this problem, there is a vaccination available for ringworm in cats. Ask your veterinarian for his opinion on its use in your situation.

Urinary Calculi

Urinary calculi trouble male cats more often than females due to the size of the passageway through which the urine exits the body. There is little agreement on whether or not castration affects the incidence of the problem. Some studies have been done, and they reveal no significant difference in the size of the urethra between neutered and unneutered males; but many veterinarians do believe there is a definite connection between castration of young males and urinary calculi. For this reason, it's generally recommended that you wait until the male is seven to nine months old to castrate it.

Feeding a diet of only dry food will often contribute to problems with urinary calculi. When fed a moist diet, such as canned food or meat, the cat gets additional moisture through the food. When eating dry food, the cat often does not drink enough additional water.

A change in the pH of the bladder, whether due to an infection or other causes, can also contribute to urinary calculi. As the pH in the bladder becomes more alkaline, salts, crystals, and calcium precipitate out, forming the calculi.

Diets high in ash and magnesium have been shown to cause a high incidence of urinary calculi—perhaps the greatest cause of calculi problems in cats.

Many times the cat has passed several smaller calculi (sometimes called "sand") before one lodges and blocks the urethra. Often the first symptoms you'll notice are straining at the litter tray with scanty results, usually with increased frequency. Dullness and loss of appetite soon follow. You can feel the distended bladder as a hard, roundish bulge in the abdomen. (Do not squeeze the bladder, because it may rupture, usually causing the death of the cat.) Take the cat to the veterinarian immediately for treatment. As the problem progresses, the cat becomes toxic from absorbing the waste material. When it becomes very ill from uremia, treatment is very difficult, and the cat often dies.

Treatment in severe cases consists of emptying the bladder, by use of a catheter (which passes through the urethra) or a direct tap (a needle inserted through the abdomen into the bladder), and flushing the urethra to dislodge the plug. Once the cat is out of danger and urinating on its own, you must place it on a strict diet that is low in magnesium and ash. Many appropriate foods are available commercially; your veterinarian can recommend one to you. Or you may make up your own, following his prescribed diet of home-made ingredients. Remember, though, that once a cat has had urinary calculi, placing it on regular commercial food again will usually result in recurring attacks of the problem.

Warfarin Poisoning

Warfarin is the principal ingredient of several popular rodent poisons. Even though it is supposedly safe for children and pets, cats can be poisoned by it. This most often happens when the cat eats the rodent bait directly or eats a large rodent with a stomachful of fresh bait. Once the bait has passed through the digestive tract and kills the rodent, it usually will not harm a cat, even if the cat eats the rodent.

Warfarin and other rodenticides contain a drug, dicoumarin, which causes hemorrhage throughout the body. Affected cats seem weak, anemic, and depressed. They do not appear to be in pain or severely distressed.

If you suspect that your cat may have had access to a rodent poison containing dicoumarin, take the cat immediately to your veterinarian. In most cases injections of vitamin K and confinement will aid in helping the blood begin to clot. In severe cases blood transfusions and fluids are also given.

Never leave rodent poison where it is at all possible for pets or children to reach it. Place it in a sturdy box, accessible only to rodents, and set it far away from pet feeding places or children's play areas.

Worms and Internal Parasites

Although cats are not severely bothered by worms as often as dogs are, there are several types that do infest them on occasion.

Hookworm

Hookworm is common in cats. These small worms are not seen in the stool, nor are they normally visible with the naked eye. Symptoms include anemia, bloody stools, diarrhea, and unthriftiness. Young kittens are the hardest hit and often die suddenly.

Roundworm

Roundworm is the most common cat parasite. This worm is visible to the naked eye and looks like a bean sprout. It is most often seen after being vomited up, often along with a hair ball. A severely infested cat will have a potbelly but remain thin despite a good diet. It will also have a poor hair coat and act listless.

Tapeworm

Tapeworm, which quite often infests cats, is carried into the cat via the flea. While cleaning itself, the cat can swallow a flea containing tapeworm larvae. Soon the cat is infested with an adult tapeworm, which can be up to 2 feet long. Cats can also get tapeworm through eating infested rabbits or mice or other rodents. Tapeworm segments are eliminated with stool and often cling to the rectal area. When just passed, they look like inchworms, only white; when dry, they look like small grains of rice. A cat with tapeworm may just appear a bit unthrifty or have digestive or nervous disorders. Some cats do not show signs of trouble but still are infested with tapeworms.

Other Parasites

There are many other worms and intestinal parasites that can and do infest cats. A few of them are threadworms, lung flukes, liver flukes, *Giardia,* coccidia, lungworms, heartworms, and *Babesia felis.* Many come from eating infested rodents. Others are picked up when the cat licks the eggs off its feet while washing. A single indoor cat is much less likely to pick up worms than is a cat from a cattery, an outdoor cat, or a cat that goes out where stray cats and other animals roam.

Treating Parasites

When you suspect your cat has intestinal parasites, be sure to take a fecal sample to your veterinarian for examination. Each worm or group of worms has one or two medications that work best on it, and some worms require rather complicated treatments. Using a "shotgun" wormer from the drugstore will do your cat no good and may even be dangerous, should the cat be severely debilitated or sick from a problem other than worms.

Every cat should have a regular fecal examination for worms and other intestinal parasites at least once a year. This examination is simple, quick, and inexpensive, and it's worth every penny. With many parasites you will not see visible damage until there's not much you can do to save the animal. Lungworms, for instance, cause scarring and infections in the respiratory tract, while many protozoa (one-celled organisms) cause ulceration in the intestinal tract, which can become infected. Many worms cause digestive upsets, sometimes severe enough to kill the cat, as they burrow into the mucous lining of the stomach and intestines. Hookworm can cause anemia, which can bring about sudden death. And large migrating worms or dead adult worms can cause plugs in blood vessels or heart attacks. The point is that the few minutes it takes to collect a small fecal sample and take it to your veterinarian could easily save your cat's health, if not its life.

SOME BASICS FOR THE LAYPERSON

ADMINISTERING DRUGS

Sooner or later, you'll be called upon to administer drugs or medications to your animals. Knowing the correct way to give these materials generally makes this very easy and not traumatic—to you or the animal!

Oral Liquid

Liquid medications administered orally are most often used either to treat gastrointestinal troubles (such as diarrhea or worms) or to provide systemic treatment for bacterial infections.

Giving farm animals liquid orally can be a challenge because of their size and strength, but there are some tricks you can use to make the job easier. Restraint is essential: You can't just chase an animal around with a drenching bottle or syringe stuck in its mouth. Also, when giving liquid orally, you need to tilt the head upward slightly. The mouth should *not* be higher than the eyes, however. If the head is tipped upward too far, large amounts of liquid can choke the animal or, worse, get into the lungs and cause inhalation pneumonia. Give small amounts at a time, allowing the patient to swallow before you give more. Keep the animal calm and unexcited to prevent gasping (which could allow droplets to get into the lungs). Many liquid medicines—especially bitter compounds, such as sulfas—are usually more readily acceptable to animals if mixed with diluted honey or molasses.

When using a drenching syringe or tip, be sure to place the end beyond the hump in the tongue; this makes the patient more prone to swallow the medication, not spit it out. Massaging the

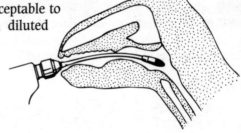

Drenching. *When giving liquid medications orally, tilt the head upward slightly. The animal's mouth should not be higher than its eyes.*

throat as the dose is delivered encourages swallowing. A glass bottle should be used only as a last resort, especially by the novice, because it can break if it's knocked against the teeth or bitten by the patient.

A dog will take liquid medication more easily if you can form a pouch with the corner of its lower lip to receive the liquid. Administer a small amount, and then tilt the dog's head back slightly and stroke its throat. When it swallows, give it the rest of the medicine in the same way.

Cats are a little harder to dose with an oral medicine. Using an eyedropper or syringe is often easier than a spoon due to the size of the mouth. If the cat is unruly, wrap it in a heavy towel to avoid scratches with the hind feet, and have an assistant hold it. To treat a very hard-to-handle cat, you can mix small amounts of oral medicine with a sticky substance, such as honey, and smear it on the nose or front paws. The cat, when cleaning itself in disgust, will lick off the medicine. Do not use this method on a very ill cat, however, as the cat will not feel like cleaning itself, and the medication will do no good on the outside of the cat.

Some oral liquid medications are meant to be mixed with the drinking water, which provides the easiest route to medicate many animals or birds. Do not use this route if the patients are very sick, though, as many times they will not drink adequate water to correctly medicate themselves. If an animal refuses its water because of the taste, try mixing some molasses or powdered cider mix with the water, even before adding the medication, to get it used to different-tasting water. Then the additive will mask the flavor of the medication. Some animals, and most birds, will take liquid medications in their water very well. Others, such as goats and horses, are quite finicky. If they are, and you cannot fool them by masking the flavor, you'll need to use another method to medicate them.

Oral Pill

Pills are often used to get oral medicine into small animals. (Under the term *pill,* we also include tablets and capsules.) It's generally quite easy to give dogs pills. While a dog is eating its other food, try offering the pill wrapped in some hamburger or, better yet, a chunk of hot dog. (This has a strong odor that masks any odor the pill may have.) Some dogs are very clever about taking medicated food, however, so keep an eye on them; they may take the meat and then spit out the pill. Most pills can be crushed, which eliminates the feel of a lump in the meat. With the wise dog, try giving a small ball of unmedicated food, quickly followed by a medicated ball, and then quickly give another unmedicated ball. In its haste to get all the meat, the dog will usually gobble up the medicated ball with no hesitation. A chunk of hot dog is great as you can cut a small slit in the center, insert the pill, and then feed it quickly. Only the very clever patient will detect your trick.

The same tricks can work for giving pills to a cat. Cats are especially careful of what they eat, so try to be particularly careful when you conceal the medication. Many times you can divide the pill (ask your veterinarian first) and put the portions into bits of tempting food. Feed each bit, leading off with a morsel of unmedicated food.

Sometimes it is necessary to give the pill by hand, as with a very sick animal that refuses to eat. And when capsules and pills come with instructions that they should not be chewed, they obviously should not be given in food. With a dog the best method is to simply push the pill down its throat as far as you can. Just putting it into the dog's mouth is not enough as it will chew or spit out the pill and may put up a fight when you try to give it more medication. If the dog is not excited and you quickly slip the pill down its throat, most dogs will instinctively swallow without a struggle.

If the dog must receive multiple pills, give only one at a time. An exception can be made for very tiny pills; but even with these, no more than two should be given together, or the dog may have some trouble swallowing. If swallowing is uncomfortable for the dog, dosing will not be easy the next time. It can help to coat each pill with butter, which not only helps the dog swallow but also makes the pills seem to taste better. (An exception to this is any of the tetracycline antibiotic family of drugs, which should not be given with dairy products, because these foods interfere with the action of the drugs. With these medicines use vegetable oil or margarine.)

Cats don't often take pills easily. If you have an assistant restrain the paws and you curl the top lip around the top canine teeth, you can quickly open the mouth, insert the pill, and push it down the throat with the thrust of one finger. Then quickly shut the mouth, and stroke the throat to encourage swallowing. This method can also work on a dog that struggles or tries to bite when being dosed.

For extremely difficult patients, there are now tablet and liquid dispensers available, which flush the medication down the animal's throat. Check with your veterinarian or in pet supply catalogs.

Oral Bolus

Because of their large size, farm animals receive a bolus rather than a small pill. The bolus (pronounced bowl-us) is usually a large, oblong pill. Again, restraint is very important in proper administration.

It's easiest to give a bolus with the aid of a balling gun. There is usually little objection from the animal, and you'll avoid the sharp teeth. Simply fit the bolus into the gun, insert it into the mouth, thrust it behind the tongue, and pop the bolus down the throat. It is usually a good idea to lubricate the bolus with shortening or vegetable oil before placing it in the balling gun. The bolus will slip down the throat easier, and when the animal comfortably swallows the bolus, it will be easier to dose the second time.

Using a balling gun. *It's important to restrain an animal before giving it medication. With smaller animals it's easiest to straddle the animal, facing in the same direction, and hold it with your knees.*

Medicated Feed

There are many medications, usually powders or crystals, that you can mix with the feed. However, medications with an objectionable taste or smell are often hard to give this way, especially to finicky animals. You can usually mask the taste by adding molasses to the feed and block the odor by smearing a strong-smelling ointment, such as Vicks VapoRub or camphorated oil, on the animal's nose.

Medication via Stomach Tube

Veterinarians often use a stomach tube to administer large quantities of liquids, particularly to large animals. When a ruminant, such as a goat or cow, is dosed with a stomach tube, a mouth speculum is frequently used to keep the animal from biting the tube. The flexible tube slides through this short, pipelike instrument, making it easier to slip the tube down the throat while protecting the tube. Horses usually receive the stomach tube through a nostril. In such cases no speculum is used. Once the tube is in the stomach, the medication is pumped down. It's critical to take care that the tube does not go into a lung. Pushing the tube down slowly while the animal swallows ensures safety. If you attempt to administer drugs yourself in this way, *never use a milk hose or garden hose.* These have sharp edges and may cut or severely injure the esophagus, resulting in death.

Intramuscular Injection

Many drugs, especially antibiotics, are administered with an intramuscular (IM) injection. It's easy to give this kind of injection, and the medicine is absorbed fairly rapidly into the bloodstream. You can use any large muscle mass for the injection, but those most often employed are on the side of the neck (for large animals) and in the hindquarters.

Restrain the animal well before preparing to give the injection to avoid injury to either the animal or you. Then clean the hair of any dirt or debris by wiping the area with a cotton ball drenched in alcohol. (I do not use the term *sterilize* for this process, because it is impossible to sterilize skin, especially skin that is covered by hair.)

With large animals it is usually easiest to take the needle off the syringe, give the animal a couple of slaps with the back of your hand, and then quickly plunge the needle into the muscle. (This is done in a quick rhythm: slap, slap, pop! The needle is put in with a motion as if you were throwing a dart.) The nerves in the skin, where the most feeling is, will still be tingling from the slaps, and the animal will not feel the needle enter the body. Then quickly reattach the needle to the syringe. To be certain you have not hit a blood vessel, draw back on the syringe. If blood enters the syringe, you are into a blood vessel and should retract or advance the needle. Then inject the drug.

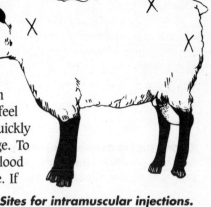

Sites for intramuscular injections. *Give intramuscular injections into a large muscle mass, as indicated. Make sure the animal is well restrained first!*

After pulling the needle out of the skin, it is often a good idea to massage the area to aid absorption and to reduce leakage through the puncture in the skin.

Intravenous Injection

The intravenous (IV) injection often is used to administer large amounts of fluids or to get a drug into the bloodstream more quickly. It requires more experience and caution to give an intravenous injection correctly than other types of injections. Only those solutions recommended for intravenous use should be given in that way as many drugs will kill when given improperly. Likewise, be sure that your equipment is clean and the drug or fluid you are giving is pure because any bits of "settled out" ingredients, dirt, or old dried blood in the intravenous set may kill your patient if injected into a vein.

An intravenous injection is usually given in the jugular vein for horses, cows, sheep, and goats. Dogs and cats most often receive an intravenous injection in the large vein in the front leg. Other veins are used on occasion, depending on the situation.

Restrain the animal very well before giving an intravenous injection. An assistant is certainly helpful. The area is usually clipped, if heavily covered by hair or wool, and cleaned with alcohol. Next the vein is usually "popped up" by using manual pressure

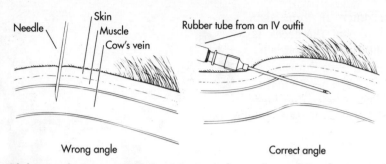

Needle | Skin | Muscle | Cow's vein | Rubber tube from an IV outfit

Wrong angle   Correct angle

Giving an intravenous injection. Insert the needle parallel to the vein to help hold it in place. Inserting the needle at a 90° angle can allow it to slip out or stick all the way through the vein.

behind the injection site or a tourniquet (you can use a rope or even hay string, tightened firmly but not enough to choke the animal). Push the needle, with a syringe attached, into the vein. When the needle enters the vein, usually with a small "pop" feeling, blood will enter the syringe when you apply a little suction by drawing back a bit on the syringe. (In cattle it is not necessary to draw back on the syringe as you'll use a larger needle into which the blood will flow easily.)

Thread the needle up through the vein, with the needle parallel to the vein. This holds it in place, should the animal make a sudden move. For long injections, placing a piece of adhesive tape across the "hub" of the needle provides added protection against accidental withdrawal. Ether—such as that used to start cars—can be sprayed on the tape to increase the tape's sticking ability on hair or skin.

Always administer an intravenous solution slowly. Some drugs can cause serious discomfort or even kill the animal if they hit the heart too rapidly. Do not let the needle slip from the vein or stick all the way through the vein to the other side. Some intravenous medications can seriously irritate muscles if they leak out of the vein, even causing the area to become necrotic and slough off.

Intraperitoneal Injection

In some cases it may not be possible to give an intravenous injection: Possibly the animal's blood pressure is too low, or the person doing the injecting is not experienced. In these cases you may

choose an intraper-
itoneal (IP) injection
(injection into the
abdominal cavity).
The material will be
absorbed rapidly, and you can
give large amounts of fluid, such
as electrolytes, in this way. It is
not as dangerous to the animal as
it might appear.

First, make sure the an-
imal is well restrained, by
an assistant, if possible. Clip
the site if it is heavily covered with hair or wool, and
then clean it well with alcohol. Next, you'll need a
long needle to penetrate the

*Site for an intraperitoneal injec-
tion. Injecting into the abdominal cavity
allows for rapid absorption, and you can
give large amounts of fluid this way. Slowly
but firmly insert a long needle through the
abdominal wall of the restrained animal.*

skin, muscle, and peritoneum (the lining of the abdomen) sufficiently to administer the drug or fluid easily. Insert the needle
slowly but firmly through the abdominal wall. Do not jab, or you
may hit an intestine or other body organ. (When you firmly but
slowly insert the needle, the internal organs will usually move out
of the way, pushed by the needle.) When the needle is in place, start
administering the drug. You may choose to use an intravenous set
if you need to give large amounts of fluid.

An intraperitoneal injection will sometimes cause temporary
abdominal cramps. These will pass as the fluid is absorbed.
Administering the drug slowly will often prevent this.

Subcutaneous Injection

Subcutaneous injection is recommended for many drugs.
Because the drug is administered just under the skin, the injection
is easy to give and usually quite painless. Take care to read labels
before choosing this route, however; drugs not meant for subcutaneous injection can cause irritation and abscesses.

Give the subcutaneous injection in an area where there is loose
skin. The neck, flank, "underarm flap," and side of the withers are
all routinely used. If you need to give large volumes of fluids, it is

best to use several injection sites rather than one as excessive irritation may result.

Before inserting the needle, clip the area if it is heavily covered by hair or wool; then clean it with alcohol. Next pull the skin up, away from the muscle, to leave a pocket. Slip the needle firmly through the skin but not into the muscle. If you pull a bit on the skin when the needle is in place, you should be able to feel it drift free.

Leaking is often a problem in subcutaneous injections due to the back pressure of the drug as it lies under the skin. So after the injection is complete, rub the site vigorously because this aids absorption and prevents leaking.

If you must give several subcutaneous injections, use a different site each time to avoid irritation.

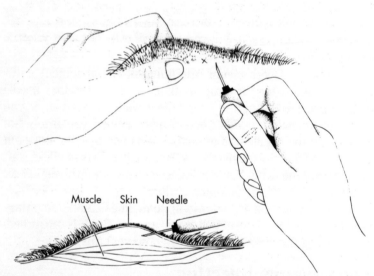

Muscle   Skin   Needle

Giving a subcutaneous injection. *Pull the loose skin away from the muscle to create a pocket. Slip the needle firmly through the skin into the pocket. After the injection remove the needle, and rub the site vigorously.*

Intradermal Injection

Intradermal injection is made into the skin as compared with under the skin in a subcutaneous injection. Intradermal injection is

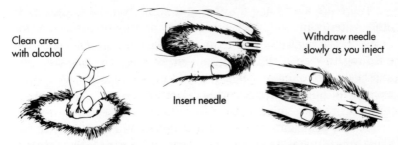

Clean area
with alcohol

Insert needle

Withdraw needle
slowly as you inject

Giving an intradermal injection. *To administer directly into the skin, clip the area very short, and wipe it with alcohol. Pinch the skin up, and slide the needle into the skin. As you inject the fluid, slowly withdraw the needle.*

most often used in certain vaccinations and in the tuberculosis test. Very few antibiotics or other drugs are administered in this way.

The area is clipped very short and then cleaned with alcohol. The skin is pinched up, and the tiny intradermal needle is slipped gently into the skin. As the drug is injected, it will raise a tiny bump, which will slowly be absorbed into the body.

Epidural Injection

This is the "spinal" often given to large animals during some obstetrical work and when the uterus has been thrown out and must be replaced. The anesthetic is administered in between the vertebrae and numbs the entire rear quarters, eliminating straining. It requires quite a bit of experience to give this injection properly: The needle must be passed between the vertebrae, and one must decide just how much anesthetic the animal needs as it is given. Too much will put the animal down, and too little will not provide adequate anesthesia. For this reason, it's best to leave this type of injection to your veterinarian.

ANTIBIOTIC COMPATIBILITY

There are certain antibiotics that enhance each other's action. These drugs are often commercially mixed or given simultaneously. Such drugs are penicillin-streptomycin, penicillin-neomycin, and neomycin-polymixin B.

There are also some drugs that are antagonistic toward each other, interfering with each other's action. This occurs when, for instance, the penicillin and tetracycline families are mixed. When used together or at the same time, or even closely following one another, each often negates the effects of the other. A typical example of this is when scouring calves are treated. Often there is terramycin in the milk replacer or terramycin is given in a scour bolus, and penicillin-streptomycin is given intramuscularly at the same time. Studies have been done that indicate the futility of such treatment: One cancels out the other. When you are using more than one antibiotic or when you are changing antibiotics, be sure that you consult your veterinarian. You'll save money and time by using the most compatible drugs.

ARTIFICIAL RESPIRATION

There are some instances where you may need to give an animal artificial respiration. Quite often it is necessary for newborn animals

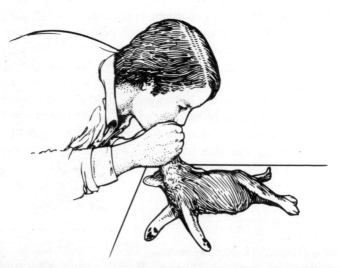

Artificial respiration on a smaller animal. When giving artificial respiration to a small animal, cup your hands around the mouth to prevent air from escaping as you blow.

that have not begun to breathe on their own, for animals that have received an electrical shock, or for those that have almost drowned.

With small animals there are two common methods. One is the mouth-to-mouth method, where you clear mucus from the airway by suction or gravity, cup your hands around the mouth, and blow directly into the airway. The amount of air needed varies with the size of the animal, but it is very important not to blow hard or force too much air into the lungs as death could result. Generally, with small animals only a tiny "puff" is all that is needed, repeated regularly but with no force. The chest should expand to natural size with each breath. Keep the mouth and throat clear of fluids and mucus; if necessary, hold the animal upside down by the hind legs. Quickly wipe the mouth clear, and then continue artificial respiration as long as there is a heartbeat.

The second method commonly used on small animals is also the one used on larger animals in many instances. Clear the animal's airway of fluid and mucus, and then lay the animal on its side. Raise the top foreleg, and hold down the bottom foreleg. Then "play" the animal like an accordion, pressing down and pulling up on the top leg every four seconds. This allows the lungs to fill and compress.

An alternative method of artificial respiration on large animals is the use of a respirator, usually also containing an aspirator, which removes fluids from the airway. In a herd situation, having a respirator available is a good safeguard. Costing about $60, this tool is a worthwhile investment.

Sometimes pain will work to get the animal breathing again when nothing else will. This is especially true of newborns. (Remember, the human doctor

Artificial respiration on a larger animal. While the animal is lying on its side, hold down the bottom foreleg. Press down and pull up on the upper foreleg to allow the lungs to compress and fill.

smacks baby's bottom at birth if breathing has not started well.) Poking a finger up the nose or down the throat, biting or pinching an ear, or slapping the chest may cause the animal to gasp out of reflex, and breathing will start. As long as there is a heartbeat, there is life and a chance to save the animal.

As soon as the animal begins to breathe, keep it warm. If the animal stopped breathing owing to an accident, consult with your veterinarian to guard against the pneumonia that can follow.

COMMON ACCIDENTS AND OTHER PROBLEMS

There are a number of problems that can happen to all animals. Also, keep in mind that some problems can affect several but not all animals, so it's worth checking other chapters if you don't find a certain condition covered here or in the chapter on your particular animal.

Bee Stings

When an animal is stung by a bee or wasp, inspect the area for the stinger. When you locate it, scrape it out using a fingernail. Don't pick it out with your fingers, because extra poison may be squeezed into the wound if the poison sac is still attached to the stinger. Then clip the hair to allow access to the sting. Often a cold pack, along with a paste made from a little baking soda mixed with water, applied to the sting will quickly relieve the pain.

In cases of severe sting, it may be necessary to give the animal an injection of antihistamine to combat the allergic reaction, which could kill the animal. This is often the case where an animal has received stings from many bees or wasps and experiences severe swelling or shocklike symptoms.

Burns

Animals most often receive burns by having hot liquid spilled on them or by stepping on a hot stove or fire. With good nursing most burns heal rapidly and well. Examine the injured area carefully as soon as possible after the burn. Clipping the hair off will be helpful. Flush the area gently with cold, soapy water, and then rinse. The cold water will help prevent the burn from becoming any more severe, and the soap will help clean the area of bacteria and dirt. If a small area is affected, daubing aloe gel on the area, repeating every hour for the first six hours, usually provides relief. Should the burn involve unclean skin or some muscle, your veterinarian may suggest using an ointment containing antibiotics and a local anesthetic.

If the burn is severe, involving large areas of skin or muscle as well as skin, rush the animal to your veterinarian. Many animals suffer shock when a large area is burned. Using sterile cloths soaked in a mild saline solution on the burn area, along with giving systemic antibiotics and fluids, will often save an animal that might have otherwise died. Good nursing is very important in severe burn cases. A high-protein diet with a good vitamin-mineral supplement will aid healing.

Poisoning

In cases of poisoning (be sure the animal was poisoned and is not just ill), call your veterinarian at once. If possible, have the product in hand so you can read the label to him. Most poison cases benefit from making the animal vomit, but read the label on the product as some chemicals should not be vomited by a poison victim.

You can make an animal vomit by giving it a couple of tablespoonsful of salt on the back of the tongue, mustard mixed with water, or warm salt water. This will get the toxic material out of the stomach quickly, preventing more from being absorbed into the system. Then rush the animal to the veterinarian. Do *not* give emetics if the animal is having convulsions. Such symptoms indicate possible strychnine poisoning. With this poison the animal's nerves are supersensitive, and even slight stimuli, such as light or a small noise, can throw it into a convulsion. Giving an emetic can cause so violent a convulsion that the animal may die.

There are many hundreds of toxic materials, many specific to a certain area; among these are poisonous plants. It is a good idea to ask your veterinarian or county Cooperative Extension Agent (usually located in your county seat) which ones are likely to be a problem in your area. Some are poisonous only at a certain time of the year; in others only one part of the plant (such as the roots or leaves) is toxic. A few plants that are toxic include chokecherries, lupines, cocklebur, bracken fern, locoweed, lechuguilla, rubberweed, milkweed, water hemlock, lambkill, castor bean, sorghum, Sudan grass, jimsonweed, buttercup, and rhubarb leaves and roots.

Lead poisoning used to be very common in animals, especially when young cattle licked and chewed at barn walls and fences that had been painted with a lead-based paint. Lead poisoning should still be considered a possibility if your buildings have old paint on them and your animals exhibit illness in the form of weakness, diarrhea, and staggering.

Household chemicals kill a surprising number of pets every day. These range from fly sprays to common cleaners and toilet bowl disinfectants. One of the most common killers of animals is ordinary automobile antifreeze, which has a sweet, enticing taste to its victims. You should always keep it in an enclosed container. Quickly mop up any spills, and wash the area well.

An amazing variety of other things also can harm your animals. Clay pigeons used in trapshooting will poison hogs, as will molds growing in corners of their feeders. Rat poisons and fly bait sometimes kill more poultry than they do vermin. Doubling up on organophosphates—for instance, using organic phosphates as a wormer and then treating the barn with a spray containing organic phosphates—has killed horses and small animals. Insecticides, such as fly sprays and flea collars, can kill an animal that has been given a general anesthetic. Chemical fertilizers and herbicides should be stored very carefully as cattle can die from eating the bags in which these toxic substances are packed, and farm and ranch cats often die from contact with them while hunting. Salt can poison, especially if too much has been accidentally mixed with the feed. Alkali poisoning is a problem in some areas.

These poisons are listed just to give you an idea of a few of the many toxic materials that can often be readily available to animals. Most have differing symptoms. If you check your animals daily and are aware of what actions are normal for them, you should be able to spot any unusual signs before an animal is past help. Obviously, keeping any poisonous chemicals and substances away from animals will do much in keeping them safe from poisoning. When in doubt about a toxic substance or possible symptoms of poisoning, call your veterinarian.

Prolapsed Eyeball

Certain traumas can cause the eyeball to prolapse or, in other words, pop out of the socket. Bumping the eye in a certain way, or severe strain, especially with such breeds of dogs as Pekingese or cattle such as the Jersey, can cause a prolapsed eye.

The two most important things here are to keep the animal calm and restrained and to try to get the eyeball back into the socket as soon as possible. An excited animal can tear the eyeball off on a fence or furniture. And the longer the eyeball is out of the socket, the more swelling occurs and the less chance there is of getting it back in.

Often you can replace the eyeball simply by holding a warm, soft, damp cloth over the eyeball and firmly but gently pressing inward. With a large animal, such as a cow or horse, make sure you take adequate restraint measures first. Also, your veterinarian should be called immediately. If you cannot replace the eyeball with one or two tries, the veterinarian must be ready to do so. Sometimes tranquilizers or general anesthetics are necessary to get the animal to relax enough to replace the eyeball. Aftercare consists of bandaging the head over a clean sanitary napkin placed over the eyeball. This keeps dirt and light out while keeping the eyeball in place until pain and swelling are gone. Antibiotics are often given to prevent infection as well as cortisone to control swelling and pain.

(Note: The prolapsed third eyelid, mentioned elsewhere in this book, is not a problem in itself but rather a symptom of tetanus or other conditions, such as an inflamed nictitating membrane. This third eyelid is the thin "skin," or membrane, in the corner of the eye.)

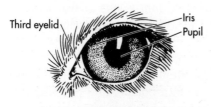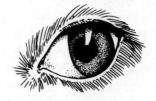

Normal eye   Eye of animal with tetanus

The third eyelid. *The third eyelid is the thin "skin," or membrane, in the corner of the eye. A prolapsed third eyelid, when the membrane extends over the eye, is a symptom of tetanus or other conditions.*

Snakebites

In various areas different snakes can be a problem with just about any animal. For more information, refer to "Snakebites" on page 328.

Urinary Tract Infection

Infections of the urinary tract, especially the bladder, are quite common, especially in small animals. Often the first symptom you will notice is increased urination, frequently with scanty results because the bladder does not have time to fill between voidings. (Do not confuse frequent urination due to heat in a female for a urinary tract infection.) An animal with an infection may run a fever and act sick. Sometimes it will vomit.

Take your animal to your veterinarian for examination as soon as you notice the first symptoms. A culture and a sensitivity test are great helps in choosing the right antibiotic from the beginning of treatment, which often lasts for two to three weeks.

Good home nursing is a must. This includes providing the animal with plenty of fresh, clean water to encourage water consumption, which flushes the bladder of bacteria.

Relapse is common, so watch the animal in the future for recurrences of this problem.

ELECTROLYTES IN THE BODY

Electrolytes are normal acids, bases, and salts found in the blood. The loss of fluid due to scours, fever, and other problems is the loss of water *and* electrolytes; there is seldom a loss of water alone. When the animal is dehydrated to a critical point, cellular death occurs. Replacing the water and the electrolytes is necessary to prevent irreversible damage. Electrolyte therapy supplies the needed water, along with sodium, magnesium, potassium, and calcium, combined with sulfates, chlorides, bicarbonate, and phosphate as well as amino acids and proteins. Electrolytes are often given intravenously over a period of several hours as a continuous drip. They are also used subcutaneously and intraperitoneally, which are easier for the layperson to administer.

For scouring calves, using oral electrolytes in the place of milk is very effective. The electrolytes replace the irritating milk, which is only making the scours worse, and at the same time, they aid in restoring the electrolyte balance in the body. Oral electrolytes can also be helpful when placed in the drinking water of birds or animals in a stressful situation.

Handling an Animal in Shock

Shock is a condition often brought about by trauma, which shows itself in reduced circulation, rapid breathing, rapid pulse, often subnormal temperature, weakness, shaking, vomiting, and prostration. It can be difficult, without running tests, to determine the difference between shock and internal bleeding, which may happen after an animal is hit by a car. Drugs given to increase blood pressure, which are needed in shock, will serve only to increase hemorrhage if there is also internal bleeding. Therefore, it is important to differentiate between the two. Remember also that shock can be brought about by pain and hemorrhage.

The cause of the shock should be determined, if at all possible. If you can remove the cause of the shock, such as severe chilling (due to falling through ice or being stuck in a snowbank, for example) or heat exhaustion, for instance, you'll greatly aid the recovery. Do not excite the animal or move it unless necessary. Before moving any injured animal, check the color of the gums and mucous membranes first. Paleness may indicate internal bleeding, and if there is internal bleeding, moving the animal might be very dangerous; consult with your veterinarian first.

If you must move a small animal, slipping a blanket under the patient like a stretcher will make moving safer. If a blanket or jacket is not available, gently grasp the skin on the back of the neck and back, lift the animal, and place it in a box or carrier or on the floor of a car. This will protect the animal, should there also be internal injuries. Leave large animals where they are, and cover them with a blanket to prevent chilling (unless, of course, it is very hot outdoors, in which case any additional heat can add to the shock).

An animal in shock needs prompt veterinary attention. There are many drugs that can combat shock and internal hemorrhage effectively, but they are of no use when the animal has been in severe shock for so long that it is past the point of no return.

The Importance
of Body Temperature

Although it will vary among individual animals, there is an average normal temperature for each species of animal. It is a good idea to have on record the normal temperature for each of your animals. Of course, if you own many animals, this may not be possible; but for the time spent, it is very worth your while.

When an infection or septicemia is present in the body, very often there will be a rise in temperature. This fever is a body defense mechanism, which tries to kill the bacteria by heat. It does not, however, work in all cases. When an animal appears sick, take its temperature before starting any treatment. If the temperature is up 1° or 2°, it should be on the decline within 24 hours of starting treatment. If it is not or if it continues to rise, you may need to change antibiotics. If the temperature is down, even slightly, you will have a good idea that the antibiotic you are using is doing its job.

Bear in mind that some fevers are caused by a viral infection, which will not be affected by any antibiotic.

A very high temperature can destroy brain cells or cause seizures, so it may be necessary to use alcohol baths or aspirin to reduce the fever until the antibiotic begins to work. Do not use these fever-reducing methods unless there is an emergency situation threatening, though, as you will not have as good an idea of how well the antibiotic is working if the fever is lowered artificially.

A subnormal temperature is very often more to worry about than a fever. A slight subnormal temperature is often a sign of shock. One degree to 2° (or more) below normal usually is a sign that the animal is dying. Make an effort to raise the temperature to near normal using heat lamps or heating pads. Just using blankets will not work, as the animal has lost the ability to produce its own heat; unless you supply artificial heat, a blanket cannot warm a hypothermic animal. When an animal's temperature has remained subnormal for some time, irreversible damage is usually done, and nothing can save it.

Taking an Animal's Temperature

Any time you notice an animal acting abnormally, take its temperature before giving any medication. Otherwise, you will never know if the animal had a temperature before the medication was given, and you won't be able to judge if the medication was effective or just unneeded. An above-normal temperature indicates a bloodstream infection or other sickness (or heat prostration). A below-normal temperature indicates shock and often a dying animal.

You can use any thermometer—even a human oral thermometer, which is most often handy—but the animal must have its temperature taken rectally. For this reason, it's best to use a veterinary rectal thermometer, which has a sturdier construction than the human oral thermometer. Shake the thermometer down to a point below

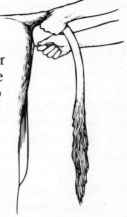

Taking the temperature.
When taking a rectal temperature, shake the thermometer down to below the normal point for that animal. Insert it halfway into the rectum while holding the tail to steady the animal.

normal for that animal. Grasp the tail, and insert the thermometer an inch or two into the rectum, depending on the size of the animal. Leave it in place for three minutes while you hold the animal quiet. Most animals are quite easy to handle during this process.

VACCINATIONS

A vaccine is made up of the agent that causes the disease. It is either live, attenuated (weakened), or dead. When administered, it encourages the host's body to produce antibodies against that specific agent. (Antibodies are a natural body defense mechanism to combat a disease or foreign protein.) After the first vaccination, the body builds up a level of protective antibodies, which, depending on the vaccine, may or may not drop after a period of time. If it drops, a booster (a second injection) is given to raise the antibody level, keeping the animal safe. Often a yearly booster is required, following the initial immunization series, to provide adequate protection. By giving these boosters, your veterinarian is not trying to "make money" but to keep your animals safe.

VIRUS OR BACTERIA?

To effectively treat a disease, you need to understand the difference between viruses and bacteria, both of which cause diseases. To complicate matters more, sometimes a disease is initially caused by one or the other, and then a secondary invader comes along, making things worse.

Viruses

Viruses reproduce themselves and are considered living, though they have no energy of their own, obtaining energy from body cells that they enter. Different viruses have preferences for different parts of the body. For example, rabies affects the central nervous system, while red nose in cattle affects the respiratory system and reproductive tract. Viruses cause damage to the body from inside a cell, so anything that will effectively kill the virus will, 99 percent of the time, damage or kill the body cells, as well. At the present time, there is no specific treatment for any viral diseases other than vaccinating against them before sickness strikes. Treatment for viral diseases consists mainly of treating the symptoms, such as diarrhea or respiratory distress, good nursing to support the patient, and allowing the disease to run its course. Antibiotics can be useful for treating secondary bacterial infections, which often occur in a stressed animal, but antibiotics do nothing to treat a viral infection.

Bacteria

Bacteria are a group of one-celled organisms that belong to the plant family. Many bacteria found in or on animals are harmless and even necessary—that is, as long as they stay in their normal place in the body. But if, for some reason, they show up where they don't belong, they can cause trouble. For example, *Escherichia coli* is a normal gut bacterium and has essential functions in the alimentary canal. If *E. coli* should suddenly be transferred to the urinary tract and then the bladder, however, the results may be cystitis or inflammation and infection of the bladder.

Bacteria cause trouble in a different way than viruses do. While viruses work from within the body cells, bacteria work outside the cells: overwhelming the body by sheer numbers or producing a toxin that is detrimental to the health of the host. Certain species of *Clostridium* bacteria, for instance, produce toxin that in turn can cause tetanus, botulism poisoning, gas gangrene, blackleg, and so forth.

Bacteria are classified in various ways. The classification is based on the way the organisms stain with the Gram stain, which is a routine stain used in all diagnostic laboratories. All bacteria are either always Gram-positive or Gram-negative. This staining characteristic is also closely connected to the susceptibility of the bacterium to a particular drug or antibiotic. Some antibiotics, such as penicillin, are primarily effective only against Gram-positive organisms. Other drugs are mainly effective against Gram-negative organisms. Then there are broad-spectrum antibiotics that are effective against both types of organisms.

However, all antibiotics effective primarily against Gram-positive organisms are not effective against *all* Gram-positive organisms, and not all antibiotics effective against Gram-negative organisms are effective against *all* Gram-negative organisms. Nor are the broad-spectrum antibiotics or antibiotic combinations effective against *all* organisms. Sensitivity tests can be run in a laboratory to determine which antibiotic is most effective against a certain organism. For example, *Staphylococcus aureus* is a common skin contaminant and is a Gram-positive organism. It should, by reason, be sensitive to penicillin, and it quite often is. But you can run into a strain of *S. aureus* that might be sensitive only to an antibiotic that is very rarely used because of its limited effectiveness.

This is why it is best, when at all possible, to have your veterinarian take a culture before you treat an infection—especially if the problem affects more than one animal in your flock or herd. The laboratory will identify the organism and then run a sensitivity test on it to determine the most effective antibiotic. This way, you can treat the infection effectively and without loss of time.

GLOSSARY OF COMMONLY USED TERMS

Abdominal cavity. The part of the body that contains such organs as the stomach, liver, kidneys, spleen, uterus (in the female), and intestines.

Abomasum. The fourth, or true, digestive stomach of a ruminant.

Abortion. The termination of a pregnancy before the due date.

Abscess. A localized collection of pus surrounded by inflamed tissue.

Acetonemia. Another name for ketosis; *see* Ketosis.

Acute. Sudden onset, often severe.

Aerobic organism. An organism that lives in the presence of oxygen.

Afterbirth. The placenta, which is expelled after the birth of a mammal.

AI. Abbreviation for artificial insemination; *see* Artificial insemination or breeding.

Alimentary canal. The tubular passageway from the mouth to the anus, which functions in digestion, absorption of food, and elimination of waste.

Amniotic fluid. The fluid surrounding the fetus in the uterus.

Anaerobic organism. An organism that lives in the absence of oxygen.

Anal glands. Two scent glands, one on either side of the rectum, which empty into the rectum during a bowel movement or at times of fright.

Anaphylactic shock. Extreme sensitivity of an animal to a drug or foreign protein, causing severe shock or death.

Anemia. A condition in which the blood is deficient in red blood cells, in hemoglobin, or in total volume, causing lack of vitality or even death.

Aneurysm. A localized, saclike dilation of a blood vessel.

Antibiotic. A substance produced by a microorganism and able, in dilute solution, to inhibit or kill another microorganism.

Antibody. A body defense substance produced in response to vaccination, maternal immunity, or previous infection and giving a degree of resistance to future infection by the same organism.

Antiserum. A serum containing antibodies against a particular disease, which is used to treat that disease.

Antivenin. An antitoxin to a venom (poison); an antiserum containing this antitoxin.

Artery. A vessel carrying blood away from the heart through the body.

Arthritis. A crippling of the joints caused by various strains or organisms; characterized by puffiness at the joints and pain.

Artificial insemination (AI) or breeding. The introduction of semen into the uterus by other than natural means.

Ascarids. Large roundworms in the intestinal tract of almost all species of animals, including humans; infestation is characterized by unthriftiness despite good diet.

Ascites. The accumulation of serous fluid in the abdominal cavity.

Aspiration pneumonia. Pneumonia caused by breathing foreign matter into the lungs, such as amniotic fluid at birth, dust, or liquid from an improperly given drench; also called inhalation pneumonia; *see* Pneumonia.

Atrophic rhinitis. A disease in pigs similar to necrotic rhinitis but without the swollen snout or face; *see* Necrotic rhinitis.

Atrophy. A decrease in size or wasting away of a body part or tissue, as happens to testicles after castration by clamping or a muscle after paralysis.

Avian. Relating to birds.

Avian leukosis. A disease in poultry affecting the nerves, eyes, and/or internal organs; characterized according to the body part affected; no treatment available.

Azoturia. A condition that may cause lameness in horses; characterized by profuse sweating, trembling, incoordination, and darkening of the urine; treated with rest, oral electrolytes, sodium bicarbonate, and injectable thiamine.

Bacteria. One-celled organisms belonging to the plant kingdom.

Bacterin. A suspension of killed bacteria used to immunize against a specific disease.

Balling gun. An inexpensive instrument used to place a large pill through an animal's mouth and down its throat.

Barrow. A castrated male pig.

Bedsore. An ulceration of tissue caused by prolonged pressure; prevented and treated by changing positions.

Benign. Nonspreading and nonrecurring.

Bitch. A female dog.

Blackhead. A disease in poultry caused by protozoa; characterized by diarrhea, weight loss, and lack of vigor.

Blackleg. A sudden-appearing disease in cattle caused by a *Clostridium* organism, which enters the body through the digestive tract or a small puncture wound; characterized by a purple-looking leg; no sure treatment; prevented by vaccination.

Blister, external. An ointment or a salve applied to the skin surface to produce heat in the area, increasing circulation to promote healing; often used in treating lameness in horses.

Blister, internal. An injection of a drug that produces heat in the area, increasing circulation to promote healing; often used in treating lameness in horses.

Bloat. An accumulation of gas in the rumen of cattle, goats, and sheep that have overeaten, have eaten grain followed by drinking water, or have indigestion; characterized by a swollen belly, staggering, panting, and finally collapse; treated with a defoaming agent, a stomach tube, or a trochar and cannula.

Blood poisoning. Another name for septicemia; *see* Septicemia.

Bluecomb. A disease in chickens caused by a virus; characterized by watery or pasty diarrhea, weight loss, a blue comb, and depression; treated with antibiotics.

Boar. An uncastrated male pig.

Bolus. A large pill given to a large animal; usually oval in shape.

Bots. Fairly large, grublike fly larvae that attach themselves to the stomach lining of horses, causing pitting and scarring; treated with a wormer.

Botulism. A type of food poisoning caused by a neurotoxin produced by the growth of *Clostridium botulinum;* characterized by diarrhea, vomiting, and weakness.

Bovine. Relating to cattle.

Bovine virus diarrhea (BVD). A viral disease in cattle; characterized by fever, loss of appetite, diarrhea, and sometimes sores around the mouth, nose, and eyes as well as drooling or foaming at the mouth; treatment is difficult; prevented by a vaccine; also known as infectious bovine diarrhea.

Bowed tendon. A condition that causes lameness in horses; caused by severe strain or overwork; characterized by the tendon below the knee bowing outward and soreness; treated with cold and rest.

Breech presentation. An abnormal birth position in which the buttocks appear first.

Brisket. The breast or lower chest of an animal.

Brucellosis. A disease caused by *Brucella* organisms; characterized and treated according to the species infected.

Buck. A male goat.

Bull lead. A clamp used to restrain the head of a cow, fitting into the nostrils.

Bull nose. A common name for necrotic rhinitis; *see* Necrotic rhinitis.

"Bump" the calf. A common manual method of determining pregnancy in cattle, usually after the fifth month. Make a fist, and gently but firmly bump into the cow's right flank; if you feel a hard, abnormal lump bump you back, there is a calf.

BVD. Abbreviation for bovine virus diarrhea; *see* Bovine virus diarrhea.

Caked bag. A bag that becomes swollen just before or after freshening, due to fluid retention; another name for udder edema.

Calcification. The process of depositing calcium salts to make something inflexible, as in the healing of a bone.

California Mastitis Test (CMT). A test used to determine if a milk-producing animal has mastitis.

Canine. Relating to the dog family.

Cannibalism. When an animal devours its own kind.

Cannula. A small tube that is inserted with a trochar into a ruminant's bloated stomach and left in place to allow gas to pass out of the body.

Capped elbow or hock. A condition that causes lameness in horses; caused by bruising; characterized by swelling on either the elbow or hock; treated with ice, cortisone, rest, and mild exercise as the lameness passes.

Caprine. Relating to goats.

Caruncles. Cup-shaped, spongy-textured lobes or "buttons" on the uterus that attach to the placenta.

Caseous lymphadenitis. A serious abscess infection in the lymph glands of sheep and goats caused by bacteria; characterized by weight loss; also called wasting disease.

Cast. A device to protect and immobilize a broken or severely injured limb. Also refers to an animal stuck in a down position, such as when a horse gets stuck down in a stall or fence or in deep snow or mud.

Castration. Removal or destruction of the testicles; neutering of a male animal.

Catheterize. To insert a tube into a body passageway or cavity to permit injection or withdrawal of fluids, as into the urethra to drain the bladder.

Caustic ointment. A paste applied in a ring around the base and on the button of a young animal's horn buds to prevent them from growing; a method of dehorning.

Cauterization. The use of a hot iron, caustic, or other agent to burn, scar, or destroy tissue; often used to stop bleeding.

Cecal worm. A worm that parasitizes the cecum of chickens and turkeys, causing inflammation of the cecum and unthriftiness; a carrier of the protozoa that cause blackhead disease; treated by good sanitation and a wormer.

Cecum. The blind pouch that begins the large intestine; resembles the appendix in a human.

Cervix. The narrow outer opening of the uterus.

Cesarean section. The removal of the fetus through an incision in the mother's abdomen and uterus.

Chorea. A nervous disorder marked by spasmodic twitching of the limbs or facial muscles and by incoordination.

Chorioptic mange. The most common type of mange found in many animals; *see* Mange.

Chromosome. A microscopic cell structure containing genes, which determine hereditary factors.

Chronic. Of often slower onset, longer duration, with often lesser symptoms; somewhat resistant to treatment.

CMT. Common abbreviation for California Mastitis Test; *see* California Mastitis Test.

Coagulant powder. A powder used to slow down and stop bleeding by causing it to clot.

Coccidia. Parasitic protozoa that can enter the digestive tract of birds and animals; infestation is often characterized by unthriftiness and diarrhea, especially in the young.

Coccidiosis. Infestation with coccidia; often treated with sulfas.

Coggins test. A blood test for swamp fever (equine infectious anemia).

Colic. A bellyache caused by overeating, eating grain and then drinking large quantities of water, drinking water while overheated, constipation, or impaction; characterized by pacing, sweating, kicking at the belly, hard breathing, frequent lying down and rising, and rolling; treated with oral medication or injections to calm the stomach and relieve the pain.

Colostrum. The first milk secreted by a mother after giving birth; characterized by high protein and necessary antibodies for the newborn.

Comminuted fracture. A smashed bone containing many fragments.

Compound fracture. A break in both bone and skin.

Congenital. A condition existing at birth but not hereditary.

Conjunctiva. A mucous membrane covering the eyeball and the inner side of the eyelid.

Conjunctivitis. Inflammation of the conjunctiva caused by irritation by foreign matter, such as dust or pollen, or occurring as a symptom of a disease; characterized by mattered, runny, or itchy eyes; often treated with an anesthetic ointment.

Constipation. Abnormally delayed or infrequent passage of dry, hardened feces.

Corns. A painful foot condition in cattle, horses, goats, and sheep characterized by a soreness in a local area. Also refers to a "growth" extending from between the toes of sheep, goats, and cattle; usually removed surgically.

Coronet. The lower part of a horse's pastern, where the horn of the hoof terminates in skin.

Cotyledons. Knobs on the placenta, or afterbirth, which connect with the caruncles on the uterus.

Creep-fed ration. A ration for growing animals meant to be fed free-choice.

Creep-feeding. A method of feeding growing young animals that allows access to feed by the young while excluding adults by the size and placement of the feeder.

Cross ties. A restraining device made of two ropes, one extending from each side of a barn aisle, that snap on the side rings of a horse's halter.

Cull. To permanently remove an animal from a herd or flock.

Cuterebra. A large fly larva that often appears in a lump with a hole in it in the neck or chin area of a cat or rabbit; treated by removing with forceps (without crushing the larva), flushing the area, and applying an antibiotic solution.

Cyanosis. A bluish or purplish discoloration of the mucous membranes or skin due to oxygen deficiency in the blood.

Cystic ovaries. Ovaries containing cysts; characterized by a female that is continually in heat; treated with hormones or surgery.

Cystitis. Inflammation of the bladder, often caused by infection.

Debeaking. Trimming back the top beak of a chick to prevent cannibalism.

Dehorning iron. An instrument used to burn (kill) the horn cells of a young goat or calf; also called disbudding iron.

Demodectic mange. A common type of mange found in animals; *see* Mange.

Dermatitis. Inflammation of the skin caused by irritation, diet, or infection.

Dermatosis. Any disease of the skin, not necessarily with inflammation.

Descenting. The removal of the major scent glands.

Dewclaw. A toelike projection on the lower leg of an animal; it does not reach the ground.

Diabetes. A disease common in dogs as well as humans; characterized by increased thirst, frequent urination, weight loss, and high blood sugar; controlled by diet, medication, and insulin injections.

Diarrhea. Abnormally frequent bowel movements with quite fluid stools.

Distemper. In dogs a very contagious disease of the central nervous system caused by a virus; characterized by running, mattered eyes, a plugged, crusty nose, diarrhea, vomiting, and twitching; treated with antiserum or globulin, antibiotics to prevent secondary infections, and good nursing; dogs may be protected against distemper by vaccination. *See also* Panleukopenia. Also a common name for strangles in horses; *see* Strangles.

Diuretic. A substance given to increase the flow of urine by drawing fluid from the body; often given for edema.

Dock. To cut off the end of a body part, such as the tails of lambs and puppies.

Doe. The correct name for a female goat, often incorrectly called a "nanny."

Downer cow. A cow unable to stand, such as a cow that has been injured during calving.

Drake. A male duck.

Drench. To give a liquid medicine to an animal.

Eastern equine encephalomyelitis (EEE). A viral disease spread from mosquitoes to birds, back to mosquitoes, then to horses and sometimes to humans; characterized by depression, incoordination, drooping lip, high fever, pushing against a wall, or being down and unable to rise; treated by isolating the animal, treating the symptoms, and providing good nursing; commonly known as sleeping sickness.

Eclampsia. A condition of low blood calcium common in a bitch with nursing puppies; characterized by incoordination, panting, and collapse; treated by weaning the puppies and giving the bitch an intravenous injection of a calcium solution.

Edema. The accumulation of fluid in tissues caused by poor circulation in an area, often due to sprain, injury, tight leg wraps, a tight udder on giving birth, or pregnancy; treated with diuretics; commonly called stocking up or caking.

EEE. Abbreviation for Eastern equine encephalomyelitis; *see* Eastern equine encephalomyelitis.

EHV. Abbreviation for equine herpesvirus; *see* Equine herpesvirus.

EIA. Abbreviation for equine infectious anemia; *see* Equine infectious anemia.

Elastrator. An instrument that places a heavy rubber band between the body and body part (such as the testicles, horns, or tail) to be removed from a young animal; the band shuts off circulation, and eventually the body part dies and falls off.

Electrolytes. Normal acids, bases, and salts found in the blood; often become imbalanced during diarrhea, fever, or severe illness.

Emasculatome. An instrument that crushes the cords and blood vessels to the testicles, causing them to atrophy and shrink up; used in the bloodless clamping, or "pinching," method of castration.

Emasculator. An instrument that crushes and cuts both the cords and the blood vessels in the testicles; used in surgical castration.

Embryotomy knife. A special small, curved knife with a small blade; used to dissect a dead fetus causing a difficult birth, without damaging the uterus.

Emetic. An agent that induces vomiting.

Emphysema. A condition of the lung characterized by frequent bouts of difficult breathing.

Enterotoxemia. A common disease in young goats, calves, and lambs caused by a bacterial infection; characterized by diarrhea, circling, convulsions, incoordination, and weakness; prevented by vaccination; also called overeating disease.

Epidural injection. An injection between the vertebrae; also known as a spinal.

Epilepsy. Disturbances in brain function; characterized by seizures, shaking, or excitement; treated by oral drugs such as Dilantin and Primidone.

Equine. Relating to the horse family.

Equine herpesvirus (EHV). A viral disease that can cause respiratory problems, nasal discharge, fever, coughing, lack of appetite, and abortion.

Equine infectious anemia (EIA). The correct name for swamp fever; *see* Swamp fever.

Equine influenza. A highly contagious viral respiratory disease in horses; characterized by abrupt onset, coughing, fever, and nasal discharge; treatment consists of treating symptoms, antibiotics to prevent/treat secondary bacterial infections, and isolation; prevented by vaccination.

Erysipelas. An acute infection in young pigs caused by bacteria, often causing damage to joints and the heart; characterized by high temperature, pain, and diamond-shaped purple blotches on the sides, belly, and back; treated with penicillin and serum.

Estrogen. A natural female hormone.

Eversion. Turning inside out, as in the eversion of the uterus.

Ewe. A female sheep.

Expectorant. A substance that clears the air passages of secretions.

Farrow. To give birth (in pigs).

Fecal. Pertaining to the bowel movement or excreta.

Feline. Relating to cats.

Feline calicivirus. A serious contagious viral disease in cats; characterized by loss of appetite, nasal discharge, and fever; prevented by vaccination.

Feline distemper. A common name for panleukopenia; *see* Panleukopenia.

Feline infectious peritonitis. A serious viral infection in cats; characterized by hind limb paralysis, diarrhea, and respiratory distress; prevented by vaccination.

Feline leukemia. A serious viral infection in cats; characterized by chronic wasting, weakness, and lack of activity; prevented by vaccination.

Fetlock. The area on the back of the first joint above the hoof.

Fetus. An unborn, developing mammal.

Firing. The method of applying a firing pin to the skin surface to produce heat, which in turn increases circulation to promote healing; used to treat lameness in horses.

Firing pin. A hot, often electric, point used in firing horses; *see* Firing.

Flatulence. A digestive upset characterized by gas in the stomach or intestines.

Float. A special file used to file down sharp edges on horses' teeth, increasing the ability to chew efficiently.

Flush. To prepare animals for breeding by putting them on full feed and lush pasture so they are gaining weight when bred to increase ovulation.

Foot rot. A bacterial infection that attacks the feet of cattle, goats, and sheep, causing a sudden lameness; usually treated with an antibiotic and local treatment of the area.

Founder. A condition often seen in goats and horses, frequently caused by overeating lush pastures or grains, drinking water when overheated, or a retained placenta; characterized by a reluctance to move, lameness, and sometimes fever; treated with antihistamines, rest, and soaking the feet in cold water; also called laminitis.

Fowl cholera. A fast-hitting bacterial disease with a high mortality rate in poultry; characterized by bluish combs and wattles, fever, increased water intake, difficult breathing, drowsiness, and emaciation; treated with sulfas and antibiotics; prevented by cleanliness, isolation of new birds, and vaccination.

Fowl typhoid. A bacterial disease in poultry; characterized by depression, ruffled feathers, and a yellowish or greenish diarrhea; treated with antibiotics, but culling and testing are the only "cure" in a flock; prevented by testing and vaccination.

Freshen. To give birth and come into milk (in dairy animals).

Frog. The triangular, elastic, horny pad in the middle of the sole of a horse's foot, which absorbs shock while the animal is moving.

Frostbite. The freezing of some part of the body, such as the ears and feet of newborn animals; characterized by stiffness, swelling, tenderness, and heat; treated by soaking in warm water, placing in warm surroundings, and injecting cortisone intramuscularly; prevention is best.

Fungus. A simple plant, lacking chlorophyll, that often causes infections in animals.

Gall. A skin sore caused by chronic irritation or pressure.

Gander. A male goose.

Gangrene. The decay of soft body tissue due to disease or lack of circulation.

Gapeworm. A parasite that migrates to the lungs and then imbeds in the trachea of poultry, causing blockage that inhibits breathing and sometimes eating; infestation is characterized by sneezing, coughing, and neck stretching; treated with thiabendazole and by controlling access to snails and slugs, which are carriers.

Gastritis. Inflammation of the mucous membrane of the stomach, often causing vomiting or bloat.

Gelding. A castrated male horse.

Genes. The parts of chromosomes carrying hereditary factors.

Gilt. A young female pig.

Globulin. A sterile solution containing many antibodies to provide passive (short-term) immunity.

Glucocorticosteroid. The cortisone that has an effect on glucose metabolism in the body; also called glucocorticoid.

Goose. A female goose.

Gouger. An instrument used to dehorn young calves and goats; also called scoops. The instrument has two round handles, each with a sharp blade that fits down over a horn button or small horn. When the handles are pulled apart quickly, the horn button is gouged out.

Gram-negative bacteria. Bacteria that do not hold the purple dye when stained by Gram's method.

Gram-positive bacteria. Bacteria that hold the purple dye when stained by Gram's method.

Gram's method. A method used in diagnostic laboratories as a means for the differential staining of bacteria, by which some species remain colored and some are decolorized by treatment with Gram's solution (iodine and the iodide of potassium) after staining with gentian violet.

Granulation. The process of the minute red granules of new capillaries forming on the surface of a wound in healing.

Grease heel. Another term for scratches in horses; *see* Scratches.

Grubs. Parasitic fly larvae that live under the skin; commonly treated with minor surgery, sprays, pour-ons, or powders.

Gruel. Any softened, moistened, easily eaten feed.

Hair ball. A wad made of hair swallowed by a cat and collected in the digestive tract; infestation is characterized by vomiting and gastric distress or constipation and intestinal blockage; treated with mineral oil or other oily remedies.

Hardware disease. A condition in cattle caused by swallowing metal objects, such as nails, wire, and bottle caps; symptoms and treatment vary depending on the location of the metal.

Heartworm. A parasite spread by mosquitoes to dogs, which infests the heart; infestation is characterized by shortness of breath, coughing, and lack of stamina; treated with extreme care with an injectable drug that kills the worms; prevented with an oral drug given during mosquito season.

Heaves. A chronic pulmonary emphysema of a horse; characterized by difficult breathing, heaving of the flanks, and a persistent cough.

Heifer. A young cow that has not had a calf.

Hematoma. A swelling due to the collection of blood under the skin; a large bruise.

Hemorrhage. Heavy or uncontrollable bleeding.

Hemorrhagic septicemia. The correct name for shipping fever in cattle; *see* Shipping fever.

Hen. An adult female chicken, duck, guinea, or turkey.

Hepatitis. Inflammation of the liver, often caused by a virus; characterized by fever, inflamed eyes, vomiting, lack of appetite, and diarrhea; commonly treated with blood transfusions, intravenous fluids, and antibiotics to prevent secondary infections; prevented by vaccination.

Hermaphrodite. Having both male and female reproductive organs and characteristics.

Hernia. A protrusion of bowel or other organ through a weak spot in the muscle or wall of the body cavity.

Hip dysplasia. A hereditary condition of the hips, most often found in purebred dogs of certain breeds.

Hobbles. A restraining device, usually made of leather, fastened around a horse's pasterns to keep the legs together, for preventing straying or kicking or for "throwing" a horse to work on it.

Hock. The prominent joint on an animal's hind leg, corresponding to the heel of a human.

Hookworm. Often severe intestinal parasite that penetrates the skin of animals, including humans; infestation is characterized by unthriftiness, diarrhea, blood in the stool, and death due to anemia; treated with a wormer and strict sanitation measures.

Hot spots. A common fungal infection in dogs, usually occurring in the summer, often mistaken for mange; characterized by sudden-appearing red spots, each with a moist, whitish center, on the neck and back, resulting in itching or tenderness; treated with an antifungal after clipping away the hair.

Hutch burn. A condition in rabbits that are kept in wooden hutches; caused by exposure to urine; characterized by the genital-anal area being red and chapped-looking and having brownish crusts; treated with a bland ointment and proper sanitation; called scab nose when the infection spreads to the nose.

Hydrophobia. A common name for rabies; *see* Rabies.

Hypocalcemia. A deficiency of calcium in the blood sometimes seen around weaning time in heavy-milking sows with large litters; characterized by weakness in the hindquarters, incoordination, and often thinness; treated by weaning the young and giving calcium injections; also commonly called posterior paralysis.

IBD. Abbreviation for infectious bovine diarrhea, also known as bovine virus diarrhea; *see* Bovine virus diarrhea.

IBR. Abbreviation for infectious bovine rhinotraceitis; *see* Infectious bovine rhinotraceitis.

IM. Abbreviation for intramuscular; *see* Intramuscular.

Impaction. The lodgment of something in a body passage or cavity, such as feces in the bowel or feed in the crop; often caused by improper feeding; treated with mineral oil.

Infectious bovine rhinotraceitis (IBR). A viral disease that can cause respiratory distress, abortion, swollen eyes, weakness, lack of appetite, and inflamed mucous membranes in the nose.

Infectious keratitis. The correct term for pinkeye; *see* Pinkeye.

Infertility. The inability to reproduce.

Inguinal. Pertaining to the groin area, such as the inguinal canal.

Inhalation pneumonia. Another term for aspiration pneumonia; *see* Aspiration pneumonia.

Intervertebral disc lesion. A back problem in dogs arising from protrusion of a spinal disc, which puts pressure on the spinal cord; caused by an injury or may be hereditary; characterized by lameness, unwillingness to stand, and finally paralysis of the hind legs; treated with drugs, good nursing, physical therapy, and occasionally surgery.

Intradermal injection. An injection into the skin, as in a tuberculosis test.

Intramedullary pin. A stainless-steel pin that is run through the marrow of the bone to repair fractures.

Intramuscular (IM). Situated in or entering a muscle, as in an intramuscular injection.

Intraperitoneal (IP). Situated in or entering the cavity of the abdomen, as in an intraperitoneal injection.

Intravenous (IV). Situated in or entering a vein, as in an intravenous injection.

IP. Abbreviation for intraperitoneal; *see* Intraperitoneal.

IV. Abbreviation for intravenous; *see* Intravenous.

Jack. A male donkey.

Jenny. A female donkey.

Johne's disease. A chronic, often fatal, inflammation of the intestines caused by bacteria; characterized by persistent diarrhea and gradual emaciation; no treatment available.

Joint ill. Arthritis caused by systemic infection, often by bacteria entering the body through the navel at birth.

Jugular vein. The large vein on each side of the neck that returns blood from the head; the site commonly used for intravenous injections in large animals.

Ketosis. A metabolic disturbance with an abnormal increase of ketone (acetone) bodies in the blood, urine, and milk; causes, symptoms, and treatments vary according to the species; also called acetonemia or pregnancy disease.

Laminitis. The correct term for founder; *see* Founder.

Laparotomy. A surgical incision into the abdominal cavity.

Leptospirosis. A bacterial disease in animals, including humans; characterized by fever, diarrhea, increased urination, bloody or discolored urine, vomiting, weakness, and inflamed mucous membranes; treated by antibiotics and good nursing; prevented by vaccination.

Lesion. An abnormal change in tissue due to injury or disease.

Lice. Various small, oval-shaped, blood-sucking, gray insects that are parasitic on warm-blooded animals; characterized by rubbing, itching, and patchy, bald spots; treated with louse powders, sprays, or dips.

Ligate. To tie off, as in surgery.

Lockjaw. A common name for tetanus; *see* Tetanus.

Luxation of the patella. The correct term for stifling; *see* Stifling.

Lyme disease. A tick-borne bacterial disease found in animals and humans; characterized by arthritislike symptoms, lack of energy, and sometimes intermittent fever and swollen lymph glands; treated with long-term antibiotics; prevented by vaccination.

Malignant. Spreading deterioration.

Mange. A persistent, contagious skin disease caused by mites that burrow into the skin; characterized by itching, scales, crusty spots, pustules, or thickened skin; treatment varies according to the animal and type of mite; also called Scab, or scabies.

Marek's disease. A contagious viral disease in chickens; characterized by internal tumors, depression, wasting, and death; no treatment available; prevented by vaccination.

Mastitis. Inflammation of the mammary gland, often caused by bacterial infection, which commonly results in changes in the milk; symptoms and treatment vary according to the type of mastitis (acute, chronic, or gangrene).

Mastitis tube. A syringe with a flexible tip, containing an antibiotic solution to inject directly into the teat canal; commonly used in the treatment of mastitis in dairy cattle or goats.

Metritis. Inflammation of the uterus, often caused by bacterial infection; often prevents conception and normal heat cycles or causes acute illness; characterized by pus and exudate in the uterus; treated with hormones, antibiotics, and surgery.

Microfilariae. The minute prelarvae of various parasites in the blood or tissue of animals and humans; commonly withdrawn by biting insects, which then reinfect animals, where the larvae become mature parasites; most commonly seen in dogs with heartworm.

Milk fever. The common name for parturient paresis in cows; caused by low blood calcium during the establishment of the milk flow in dairy animals that have recently given birth; characterized by an ascending paralysis beginning with the hind legs, no fever, and often sudden collapse; treated with a calcium solution given intravenously.

Milk vein. A very large blood vessel on each side of a dairy animal's underside, running forward of the udder.

Mites. Small parasites that feed on blood.

Molt. To periodically shed hair, feathers, shell, or an outer layer.

Navicular disease. A condition that causes lameness in horses, due to fracture and often necrosis of one of the small bones in the foot; frequently caused by trauma, hard work on unyielding surfaces, or faulty conformation; characterized by unnatural stance, short strides, and later narrow, long hooves; no permanent treatment.

Neck rope. A strong rope with a loop with a ring tied in it about 2 feet up from the snap; used with a halter to tie a horse.

Necro. A common term for necrotic enteritis; *see* Necrotic enteritis.

Necrotic. Pertaining to dead tissue.

Necrotic enteritis. Inflammation and decay of tissue in pigs caused by dietary deficiency or bacterial infection; characterized by lack of appetite and energy, high temperature, and diarrhea; treated by improving the diet and giving antibiotics or sulfa drugs early in the course of the disease; also called necro.

Necrotic rhinitis. A condition in pigs caused by an organism introduced through an injury; characterized by a swollen snout or face, a nasal discharge, sneezing, or occasional bleeding; treated with antibiotics or sulfas; also called bull nose; *see also* Atrophic rhinitis.

Neural. Pertaining to the nerves.

Neuter. To remove the reproductive capacity of an animal; *see* Castration and Spaying.

Newcastle disease. A sudden-appearing, quick-spreading viral disease in poultry; characterized by respiratory distress followed by nervous disorders and then death; no treatment available; prevented by vaccination.

Nictitating membrane. A thin membrane at the inner corner or beneath the lower lid of the eye; also called the third eyelid.

Ocular. Pertaining to the eye.

Oocyst. An encysted fertilized egg of certain one-celled animal parasites.

Ophthalmic. Relating to the eye; for use on or in the eye, such as an ophthalmic ointment.

Osteomyelitis. Inflammation of the bone, often caused by infection.

Ovariohysterectomy. The removal of the ovaries and uterus; commonly called spaying in animals.

Overeating disease. A common name for enterotoxemia; *see* Enterotoxemia.

Oxytocin. A hormone commonly used to aid new mothers having difficulty letting down their milk or to cause uterine contractions.

Panleukopenia. A serious, contagious, quick-striking, high-mortality viral disease in cats; characterized by diarrhea, vomiting, weakness, depression, and quick death; treated with good nursing and antibiotics to prevent secondary infections; prevented by vaccination; also called feline distemper.

Parasite. An organism living in or on another organism, which depends on its host for support and/or existence without making a useful return and usually causing injury; examples include ticks, lice, and worms.

Parenteral. Situated or occurring outside the intestines; introduced other than by way of the intestines, such as intravenously or intramuscularly.

Parvovirus. A serious viral disease in dogs; characterized by severe diarrhea, often in young dogs; treated with antibiotics to prevent secondary infection, along with fluids and good nursing; prevented by vaccination.

Pastern. The part of a horse's lower leg extending from the fetlock to the hoof.

Pasteurellosis. The correct term for snuffles in rabbits; *see* Snuffles.

Patella. The kneecap.

Pediculosis. Infestation with lice.

Pen-strep. Shortened form for penicillin-streptomycin, a common broad-spectrum antibiotic combination.

Pericardium. The membrane that encloses the heart and its surrounding blood vessels.

Peritoneal cavity. The membrane lining the abdomen.

Peritonitis. Inflammation of the abdominal membrane caused by various means, including infection, trauma, and retained afterbirth; commonly treated with antibiotics.

Phenol poisoning. A common form of household cleaner poisoning in cats; characterized by gastric upset and death in severe cases; treated by inducing vomiting, giving fluids parenterally, and good nursing.

Pinkeye. An infection commonly seen in cattle, spread by flies; characterized by watery eyes that may become bloodshot and severely irritated; treated with eye powders and solutions containing antibiotics; prevented by vaccination; also called infectious keratitis.

Pinworms. Intestinal parasites that cause intense itching around the anus; common in horses; treated with a wormer.

Placenta. The membrane that unites the fetus with the uterus.

Pneumonia. A disease of the lungs commonly caused by bacterial or viral infection, initiated by stress; characterized by fever, difficult breathing, coughing, and lack of appetite; treated with antibiotics, often expectorants, and good nursing; *see also* Aspiration pneumonia.

Pneumonitis. A serious contagious viral disease in cats; characterized by sneezing, coughing, a discharge from the eyes and nose, fever, and weight loss; treated with good nursing, antibiotics to prevent secondary infections, and isolation; prevented by vaccination.

Polled. Having no horns as a result of heredity.

Posterior presentation. Another term for rear presentation; *see* Rear presentation.

Poult. A young turkey.

Pregnancy disease. A common term for ketosis, often used in reference to sheep; *see* Ketosis.

Prolapse. The dropping down or slipping of a body part from its usual position.

Prolapsed eyeball. A condition, caused by trauma, in which the eyeball pops out of its socket; treated by replacing the eyeball; aftercare consists of bandaging the head and giving antibiotics to prevent infection and cortisone or aspirin to prevent swelling and pain.

Protozoa. One-celled organisms.

Proud flesh. An excessive granulation, resulting in a tumorlike growth, produced in the healing of a wound; characterized by oozing, bleeding easily, enlarging, and being easily injured; treated surgically or with drying agents.

Pullet. A young female chicken.

Pullorum. A destructive poultry disease caused by a bacterial infection; characterized by diarrhea, huddling together, and droopiness; treated with sulfas.

Pyometra. An infection of the uterus; characterized by pus in the uterus, lack of heat cycles, and sometimes fever and extreme illness; treated with hormones, antibiotics, and sometimes surgery.

Pyrethrin. A plant-derived insecticide.

Quarter crack. Another term for sand crack; *see* Sand crack.

Queen. A female cat.

Rabies. A serious viral disease of mammals, including humans, which is spread by the high concentration of the virus in the saliva of infected animals; characterized by personality change, aggressive behavior, or unusually friendly or quiet behavior; no treatment available once the symptoms show; prevented by vaccination; also called hydrophobia.

Rear presentation. A less frequent, but still normal, delivery position of a young animal; backward, with the hind feet coming first; also called posterior presentation.

Retained corpus luteum. A reddish yellow mass of tissue forming from a ruptured cyst in the ovary, preventing a female from having heat cycles; commonly treated with estrogen injections.

Retained placenta. A condition in which the placenta has not been expelled at birth or shortly thereafter; indicated by tissue hanging out of the vulva or being retained internally, which often causes uterine infections; treated by manual removal (in large animals), injections of hormones, and antibiotic or sulfa boluses, powders, or infusions.

Reticulum. The second stomach of a ruminant.

Rhinopneumonitis. A contagious equine viral infection; characterized either by respiratory symptoms, fever, and lack of appetite or by abortions in bred mares between the 7th and 11th months of gestation; treatment consists of antibiotics to prevent secondary bacterial infections, treating the symptoms, and good nursing; prevented by vaccination.

Rhinotracheitis. A contagious viral disease in cats; characterized by a discharge from the eyes and nose, sneezing, and coughing; treated by antibiotics to prevent/treat secondary bacterial infections, treatment of the symptoms, and good nursing; prevented by vaccination.

Rickets. A condition caused by failure to assimilate and use calcium and phosphorus, due to poor diet, inadequate sunlight, or vitamin D deficiency; characterized by soft, often deformed bones, especially in young, growing animals.

Ringbone. A condition that causes lameness in horses; characterized by swelling or ridges in the bone of the pastern area; brought on by trauma, hard work, or arthritis; treated with pasture rest and commonly cortisone or Butazolidin.

Rooter. A hard ridge of cartilage, near the snout, that a pig roots with.

Rotenone. A plant-derived insecticide.

Roundworm. The most common internal parasite in most animals; quite large, white, and tapered at both ends; seen when coughed up or in the stool; treated with a wormer.

Rumen. The large first stomach of a ruminant.

Rumenotomy. A surgical incision into the rumen.

Ruminant. An animal that chews a cud, such as a cow, goat, or sheep.

Ruptured pig. A pig with an inherited defect characterized by an enlargement and softness in the testicle(s) due to the presence of intestines in the scrotum along with the testicle(s); treated surgically.

Saddle sore. An irritation that develops on the back of a horse at a point of pressure; caused by an ill-fitting saddle or trauma from hard use; treated by resting the horse and correcting the condition that caused the problem.

Sand crack. A crack in the hoof of a horse, sometimes with lameness; treated with moisture, a hoof dressing, and sometimes corrective shoeing; also called quarter crack.

Sarcoptic mange. A type of common mange; *see* Mange.

Scab, or scabies. Another term for mange; *see* Mange.

Scab nose. Hutch burn infection of the nose; *see* Hutch burn.

Scirrhous cord. A buildup in the scrotum of a castrated animal, containing fibrous scar tissue; caused by not removing part of the tunic; treated by blunt dissection and surgical removal.

Scoops. Another name for a gouger-type dehorner; *see* Gouger.

Scours. Severe diarrhea in animals.

Scratches. A condition appearing on the back of a horse's pastern; characterized by sores or roughness, swelling, tenderness, lameness, and crusts of dried serum; treated with daily washings, hair clipping, and alternate use of astringent and antibiotic ointment; also called grease heel.

Scrotum. The external sac, or pouch, of skin containing the testicles.

Scurs. Misshapen horns, often small, knotted, and twisted; often caused by injury to the horn bud by improper dehorning.

Septicemia. A bloodstream infection; characterized by chills, fever, and weakness; treated by antibiotics and good nursing; also called blood poisoning.

Septum. A dividing wall or membrane between body spaces or masses of soft tissue, as between the nostrils or testicles.

Sheath. The tubular fold of skin into which the penis is retracted.

Shipping fever. A common term for a pneumonia complex in cattle, horses, and goats; often accompanied by diarrhea; caused by stress but not always from shipping; also called hemorrhagic septicemia.

Shock. A condition brought about by trauma that results in reduced circulation, rapid breathing, rapid pulse, subnormal temperature, weakness, vomiting, and prostration; must be treated by a veterinarian immediately.

Simple fracture. A break in the bone without a break in the skin; a break without secondary complications.

Slicker. A flat grooming brush with bent metal pins.

Snuffles. A common contagious bacterial disease in rabbits; characterized by sneezing, wheezing, coughing, and running eyes; treated with antibiotics, proper nutrition, and good nursing; also called pasteurellosis.

Sore hocks. Chaffed or bruised hocks in rabbits that may become infected; characterized by bald, red, scabby, or swollen hocks; treated with a sulfa or an antibiotic plus an ointment or powder, as well as removal from harsh footing.

Soremouth. A contagious viral disease in sheep or goats; characterized by swollen lips with scabs that may extend into the mouth and may be on the feet, between the toes, and on the nose; treated by keeping the animal's strength up with moist foods until the virus runs its course; prevented by vaccination.

Sow. An adult female pig.

Spaying. The removal of the ovaries and uterus; neutering a female animal; technically called ovariohysterectomy.

Speculum. An instrument inserted into a body passage for inspection or medication, as a mouth speculum used for dental work or a stomach tube.

Splints. A condition that causes lameness in horses; caused by hard work on hard or rough surfaces, blows, or injuries; characterized by small inflamed spots; treated with pasture rest and liniments.

Sprain. A sudden or violent twist or wrench of a joint, with stretching or tearing of ligaments; characterized by lameness, heat, and tenderness; when fresh, treated with cold water or ice, alcohol rubs, cooling liniment, and cortisone injections; after swelling has occurred, treated with heat, heating liniment, hot udder ointment, and massage.

Stanchion. A device that fits loosely around an animal's neck and limits forward and backward motion.

Stifle. The joint above the hock in the hind leg of an animal that corresponds to the knee in a human.

Stifling. A condition that causes lameness in animals; caused by a conformation weakness, often hereditary; characterized by a hind leg being "stuck" straight; treated by replacing the dislocation; also called luxation of the patella.

Stocking up. A term for edema in horses; *see* Edema.

Stool. A bowel movement.

Strangles. A contagious disease in horses caused by bacterial infection; characterized by heavy mucus secretions from the nose, cough, fever, and enlargement or abscess of the lymph glands between the lower jaw; treated by isolation and good nursing.

Stress. A physical or mental disruption upsetting the well-being of an animal, such as moving, changes in the weather, a switch in feed, or being chased by predators.

Strongyles. A group of roundworms that infest the intestinal tract of horses; larvae migrate in the bloodstream, causing scarring of the vessel walls and parasitic thrombosis; treated with a wormer.

Strychnine poisoning. Poisoning characterized by trembling, panting, and acting nervously, followed by convulsions; treated with a general anesthetic, fluids, and rest.

Subcutaneous injection. An injection given just under the skin.

Suture. To sew (verb); the material used for closing wounds (noun).

Swamp fever. The common term for equine infectious anemia; a viral disease in horses spread by biting insects; symptoms vary but generally include recurrent bouts of illness; no treatment or vaccine available.

Syringe. An instrument used to inject into or to remove fluid from the body.

Systemic. Throughout the body, as opposed to local (occurring in one area).

Tapeworms. A large, flat, long, segmented parasite that enters the digestive tract of animals, including humans; commonly ingested with a flea containing tapeworm larvae; seen as white rice-like pieces in the stool or around the anus; treated with a wormer.

TB. Abbreviation for tuberculosis; *see* Tuberculosis.

Tendonotomy. Surgery on the tendons.

Tetanus. A bacterial disease that causes poor coordination, stiffness in the rear limbs, and inability to eat and drink; also called lockjaw.

TGE. Abbreviation for transmissible gastroenteritis; *see* Transmissible gastroenteritis.

Third eyelid. A term for the nictitating membrane; *see* Nictitating membrane.

Thoracic cavity. The area between the neck and abdomen where the heart and lungs lie.

Thrombosis. The formation or presence of a blood clot or blockage in a blood vessel.

Thrush. A diseased condition of the feet, causing lameness; characterized by pus and a foul odor; treated with drying agents, improved cleanliness, and foot soaks.

Ticks. Any of numerous blood-sucking, flat, parasitic creatures that attach themselves to warm-blooded vertebrates; treated with a dip, spray, or powder insecticide.

Tonsillitis. Inflammation of the tonsils, often caused by bacterial infection; characterized by coughing, gagging, vomiting, lack of appetite, fever, and dullness; treated with an antibiotic, cortisone, and good nursing.

Torsion. Twisting, as when the uterus twists on itself, preventing the birth of an animal.

Transmissible gastroenteritis (TGE). A rapidly spread, contagious viral disease in pigs; characterized by diarrhea, vomiting, severe dehydration, and weight loss; prevented by vaccination.

Trauma. A wound or stress.

Trochar. An awl-shaped, pointed instrument used to form a small hole and insert a tube (cannula) into an animal to allow the passage of gas, as in bloat in cattle.

Tuberculosis (TB). A contagious bacterial disease in animals and humans; characteristics vary according to the species.

Tumor. An abnormal mass of tissue that is not inflamed, in which the multiplication of cells is uncontrolled and progressive; also called neoplasm.

Tunic. The tough, white membrane surrounding the testicle.

Twitch. A restraining device for horses, slipped over the upper lip and tightened.

Udder. The organ of milk production; mammary gland.

Udder edema. The correct term for caked bag; *see* Caked bag.

Umbilical. Pertaining to the area or attachment of the cord between the uterus and fetus.

Unthriftiness. The condition of not doing well; characterized by a dull coat, thinness, and dullness of spirit.

Urea. A soluble, weakly basic nitrogenous compound that is the chief solid component of mammalian urine; used as an animal protein supplement and ingredient in some commonly used medications.

Uremic poisoning. A toxic condition commonly seen in kidney disease or failure; caused by accumulation in the blood of constituents normally eliminated in the urine; also called uremia.

Urinary calculi. Deposits of calcium carbonate, calcium, sodium, calcium phosphate, or cystine in the urinary tract that can obstruct urination, making it difficult or impossible.

Urinary incontinence. The inability to completely control urination; characterized by dribbling urine.

Uterus. The muscular, fleshy pouch in the female in which the fetus grows.

Vaccine. A suspension of live, killed, or attenuated (weakened) virus or bacteria administered to the body to build up immunity to diseases caused by those organisms.

Vagina. The canal in the female that leads from the uterus to the vulva.

Vaginitis. Inflammation of the vaginal walls, often caused by a bacterial or viral infection.

VEE. Abbreviation for Venezuelan equine encephalomyelitis; *see* Venezuelan equine encephalomyelitis.

Venezuelan equine encephalomyelitis (VEE). An equine disease similar to Eastern equine encephalomyelitis but not commonly found in the United States; *see* Eastern equine encephalomyelitis.

Virus. A microorganism that reproduces itself and obtains its energy from the body cells it enters, causing damage to the cells from within.

Visceral. Pertaining to the liver, kidneys, or other body organs.

Vulva. The external parts of the female genital organs; also the opening between the projecting parts of the external organs.

Warfarin. A crystalline anticoagulant compound used in a rodent poison.

Warfarin poisoning. Poisoning commonly seen in cats that eat the rodent poison or ingest rodents with a stomachful of fresh poison; causes internal hemorrhages; characterized by weakness, anemia, and depression; treated by a veterinarian with vitamin K, fluids, and confinement.

Wart. A horny projection on the skin caused by a virus; commonly treated with a wart vaccine.

Wasting disease. A common term for caseous lymphadenitis; *see* Caseous lymphadenitis.

WEE. Abbreviation for Western equine encephalomyelitis; *see* Western equine encephalomyelitis.

Western equine encephalomyelitis (WEE). An equine disease similar to Eastern equine encephalomyelitis but found mainly in the western and midwestern United States; *see* Eastern equine encephalomyelitis.

Wether. A castrated male goat or sheep.

Whelp. To give birth (in dogs).

Whipworm. A common parasitic worm of the cecum in dogs; characterized by a liquid, foul-smelling stool; treated with a wormer.

Wind puffs. A condition that causes lameness in horses; caused by strain; characterized by puffy swellings on the lower leg; treated with cold packs, rest, and astringents.

Withers. The high point just behind the neck of an animal.

RECOMMENDED READING

Brennan, Mary L., and Norma Eckroate. *The Natural Dog: A Complete Guide for Caring Owners.* New York: NAL Dutton, 1994.

Carlson, Delbert G., James M. Griffin, and Lisa Carlson. *Cat Owner's Home Veterinary Handbook.* New York: Howell Book House, 1995.

Damerow, Gail. *The Chicken Health Handbook.* Pownal, Vt.: Storey Communications, 1994.

———. *Your Chickens.* Pownal, Vt.: Storey Communications, 1993.

———. *Your Goats.* Pownal, Vt.: Storey Communications, 1993.

Edney, Andrew. *Complete Cat Care Manual.* London: Dorling-Kindersley, 1992.

Fogle, Bruce. *Complete Dog Care Manual.* London: Dorling-Kindersley, 1993.

Frazier, Anitra, and Norma Eckroate. *The New Natural Cat: A Complete Guide for Finicky Owners.* New York: NAL Dutton, 1990.

Griffin, James M. and Tom Gore. *Horse Owner's Veterinary Handbook.* New York: Howell Book House, 1989.

Hawcroft, Tim. *A–Z of Horse Diseases and Health Problems: Signs, Diagnoses, Causes, and Treatment.* New York: Howell Book House, 1990.

Haynes, N. Bruce. *Keeping Livestock Healthy: A Veterinary Guide to Horses, Cattle, Pigs, Goats & Sheep.* 3rd ed. Pownal, Vt.: Garden Way Publishing Company, 1994.

Hill, Cherry. *Your Pony, Your Horse.* Pownal, Vt.: Storey Comunications, 1995.

Kanable, Ann. *Raising Rabbits.* Emmaus, Pa.: Rodale Press, 1977.

Lose, M. Phyllis. *Blessed are the Broodmares.* New York: Howell Book House, 1991.

———. *The Merck Veterinary Manual.* 7th ed. Rahway, N.J.: Merck & Company, 1991.

Luttmann, Rick. *Chickens in Your Backyard: A Beginner's Guide.* Emmaus, Pa.: Rodale Press, 1976.

Marder, Amy. *Your Healthy Pet.* Emmaus, Pa.: Rodale Press, 1994.

Morrison, Frank B. *Feeds and Feeding.* 9th edition. Clinton, Iowa: Morrison Publishing Company, 1961.

Pitcairn, Richard H., and Susan Hubble Pitcairn. *Dr. Pitcairn's Complete Guide to Natural Health for Dogs and Cats.* 2nd ed. Emmaus, Pa.: Rodale Press, 1995.

Prevention Magazine Health Books Editors. *The Doctors Book of Home Remedies for Dogs and Cats.* Emmaus, Pa.: Rodale Press, 1996.

Rooney, James R. *The Lame Horse.* Ossining, N.Y.: Breakthrough Publications, 1986.

Searle, Nancy. *Your Rabbit.* Pownal, Vt.: Storey Communications, 1992.

Siegal, Mordecai. *The Cornell Book of Cats.* 2nd ed. New York: Random House, 1997.

Simmons, Paula, and Darrell L. Salsbury. *Your Sheep.* Pownal, Vt.: Storey Communications, 1992.

Storer, Pat. *Your Puppy, Your Dog.* Pownal, Vt.: Storey Communications, 1997.

INDEX

Note: Page numbers in *italics* refer to tables.
Boldface references
indicate illustrations.

H

NOTES